SLEEP AND
BIOLOGICAL RHYTHMS

SLEEP AND BIOLOGICAL RHYTHMS

Basic Mechanisms and Applications to Psychiatry

Edited by

Jacques Montplaisir
Roger Godbout

Département de Psychiatrie
Université de Montréal
Montréal (Québec) Canada

New York   Oxford
OXFORD UNIVERSITY PRESS   1990

Oxford University Press

Oxford   New York   Toronto
Delhi   Bombay   Calcutta   Madras   Karachi
Petaling Jaya   Singapore   Hong Kong   Tokyo
Nairobi   Dar es Salaam   Cape Town
Melbourne   Auckland

and associated companies in
Berlin   Ibadan

Library of Congress Cataloging-in-Publication Data
Sleep and biological rhythms : basic mechanisms and applications to
psychiatry / edited by Jacques Montplaisir and Roger Godbout.
p. cm.   Includes bibliographical references.
ISBN 0-19-505825-9
1. Sleep-wake cycle—Congresses.
2. Sleep disorders—Congresses.
3. Biological rhythms—Congresses.
I. Montplaisir, Jacques. II. Godbout, Roger.
[DNLM: 1. Biological Clocks. 2. Periodicity. 3. Sleep—physiology.
WL 108 S608] QP425.S658   1990   612.8'21—dc20
DNLM/DLC   for Library of Congress   89-70941

Based on proceedings of the 10th symposium of the
Centre de recherche en sciences neurologiques,
Université de Montréal, 1988.

987654321

Printed in the United States of America.
on acid-free paper

Foreword

This work is very timely since there have been remarkable advances during recent years in our understanding of the anatomical, neurochemical, neurophysiological, and behavioral mechanisms involved. In addition, these advances in basic mechanisms have made possible a renewed appreciation of relationships between sleep and various mental and behavioral disorders in man.

These rapid developments have been made possible by many technological advances in neuroscience, particularly the study of the neurochemistry of the brain in relation to states of sleep and waking, and "chemocytoarchitectonics" of the brain, for example, techniques which make possible the mapping of neurochemically specific nuclei and pathways which have local and diffuse molecular controls on widespread neuronal circuits involved in states of consciousness.

These revolutionary advances in neuroscience, together with improvements in microelectrophysiological techniques which permit the recording of the electrical activity of single cells throughout the CNS in anaesthetized animals, asleep and awake, make it possible to correlate the electrical activity of single cells with behavior, states of reactivity, and consciousness.

Thus we now have a clearer picture of both the electrical and chemical or molecular systems of control and communication in the brain and their relationship to behavior. The importance of these developments, of course, surpasses the subject of this book. The state of reactivity of the brain to environmental stimuli depends more on the reactive state of the brain (sleep or waking, hungry or satiated, afraid or angry, and so forth) than it does on environmental stimuli. It becomes important, therefore, to understand not only the controls involved in the determination of all states of reactivity, such as those in sleep and waking and biological rhythms, but to begin to understand those brain mechanisms underlying behavior and conscious mental life. This book also far exceeds the restrictions of its subject since it sheds light on the nature of mechanisms of control for the reactivity of the brain as a whole in many different situations, so important for our understanding.

I first became interested in brain mechanisms of sleep and waking in 1934. Looking back over fifty years, I can assure you that it was most exciting to see the first tracings of the electrical activity of the human brain in the EEG and to realize that we now have before our eyes an objective record of the stages of sleep and waking in man.

I remember being invited to Alfred Loomis's laboratories in Tuxedo Park, New York, together with Hal Davis, Newton Harvey, G. Hobart, and others to witness the first all-night EEG tracings being carried out there. We were invited to witness a memorable recording of sleep from the brain of Albert Einstein. Newton Harvey had brought Einstein up from Princeton just for this recording. Einstein was also very much interested in seeing the changes in the brain waves during sleep and arousal. In fact he was so interested that we had great trouble getting him to fall asleep for his own recording.

Finally, well after midnight, he did fall asleep and showed slow waves and spindles characteristic of normal light sleep. After about thirty minutes we noted that the slow waves disappeared to be replaced by low voltage fast activity. (We did not know of REM sleep at the time.) Suddenly he woke and sat up in bed asking for a telephone. He said he had to call Princeton; he had just discovered a mistake he had made in the calculations of the day before and must tell his associates right away, although it was after midnight at the time. The EEG had predicted the arousal and mental activity which preceded his overt waking behavior.

In our own laboratories at Brown University in Providence, Rhode Island, we had observed and recorded the dynamic changes in the electrical activity of all parts of the brain implanted with electrodes in freely moving cats. The EEG showed large slow waves and spindles similar to the sleep patterns seen in man. We also found occasional interruptions in this pattern with a change to rapid waves in spite of apparently continued sleep behavior. It was not as dramatic as Einstein's calculations, but just as much a sign of arousal which we learned to heed during our experiments.

Any stimulus presented to the alert cat caused changes in the electrical activity of all brain areas, not only in the sensory receiving area for the kind of stimulus being presented. Thus we were observing the general arousal or attentive response of the brain as a whole fifteen years before Morruzzi and Magoun had described the ascending reticular activating system of the brain stem. We soon learned that Penfield, in his Harvey lecture of 1936, proposed that there must be a system of neurones in diencephalon and brain stem which was the "essential substratum of consciousness" which he later called the "centrencephalic system." And Bremer had described his "cerveau isolé" preparation pointing to the importance of the brain stem in the control of waking behavior.

We now know that these early conceptions were far too simple, although they contained some important principles which guided much of the research that followed, some of which is described in this book.

I am particularly glad to see that the organizers of this symposium have linked their studies of sleep and biological rhythms with mental states of concern to psychiatry. This involves not only the effects of sleep mechanisms on mental states, but also the effects of mental states on sleep mechanisms, adding a new dimension to our understanding.

I would like to close on a more personal note of thanks to my first graduate student at the University of Montréal, Dr. Jacques Montplaisir, for his excellent organization of this symposium with his colleague Roger Godbout, and for their kind invitation to write this foreword on a subject which has been a lifelong interest for me in my adventures in neuroscience.

Herbert H. Jasper

Centre de Recherches en
Sciences Neurologiques
Université de Montréal

Acknowledgments

The Tenth Symposium of the Centre de recherche en sciences neurologiques was cosponsored by the Département de Psychiatrie of the Université de Montréal. We are grateful for the financial support received from the Faculté de Médecine of the Université de Montréal, Rhone-Poulenc Pharma, Squibb Canada, and Upjohn Canada. We also thank the technical and secretarial staffs of the Département de Physiologie and of the Centre de Recherche for their skillful assistance. The invaluable help of Ms. Helene Auzat is particularly acknowledged.

Contents

Contributors

James S. Allan
Center for Circadian and Sleep Disorders
Medicine
Department of Medicine, Division of
Endocrinology
Harvard Medical School
Boston, Massachusetts

Marc-André Bédard
Centre d'Etude du Sommeil
Hôpital du Sacré-Coeur
Montréal, Québec

Diane Boivin
Centre d'Etude du Sommeil
Hôpital du Sacré-Coeur
Montréal, Québec

Roger Broughton
Department of Neurology
University of Ottawa School of Medicine
Ottawa, Ontario

Alan B. Cady
Department of Physiology and Biophysics
University of Tennessee, Memphis
Memphis, Tennessee

Charles A. Czeisler
Center for Circadian and Sleep Disorders
Medicine
Department of Medicine, Division of
Endocrinology
Harvard Medical School
Boston, Massachusetts

Joseph De Koninck
School of Psychology
University of Ottawa
Ottawa, Ontario

Wayne Dunham
Department of Neurology
University of Ottawa School of Medicine
Ottawa, Ontario

Pierre Gagnon
Service de Psychologie
Centre Hospitalier Pierre-Janet
Hull, Québec

J. Christian Gillin
San Diego Veterans Administration
Medical Center
Department of Psychiatry
University of California, San Diego
La Jolla, California

Roger Godbout
Centre d'Etude du Sommeil
Hôpital du Sacré-Coeur
Montréal, Québec

Lars Johannsen
Department of Physiology and Biophysics
University of Tennessee, Memphis
Memphis, Tennessee

James M. Krueger
Department of Physiology and Biophysics
University of Tennessee, Memphis
Memphis, Tennessee

Richard E. Kronauer
Harvard University
Division of Applied Sciences
Cambridge, Massachusetts

Odile Lapierre
Centre d'Etude du Sommeil
Hôpital du Sacré-Coeur
Montréal, Québec

Alfred J. Lewy
Sleep and Mood Disorders Laboratory
Department of Psychiatry
The Oregon Health Sciences University
Portland, Oregon

Jeanine Majde
Office of Naval Research
Arlington, Virginia

Wallace B. Mendelson
Department of Psychiatry
Health Sciences Center, School of
Medicine
State University of New York, Stony
Brook
Stony Brook, New York

Robert W. McCarley
Department of Psychiatry
Director, Neuroscience Laboratory
Harvard Medical School
Boston, Massachusetts

Jacques Montplaisir
Centre d'Etude du Sommeil
Hôpital du Sacré-Coeur
Montréal, Québec

Dr. Robert Y. Moore
Department of Neurology
Health Sciences Center, School of
Medicine
State University of New York, Stony
Brook
Stony Brook, New York

Ferenc Obál, Jr.
Department of Physiology and Biophysics
University of Tennessee, Memphis
Memphis, Tennessee

Denis Paré
Laboratoire de Neurophysiologie
Faculté de Médecine
Université Laval
Québec, Québec

Benjamin Rusak
Department of Psychology
Dalhousie University
Halifax, Nova Scotia

Robert L. Sack
Sleep and Mood Disorders Laboratory
Department of Psychiatry
The Oregon Health Sciences University
Portland, Oregon

David S. Schlager
New York State Psychiatric Institute and
Columbia University
New York, New York

P. Shiromani
San Diego Veterans Administration
Medical Center
Department of Psychiatry
University of California, San Diego
La Jolla, California

Clifford M. Singer
Sleep and Mood Disorders Clinic
Department of Psychiatry
The Oregon Health Services University
Portland, Oregon

Claudio Stampi
Department of Neurology
University of Ottawa School of Medicine
Ottawa, Ontario

Mircea Steriade
Laboratoire de Neurophysiologie
Faculté de Médecine
Université Laval
Québec, Québec

Michael Terman
New York State Psychiatric Institute
and Columbia University
New York, New York

Linda Toth
Department of Physiology and Biophysics
University of Tennessee, Memphis
Memphis, Tennessee

Thomas A. Wehr
Clinical Psychobiology Branch
Intramural Research Program
National Institute of Mental Health
Bethesda, Maryland

Abbreviations

ACh acetylcholine
AChE acetylcholinesterase
ACTH adrenocorticotropic hormone
A-D advance-delay
AVS analog vigilance scale
BAT brown adipose tissue
BRAC basic rest-activity cycle
BFR bulbar reticular formation
CGI clinical global impressions scale
ChAT choline acetyltransferase
CLIP corticotropin-like intermediate lobe peptide
CNS central nervous system
CRF corticotropin-releasing factor
CRIT cholinergic REM induction test
4CRTT Four choice reaction time test
CSF cerebrospinal fluid
DA dopamine
DAB diaminobenzidine
DIMS disorders of initiating and maintaining sleep
DLMO dim light melatonin onset
DR dorsal raphe
DSIP delta sleep-inducing peptide
ECPmin minimum of a harmonic regression curve
EDS excessive daytime somnolence
EEG electroencephalogram
EMG electromyogram
EMP eye movement potential
EOG elctrooculogram
FEO food-entrainable oscillator
FR free run
FTG gigantocellular tegmental field
GABA gamma-aminobutyric acid

GH growth hormone
GHB gamma-hydroxybutyric acid
GRF GH-releasing factor
HAM-D Hamilton depression rating scale
5HT serotonin
ICV intracerebroventricularly
IFN interferon
IL-1 interleukin-1
IPSP inhibitory postsynaptic potential
IV intravenously
LC locus coeruleus
LD light-dark
LDT laterodorsal tegmental nucleus
LG(N) lateral geniculate (nuclei)
LPS lipopolysaccharide
LTS low threshold spike
MAOI monoamine oxidase inhibitor
MDP muramyl dipeptide
α-MSH melanocyte-stimulating hormone
MP muramyl peptide
mPRF medial PRF
MRF mesencephalic reticular formation
MSLT multiple sleep latency test
MWT maintenance of wakefulness test
NPY neuropeptide Y
NREM non-REM
PAP peroxydase-antiperoxydase
PB peribrachial
PFTG pontine FTG
PG prostaglandin
PGO pontogeniculooccipital
PHA-L phaseolus vulgaris leukocoaggluttinin

PHI histidine-isoleucine containing peptide

PMS periodic movements during sleep

Poly(I:C) polyriboinosinic: polyribocytidylic acid

PPT pedunculopontine tegmental nucleus

PRC phase response curve

PRF pontine reticular formation

PRL prolactine

PSD partial sleep deprivation

PSP postsynaptic potentials

PVN paraventricular nuclei

REM rapid eye movement

RF reticular formation

RHT retinohypothalamic tract

RLS restless legs syndrome

SAD seasonal affective disorder

SCN suprachiasmatic nuclei

SF sleep factor

SIGH structured interview guide for the HAM-D

SIGH-SAD SIGH version adapted for SAD

SNr substantia nigra pars reticulata

SOM somatostatin

SOREMP sleep onset REM period

SRSD selective REM sleep deprivation

SWS slow wave sleep

TAD tricyclic antidepressant

TMB tetramethyl-benzidine

TNF tumor necrosis factor

TSD total sleep deprivation

TSH thyroid-stimulating hormone, or thyrotropin

TTX tetrodotoxin

VIP vasoactive intestinal peptide

VMH ventromedial nuclei of the hypothalamus

W waking

WASO wakefulness after sleep onset

WAT Wilkinson addition test

WGA-HRP wheat germ agglutinin-horseradish peroxidase

I

BIOLOGICAL RHYTHMS

The Circadian System
and Sleep–Wake Behavior

ROBERT Y. MOORE

Circadian rhythms are a fundamental adaptation to the solar cycle of light and dark. In mammals they are expressed in a number of physiological and behavioral functions including cycles of sleep and wakefulness. Indeed, mammals may be classified into two broad groups on the basis of the temporal distribution of sleep–wake behavior. Diurnal mammals are awake during the day and sleep at night, whereas nocturnal animals are asleep during the day and awake at night. These patterns of behavior have evolved to permit a maximum adaptation with respect to both survival and reproduction. For behavioral rhythms to be successful, they must be synchronized with a series of cellular and physiological rhythms. In mammals the organization of circadian function is accomplished by a set of neural structures that I shall designate the circadian system. This system has two principal functions derived from the properties of circadian rhythms, generation by endogenous pacemakers and entrainment by environmental stimuli, particularly the light–dark cycle. The circadian system in mammals is a part of the central nervous system and its basic organization is presented diagrammatically in Figure 1-1. Three essential components comprise the system: photoreceptors and visual pathways to mediate entrainment, pacemaker(s), and efferent projections from the pacemaker to couple its activity to systems that exhibit circadian function. In the sections that follow I shall present a brief overview of the functional organization of the circadian system and propose a set of relations that would provide the coupling between it and systems that participate in the generation of sleep and waking to permit their expression in a circadian manner.

PACEMAKER(S)

The current period of intensive investigation of the neural mechanisms of circadian function was largely initiated by the discovery of a pacemaker in the mammalian brain, the suprachiasmatic nuclei (SCN) of the hypothalamus. The SCN lies in the anterior hypothalamus immediately above the optic chiasm (6,18). In most mammals the SCN are very distinctive and readily recognized (3,30; Fig. 1-2), but their participation in

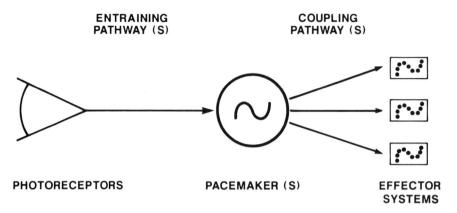

Figure 1-1 Diagram illustrating the essential elements of a circadian neural system.

circadian function was not suspected until the demonstration of a direct retinohypothal-amic projection terminating in the SCN (11,23). This was followed almost immediate-ly by two papers demonstrating that SCN ablation abolished circadian rhythms (22,42). Loss of circadian function could reflect either an effect on pacemaker function or an interruption of effector mechanisms for expression of circadian function. However, there is now substantial evidence supporting the view that the SCN is a circadian

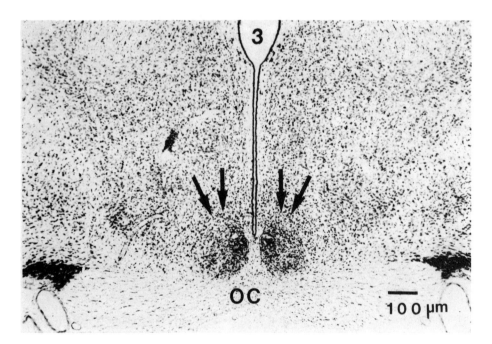

Figure 1-2 The suprachiasmatic nuclei (SCN) in the rat brain. Coronal section prepared with a Nissl stain. The SCN are designated by the double arrows. They are small, round nuclei adjacent to the third ventricle (3) and above the optic chiasm (OC).

pacemaker and that the effects of SCN ablation reflect a loss of pacemaker activity. This includes a large number of studies that have demonstrated loss of circadian function following SCN ablation (cf. 19,31 for review). As noted, this is not sufficient evidence to prove that the SCN is a pacemaker but the reproducibility of the effect, its generality among rhythms and its permanence (25) are in accord with what one would expect if SCN lesions did, indeed, remove a circadian pacemaker.

In addition, there are two other lines of evidence that support the interpretation that the SCN is a circadian pacemaker. First, the SCN exhibits rhythms in functional activity in isolation from other parts of the brain. A rhythm in multiunit activity was demonstrated in the SCN, isolated form the remainder of the brain in intact, freely moving animals (13,14). In this study the SCN, exhibiting neuronal rhythmicity, was in a hypothalamic island but the animal was arrhythmic because the knife cuts isolating the SCN had severed its connections with other brain areas. Similarly, several investigators have demonstrated that rhythms in single unit activity are preserved in the SCN in hypothalamic slices studied *in vitro* (9,10,39,41). In these studies, like those of Inouye and Kawamaura (13,14), the rhythm is expressed as high firing rates during subjective day and low firing rates during subjective night. Further, the rhythm in firing rate is found only in the SCN, not in adjacent areas. These data are confirmed by studies of glucose metabolism using the 2-deoxyglucose method both *in vivo* and *in vitro* (26,33,34,39). Glucose utilization is high during subjective day and low during subjective night in the SCN but not in other brain areas (34).

The second line of evidence that supports the view that the SCN is a circadian pacemaker comes from neural transplantation studies. If fetal anterior hypothalamus, containing the SCN, is transplanted into the rostral third ventricle in adult animals rendered arrhythmic by SCN lesions, it will restore rhythmicity (1,17,32). This effect appears dependent on the presence of SCN in the transplant (17). These data taken together clearly indicate that the SCN is a circadian pacemaker in the mammalian brain. In addition, they indicate that it is the principal pacemaker but there are further data (cf. Rusak, this volume) that support the view that other circadian pacemakers are present that may function independently of the SCN.

ENTRAINING PATHWAYS

The term entrainment connotes a resetting of pacemaker function by environmental stimuli. The pathways that mediate this are termed entraining pathways. Although it seems likely that all neural input to the SCN subserves entrainment, the principal entraining stimulus is the light–dark cycle. Hence, the major entraining pathways would be expected to be visual. The function of these pathways is to set the phase of the pacemaker to correspond to the precise timing of the light–dark cycle. Two visual pathways participate in entrainment. The retinohypothalamic tract arises from retinal ganglion cells and terminates in the anterior hypothalamus. Although early studies indicated a distribution limited to the SCN (11,23), recent work has demonstrated more widespread projections, particularly to the anterior hypothalamic area, the paraventricular nucleus and the lateral hypothalamic area (16). Ablation of all visual pathways beyond the optic chiasm produces animals that lack pupillary light reflexes and are behaviorally blind but show normally entrained circadian rhythms (20). In

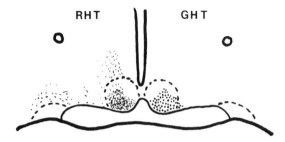

Figure 1-3 Diagrams showing the distribution of the retinohypothalamic tract (RHT) and the geniculohypothalamic tract (GHT) in the rat SCN.

contrast, lesions that undercut the SCN, ablating retinohypothalamic projections and, perhaps, secondary visual projections from the lateral geniculate nucleus, abolish entrainment (15). These observations indicate that the retinohypothalamic projection is sufficient to mediate entrainment. It is not clearly established that it is necessary for entrainment. That is, it is not known whether other SCN afferents can mediate entrainment in the absence of the retinohypothalamic tract.

The second visual pathway arises in the intergeniculate leaflet of the lateral geniculate complex and projects to the SCN in a pattern and distribution that overlap the retinohypothalamic projection (5,24). A portion of the projection is from neuropeptide Y (NPY)-containing neurons. These neurons project back through the optic tract to the SCN. Unlike the retinohypothalamic projections, the geniculohypothalamic tract projects only to the SCN. In addition, there is a commissural pathway that interconnects the two intergeniculate leaflets. Projections from the SCN and adjacent hypothalamus to the intergeniculate leaflet also have been described (4). The pattern of retinal and geniculate projections to the SCN is shown in Figure 1-3.

DEVELOPMENT—INSIGHTS INTO CIRCADIAN MECHANISMS

Although behavioral and hormonal circadian rhythms develop predominantly postnatally (cf. Davis, 7 for review), the SCN exhibits a rhythm in glucose utilization (28,29) and in firing rate (38) that appears prenatally in the rat. Neurons that make up the SCN are generated from the diencephalic germinal epithelium on embryonic days 14–17 (E14–17; 2). The rhythm in glucose utilization is present shortly thereafter, on E19, and is entrained to maternal rhythmicity (27–29). Its development is not dependent, however, on the presence of maternal rhythms as fetal SCN rhythms develop normally in pups of mothers rendered arrhythmic by SCN ablation during gestation (29,40). The early development of the rhythm in glucose utilization has interesting implications when placed in the context of the development of the circadian system. The earliest functional rhythm to develop, other than those in the SCN itself, is the rhythm in pineal content of the enzyme serotonin-*N*-acetyltransferase (8), which first appears at postnatal day 4. The development of the rhythm and its response to environmental light indicate that the SCN is innervated by the retinohypothalamic tract and functions as a pacemaker with efferent projections to effector systems by postnatal day 4. However, at

E19 when the SCN rhythm in glucose metabolism first develops, the SCN is extremely immature and contains very poorly developed neurons and few synapses (21). Indeed, there is less than one synapse per neuron indicating that the SCN would be unable to function as a network of interconnected neurons (21). This renders it unlikely that circadian function is a network property. Rather, it would seem more likely that the SCN is comprised of individual neuronal oscillators that are coupled in the developmental period by a nonsynaptic mechanism and subsequently develop conventional connections both within the nucleus and to effector areas. This view of SCN organization is further supported by studies in the adult, which show that tetrodotoxin administration, both *in vivo* (36) and *in vitro* (37), has no effect on intrinsic clock function in the SCN while eliminating neuronal functions mediated by sodium-dependent action potentials.

THE CIRCADIAN SYSTEM AND SLEEP

Sleep–wake behavior is expressed in a circadian pattern that reflects the basic adaptation of the organism under study. Nocturnal animals sleep during the day and are awake at night. Diurnal animals are awake during the day and sleep at night. The timing of highest glucose utilization in the SCN is the same in both nocturnal and diurnal mammals (35) indicating that the timing of pacemaker activity is a uniform property and that the typical patterns of behavior are determined in the sleep–wake system beyond the level of the SCN. The SCN is clearly critical for expression of sleep–wake circadian rhythmicity; SCN ablation does not alter the amount of REM or slow wave sleep but results in the random distribution of these sleep states with waking through the 24-hr period (12).

   The pathways involved in coupling SCN function with systems expressing circadian rhythms have not been studied extensively and this is particularly true for sleep.

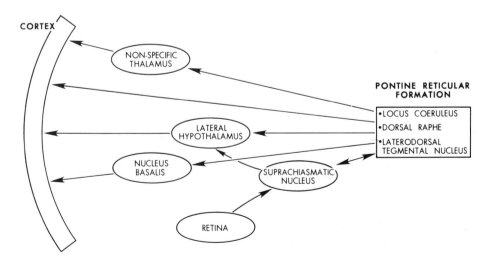

Figure 1-4 Diagram showing the anatomical interrelations of the SCN with structures involved with generation and expression of sleep and waking behaviors.

SCN efferents are well known (43) but their major sites of termination are within the hypothalamus and none project directly to the brainstem areas that have been shown to participate in the generation of REM and slow wave sleep. Nevertheless a potential set of pathways that might participate in the circadian regulation of sleep–wake behavior can be constructed and this is shown diagrammatically in Figure 1-4. As noted, the SCN receives visual input both directly and indirectly from the retina. The principal projections of the SCN are to the adjacent anterior hypothalamic area and to the retrochiasmatic area with smaller projections to the lateral hypothalamic area, tuberal hypothalamus, basal forebrain and midline thalamus (43). There are extensive inter-connections between the anterior hypothalamic area, retrochiasmatic area and lateral hypothalamic area and the pontine and isthmic reticular formation, including the locus coeruleus, dosal raphe and laterodorsal tegmental nucleus. The widespread projections of these reticular formation nuclei to cortex, either directly or through the nonspecific thalamic nuclei, lateral hypothalamus or nucleus basalis, are well known. Thus, there are specific pathways by which the circadian system, and particularly the SCN, can regulate the function of those areas directly responsible for the expression of sleep and waking behavior.

ACKNOWLEDGMENTS

The research reported in this review from my laboratory was supported by NIH Grant NS-16304.

REFERENCES

1. Aguiler-Roblero R, Garcia-Hernandez F, Fernandez-Cancino F, Bernudez-Rattoni F., Fetal suprachiasmatic nucleus transplants: Diurnal rhythm recovery of lesioned rats. *Brain Res* 1984; 311:353–357.
2. Altman J, Bayer SA. The development of the rat hypothalamus. *Adv Anat Embryol Cell Biol* 1986; 100:1–178.
3. Bleier R. *The Hypothalamus of the Cat.* Johns Hopkins, Baltimore, 1961.
4. Card JP, Moore RY. Organization of lateral geniculate-hypothalamic connections in the rat. *J Comp Neurol,* 1989; 284:135–147.
5. Card JP, Moore RY. Ventral lateral geniculate nucleus efferents to the rat suprachiasmatic nucleus exhibit avian pancreatic polypeptide-like immunoreactivity. *J Comp Neurol* 1982; 206:390–396.
6. Cassone VN, Speh JC, Card JP, Moore RY. Comparative anatomy of the mammalian hypothalamic suprachiasmatic nucleus. *J Bio Rhythms* 1988; 3:71–92.
7. Davis FC. Ontogeny of circadian rhythms. In J Aschoff (ed.), *Handbook of Behavioral Neurobiology,* Vol. 4, *Biological Rhythms.* Plenum, New York, 1981: 257–276.
8. Ellison N, Weller JL, Klein DC. Development of a circadian rhythm in the activity of pineal serotonin-N-acetyltransferase. *J Neurochem* 1972; 19:1335–1341.
9. Green D, Gillette R. Circadian rhythm of firing rate recorded single cells in the rat su-prachiasmatic brain slice. *Brain Res* 1982; 245:198–200.
10. Groos GA, Hendricks J. Circadian rhythm of firing rate recorded from single cells in the rat suprachiasmatic brain slice. *Neurosci Lett* 1982; 34:283–288.
11. Hendrickson AE, Wagoner N, Cowan WM. Autoradiographic and electron microscopic study of retinohypothalamic projections. *Z Zellforsch Mikrosk Anat* 1972; 125:1–26.

12. Ibuka N, Inouye S-I, Kawamura H. Analysis of sleep-wakefulness rhythms in male rats after suprachiasmatic nucleus lesions and ocular enucleation. *Brain Res* 1977; 122:33–47.
13. Inouye ST, Kawamura H. Persistence of circadian rhythmicity in a mammalian hypothalamic 'island' containing the suprachiasmatic nucleus. *Proc Natl Acad Sci USA* 1979; 76:5962–5966.
14. Inouye ST, Kawamura H. Characteristics of a circadian pacemaker in the suprachiasmatic nucleus. *J Comp Physiol* 1982; A146:143–160.
15. Johnson RF, Moore RY, Morin LP. Loss of entrainment and anatomical plasticity after lesions of the hamster retinohypothalamic tract. *Brain Res* 1988; 460:297–313.
16. Johnson RF, Morin LP, Moore RY. Retinohypothalamic projections in the hamster and rat demonstrated using cholera toxin. *Brain Res* 1988; 462:301–312.
17. Lehman MN, Silver R, Gladstone WR, Kahn RM, Gibson M, Bittman EL. Circadian rhythmicity restored by neural transplant. Immunocytochemical characterization of graft and its interaction into host brain. *J Neurosci* 1987; 7:1626–1638.
18. Moore RY. Retinohypothalamic projection in mammals: A comparative study. *Brain Res* 1973; 49:403–409.
19. Moore RY. Organization and function of a central nervous system circadian oscillator: The suprachiasmatic hypothalamic nucleus. *Fed Proc* 1983; 42:2783–2789.
20. Moore RY, Klein DC. Visual pathways and the central neural control of a circadian rhythm in pineal serotonin N-acetyltransferase activity. *Brain Res* 1974; 71:17–33.
21. Moore RY, Bernstein ME. Synaptogenesis in the rat suprachiasmatic nucleus demonstrated by electron microscopy and synapsin I immunoreactivity. *J Neurosci,* 1989; 9:2151–2162.
22. Moore RY, Eichler VB. Loss of a circadian adrenal corticosterone rhythm following suprachiasmatic lesions in the rat. *Brain Res* 1972; 42:201–206.
23. Moore RY, Lenn NJ. A retinohypothalamic projection in the rat. *J Comp Neurol* 1972; 142:1–14.
24. Moore RY, Gustason EL, Card JP. Identical immunoreactivity of afferents to the rat suprachiasmatic nucleus with antisera against avian pancreatic polypeptide, molluscan cardioexcitatory peptide and neuropeptide Y. *Cell Tissue Res* 1984; 236:41–46.
25. Mosko SS, Moore RY. Neonatal suprachiasmatic nucleus ablation: Absence of functional and morphological plasticity. *Proc Natl Acad Sci USA* 1978; 75:6243–6246.
26. Newman GC, Hospod FE. Rhythm of suprachiasmatic nucleus 2-deoxyglucose uptake in vitro. *Brain Res* 1986; 381:345–350.
27. Reppert SM. Maternal entrainment of the developing circadian system *Ann NY Acad Sci* 1985; 453:162–169.
28. Reppert SM, Schwartz WJ. Maternal coordination of the fetal biological clock in utero. *Science* 1983; 220:969–971.
29. Reppert SM, Schwartz WJ. Maternal suprachiasmatic nuclei are necessary for maternal coordination of the developing circadian system. *J Neurosci* 1986; 6:2724–2729.
30. Rioch DM, Wislocki G, O'Leary JL. A precis of preoptic hypothalamic and hypophysiol anatomy with atlas. *Assoc Res Nerv Ment Dis* 1940; 20:3–30.
31. Rusak B, Zucker I. Neural regulation of circadian rhythms. *Physiol Rev* 1979; 59:449–526.
32. Sawaki Y, Nihommatsu I, Kawamura H. Transplantation of the neonatal suprachiasmatic nuclei into rats with complete bilateral suprachiasmatic lesions. *Neurosci Res* 1984; I:67–72.
33. Schwartz WJ, Gainer H. Suprachiasmatic nucleus: Use of ^{14}C-labeled deoxyglucose uptake as a functional marker. *Science* 1977; 197:1089–1091.
34. Schwartz WJ, Davidsen LC, Smith CB. In vivo metabolic activity of a putative circadian of the rat suprachiasmatic nucleus. *J Comp Neurol* 1980; 189:157–167.
35. Schwartz WJ, Reppert SM, Eagen SM, Moore-Ede MC. In vivo metabolic activity of the suprachiasmatic nuclei: A comparative study. *Brain Res* 1983; 74:184–187.

36. Schwartz WJ, Gross RA, Morton MT. The suprachiasmatic nuclei contain a tetrodotoxin-resistant circadian pacemaker. *Proc Natl Acad Sci USA* 1987; 84:1694–1698.
37. Shibata S, Moore RY. Tetrodotoxin does not effect circadian rhythms in neuronal activity and metabolism in hamster suprachiasmatic nucleus *in vitro*. *Brain Res* 1988; submitted.
38. Shibata S, Moore RY. Development of neuronal activity in the rat suprachiasmatic nucleus. *Brain Res* 1987; 34:311–315.
39. Shibata S, Moore RY. Electrical and metabolic activity of suprachiasmatic nucleus neurons in hamster hypothalamic slices. *Brain Res* 1988; 438:374–378.
40. Shibata S, Moore RY. Development of a fetal circadian rhythm after disruption of the maternal circadian system. *Dev Brain Res* 1988; 41:313–317.
41. Shibata S, Oomura Y, Kita H, Hattori K. Circadian rhythmic changes of neuronal activity in the suprachiasmatic nucleus of the rat hypothalamic slice. *Brain Res* 1982; 247:154–158.
42. Stephan FK, Zucker I. Circadian rhythms in drinking behavior and locomotor activity of rats are eliminated by hypothalamic lesions. *Proc Natl Acad Sci USA* 1972; 69:1583–1586.
43. Watts AG, Swanson LW, Sanchez-Watts G. Efferent projections of the suprachiasmatic nucleus. I. Studies using anterograde transport of Phaseolus vulgaris leucoagglutinin in the rat. *J Comp Neurol* 1987; 258:204–229.

2

Biological Rhythms: From Physiology to Behavior

BENJAMIN RUSAK

A system that generates daily (circadian) rhythms can be modeled as consisting of a central pacemaker mechanism, an afferent system bringing photic entrainment information to the pacemaker, and an efferent system conveying a rhythmic signal to mechanisms that control physiological and behavioral functions (Fig. 2-1). This model has the formal structure of an open-loop control system, since the output of the effectors does not feed back to and influence the central timer. In addition, although the physical mechanism of the circadian clock may not be fully understood, it is clear that the actual occurrence of an overt rhythm is not a critical step in the physiological timing loop underlying circadian rhythmicity. The classic work that contributed to this view of the circadian system includes Richter's demonstration that merely inhibiting the expression of overt activity did not in any way influence the timer underlying the activity rhythm (30).

A more modern version is the demonstration that infusions of tetrodotoxin (TTX, a sodium channel blocker that prevents the production of sodium-dependent action potentials) into the putative mammalian pacemaker (the suprachiasmatic nuclei, SCN) disrupt the overt activity rhythms of rats, but do not alter the predicted phase of the rhythm after the TTX is washed out (39). TTX appears to prevent communication to the effector systems by efferent neurons in the SCN, but that lack of communication has no influence on how the central clock keeps time. The timing information appears to be inherent in the clock and not dependent on a loop of feedback from the effectors. It is, in fact, now traditional in primers on circadian rhythms to contrast circadian regulatory mechanisms characterized by an open-loop structure to homeostatic regulators, which are characterized by a closed-loop structure, that is, one critically dependent on feedback information.

The purpose of this chapter is to review recent studies that suggest that the orthodox view of the structure and function of mammalian circadian systems requires revision. In particular, I will address the following issues: (a) the internal complexity of the pacemaking system, (b) its susceptibility to environmental factors other than photic cues, and (c) the possibility of feedback sensitivity in the pacemaking system.

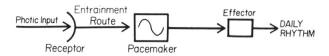

Figure 2-1 A model of a system for circadian rhythm generation. The symbol above "pace-maker" represents a self-sustained oscillator mechanism that is synchronized by afferent infor-mation from the photic entrainment route, and that regulates motor systems that generate overt rhythms. This is an open-loop control system since neither the output of the effector nor the consequences of overt rhythms feed back on the central pacemaker. [Modified from Rusak (33).]

HIERARCHIES AND GATES

The idea that circadian systems are structurally complex is not a new one. Pittendrigh (28) long ago compared animals to living clockshops, implying that they contain multiple timing mechanisms. He and his colleagues identified, for example, a hier-archy of oscillators regulating eclosion in drosophilid flies (29). In rodents, a detailed analysis of the behavior of the circadian system and its responsiveness to various lighting conditions led to the formulation of a pacemaker model involving a pair of mutually coupled oscillators (9,29).

Physiological analyses that proceeded in parallel to the development of models of circadian organization led to the identification of particular structures as representing the components of formal models. In mammals, the critical step was the identification of the SCN as the putative pacemaker for the circadian system (24,45). Various lines of evidence support the identification of the SCN as the pacemaker (16,34,36), but recent physiological and behavioral analyses of the system have raised unexpected questions about the internal structure of the pacemaking system.

Ablation of the SCN results in the loss of a number of behavioral and physiologi-cal circadian rhythms in mammals, but the consequences of the lesions are not simple. In hamsters, very complex behavioral patterns can develop after SCN ablation (32). These patterns appear to reflect the expression of a number of circadian oscillators that become dissociated from one another. Each of these oscillators, which must lie outside the SCN, appears able to promote the expression of overt activity, more or less independently. The lack of expression of a coherent circadian rhythm after SCN abla-tion suggests that the lesions result in the loss of an integrative function normally served by the SCN. The SCN may serve their function as pacemaker by maintaining stable phase relations among (i.e., entraining) a population of "component" oscillators that are hierarchically regulated by its output. In the absence of the SCN or an adequate external synchronizer, they lose mutual synchrony and a pattern of dissociated activity bouts results (32,33). A similar synchronizing role had earlier been suggested for the sparrow pineal gland (12).

The behavioral rhythms of intact hamsters housed in constant conditions for many months show features that can also be interpreted as reflecting the existence of multiple circadian oscillators (10). In these records, bouts of activity scan through the active or *alpha* phase, appearing and disappearing at the boundaries of the *alpha* phase. Davis and Menaker (10) interpreted their data as indicating that the SCN may act as a gating pacemaker, restricting the expression of overt activity to a portion of its own cycle, namely the daily *alpha* phase. In their model, the gating function does not involve entrainment of the subordinate oscillator systems they refer to as "bout" oscillators. These oscillators are assumed to have the following characteristics: they freerun at all times, they have access to motor systems involved in the expression of overt activity, and they achieve behavioral expression only when their active phases coincide with the pacemaker's *alpha*. SCN ablation is then seen as eliminating the gating pacemaker and permitting the overt expression of the bout oscillators at all times. The result is a pattern of dissociated circadian components, with no integrated expression of a circadian activity rhythm.

Both the "entraining" and "gating" pacemaker hypotheses imply that the SCN do not function alone to regulate circadian rhythmicity, but that they are a critical part of an oscillator hierarchy. A study by Schulz et al. (38) of the timing of rapid eye movement (REM) sleep in humans included data that provide some support for each model, but especially for the gating pacemaker model. Schulz et al. (38) presented a record of REM occurrences in a person during a month of consecutive nightly sleep recordings in the laboratory. The first nocturnal REM episode (which was usually brief) appeared to be tied loosely to the time of sleep onset. This timing presumably reflects entrainment of a mechanism controlling REM onset to photic or nonphotic 24-hr cues, perhaps even to sleep onset itself. But later REM episodes scanned the night with a circadian period, unentrained, but gated in their expression by the sleep phase. These data imply that the regulation of REM sleep might include a mechanism that is weakly entrained by the dominant pacemaker controlling the rest–activity cycle (the SCN), as well as a population of freerunning oscillators which are gated in their overt expression by the pacemaker.

Although the evidence on regulation of REM sleep is limited, the general point made by these data is that a single pacemaker system can accomplish its regulatory function by interacting in different ways with lower order components of the circadian system. The evidence for how the SCN-based pacemaker controls the expression of circadian rhythms in functions other than REM sleep is even more limited. It remains to be established whether other rhythms are regulated directly by the SCN, via inter-vening oscillators that are entrained or gated by the SCN, or by other mechanisms.

FOOD ENTRAINMENT

If circadian oscillators exist outside the SCN, there is at least the possibility that some circadian rhythms might survive SCN ablation. This has been a controversial topic for several years. There have, for example, been a number of reports of both the abolition and the survival of body temperature rhythms after SCN ablation (e.g., 11,31,37). But for other rhythms, the evidence for survival after SCN ablation seems clearcut. Terman and Terman (46), for example, have reported persistence of a circadian rhythm of photic detection sensitivity after SCN destruction, indicating that either the eye or another part of the visual system continues to express an intact rhythm without the SCN.

By far the most extensively studied rhythm that survives SCN destruction is the rhythm of increased activity generated by rats in anticipation of a daily phase of restricted food availability. The phenomenon is that when rats are restricted to a temporally limited food supply at a time of day at which they are normally inactive, they develop a bout of activity that anticipates that daily phase (4). The evidence is now overwhelming that the underlying mechanism generating this anticipatory activity is a circadian oscillator, generally referred to as a food-entrainable oscillator (FEO), which is separate from the SCN (5,41).

The evidence for oscillator properties in the food-entrainable mechanism can be summarized briefly as follows: (a) Rats can anticipate circadian but not noncircadian cycles of availability. (b) The food-entrained rhythm persists with a circadian period for several cycles after removal of all food. (c) The rhythm shows transients in response to abrupt shifts in the feeding time. (d) An appropriately phased "anticipatory" rhythm can recur during starvation instituted many days after a return to free-feeding (5,7,41). The evidence that this oscillator is separate from the SCN includes the following: (a) Food-entrained activity can express one period, while the activity rhythm regulated by the SCN continues to freerun with a different period. (b) The oscillator-like features of persistence, transients, and limited entrainment range are manifest in rats that can be demonstrated both anatomically and functionally to have complete SCN lesions (5,44).

These observations imply that the stimuli associated with food restriction operate on the FEO rather than on the SCN. One point I will return to, however, is that there are a few instances in which food restriction schedules appear to have altered or even entrained the SCN-based pacemaker in rats and monkeys. In each case, entrainment occurred only when the periods of the pacemaker and the restriction schedule were very similar (3,43). Taken together with evidence that SCN neural activity is not normally altered by food restriction schedules (14), this finding suggests that the SCN and FEO communicate directly with each other.

The physiological identity of the FEO is still not known. Early studies (15) suggested that it resides in the ventromedial nuclei of the hypothalamus (VMH), because VMH lesions eliminated anticipatory activity. More recent work by Mistlberger and Rechtschaffen (21) showed clearly, however, that the loss is transient. Months after a lesion that severely disrupted or eliminated anticipation, normal anticipatory rhythms were again manifest. Mistlberger and Rusak (23) examined two other hypothalamic sites that met the criteria of being intimately related to the control of food intake and being connected to the SCN: the lateral hypothalamus and the paraventricular nuclei (PVN). Anticipatory activity survived after either lesion, so neither structure appears to contain the unique substrate for the FEO. It is possible that food anticipation depends on a single oscillator that is localized to a still-unidentified site; alternatively, a variety of hypothalamic (or other) structures may contribute to generation of anticipatory rhythms, and the function can, therefore, survive extensive neural damage.

The PVN-ablated rats in the study by Mistlberger and Rusak (23) provided an interesting lesson on the analysis of anticipatory rhythms. Some of them showed no anticipatory increase in activity soon after the lesion, as measured by movement of the tilt-floor of their cages. When retested over 10 months later, unlike VMH-ablated rats, some still failed to increase activity before the feeding time. Yet, direct observation indicated that they were often waiting at their food hoppers before the food arrived. We tested whether measures of nose-poking into the food hopper might give a different result from measures of tilt-floor movements. We found that all animals tested increased nose-poking into the food hopper in anticipation of the daily feeding time, including those that showed little or no anticipation as assessed by general increases in activity. The measure used to test for anticipatory activity may critically affect the answer obtained (cf. 3).

The function of the FEO has typically been studied in very hungry rats. Hunger, in fact, has generally been considered an essential precondition for the expression of the FEO in overt behavior. Rats that show anticipation to a feeding schedule lose the anticipatory component as soon as free food is restored and they are no longer hungry. Days, or even weeks, later they show appropriately timed recovery of the anticipatory activity when they are simply food deprived for 24–48 hr (7). There are a variety of ideas about why hunger should be important in the expression of this oscillator, but these hypotheses should be regarded with caution, since it appears that the linkage of the FEO to food deprivation is not absolute. Mistlberger and Rusak (22) have shown that similar anticipatory activity can be generated in rats that are never food deprived by giving them access to a very attractive, fatty food for a limited time during the daily light phase, and allowing them free access to their regular diet at all times (Fig. 2-2A and B).

These data suggest that regular food for a hungry rat or an unusually attractive food for a free-feeding animal have some feature in common, other than hunger, that permits both entrainment and overt expression of the FEO. One possibility is that the availability or consumption of the food might in each case generate intense activity ("arousal") in the rat; the arousal itself might be the effective agent (cf. 25). If that were so, any stimulus that activates rats on a regular daily basis might be adequate to entrain the oscillator. This oscillator might then be best referred to as "arousal sensitive"; it is called food entrainable simply because of the historical accident that temporally restricted feeding was the "arousing" stimulus first used to affect and entrain it.

This simple explanatory hypothesis may not be completely adequate. Rats that have temporally restricted access to an attractive but non-nutritive food do not show anticipation, even though they eat the food readily (22; Fig. 2-2C). Apparently some features of the nutritional content of the restricted meal are also important. Similarly, water-deprived rats given limited daily access to water are highly aroused by its arrival and consumption, yet anticipatory activity does not usually develop (20).

One possibility is that nutritive meals contain an element critical for oscillator entrainment. Another is that general activity, such as we have usually measured, is readily connected to food availability, but it is the wrong behavior to attempt to link to other stimuli. It is now generally acknowledged in the ethological and learning literature that there are strong, pre-existing biological constraints on the relations that particular species can learn among stimuli and responses (18,40).

Hamsters, for example, can readily learn to increase the frequency of some behaviors when food is presented contingently on the performance of these behaviors, but other behaviors are difficult or impossible to influence with food reward (40). Whether food anticipation is a "learned" response in the technical sense, or depends on the phase shifting of oscillators, is probably irrelevant to this argument. In either case, a stimulus–response linkage must be established, and the types of linkages that

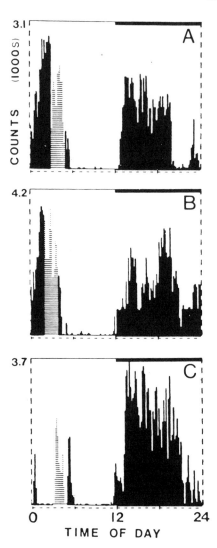

Figure 2-2 Histograms showing the 24-hr patterns of activity summed across 8 consecutive days of restricted access to an attractive diet while rats had free access to their regular diet. The data shown in gray indicates the time the restricted diet was available, and the dark bar above each record shows the daily dark phase of the light–dark cycle. (A) A rat with free access to a sweet, fatty diet during the 2 hr indicated. The rat shows a strong anticipatory increase in activity before the food becomes available. (B) A rat with access to a limited amount (4 g) of the same diet also shows anticipation. (C) A rat with unlimited access to a nonnutritive, sweet diet fails to show anticipation. [From Mistlberger and Rusak (22).]

can be established readily may be limited and characteristic of each species. Increased running activity may be linked easily to the opportunity for food consumption, but not to drinking or other biologically important opportunities.

The use of response measures other than general activity might reveal that rats are aware of the timing of all of the arousing events that have so far been tested, but that they are not prepared to express that knowledge as increased general activity. This finding would be consistent with two sets of observations. One is the report by Aschoff and von Goetz (3) that monkeys may show anticipatory manipulation of a food cup, without showing anticipatory increases in general locomotion. (In fact, locomotion decreased as the monkeys stopped climbing to manipulate the food cup.) The second is the observation that PVN-ablated rats, who became generally lethargic after the lesions and failed to increase activity in anticipation of feeding, still revealed knowledge of the timing of food availability in their nose-poking behavior (23). Until the appropriate studies are done to fully test the possibility of anticipation in other behaviors, we must conclude tentatively that not all arousing stimuli are equally effective as entraining cues for the FEO.

HOARDING ENTRAINMENT

We wondered whether a mechanism analogous to the FEO is characteristic of the circadian system of mammals other than rats. The hamster circadian system is arguably the best studied among mammals, but we do not know if it includes an FEO. The reason we do not know is that hamsters do not readily tolerate even moderate temporal restrictions on their food intake. They do not seem to be able to gorge themselves in a brief interval, and probably deal with potential food shortages by hoarding food opportunistically whenever they find it, rather than, as rats do, by consuming it opportunistically. We asked, therefore, whether hamsters might reveal a mechanism similar to the FEO of rats if they were given a limited daily opportunity to hoard rather than eat food. We expected that hamsters might manifest an activity rhythm that anticipated the daily hoarding time as well as a normal freerunning activity pattern.

Hamsters were housed in constant dim illumination and allowed to leave their home cages once daily for 30 min. During that interval they could retrieve seeds from an open-field attached by a tunnel to their home cage (35). We found that no intact hamster ever showed a separate hoarding-entrained activity component along with its main activity bout. The surprising observation was that 6 of 10 hamsters instead showed entrainment of their main activity bout, presumably driven by the SCN, to the hoarding time. We assessed whether this was true entrainment by phase shifts or by releasing animals to freerun after apparent entrainment (Fig. 2-3). But as an additional check on whether the SCN-based pacemaker was being entrained, we attempted SCN lesions in three of the six entrained hamsters.

In two animals, the lesions were incomplete. We know from earlier studies (27) that partial SCN damage shortens the freerunning period expressed by the surviving tissue. These animals showed two responses, both consistent with a shortened period. One showed a gradual phase advance of the rhythm, which then entrained at a more positive phase position, as one would predict for a shorter period oscillator. The other eventually expressed a very short-period freerun that failed to re-entrain but showed relative coordination to the hoarding time (Fig. 2-3A). The 24-hr periodicity of hoarding opportunities appeared to fall outside the entrainment range of the damaged SCN pacemaker under the influence of the presumably rather weak entraining cues provided by the hoarding opportunity.

The third ablated hamster had a complete lesion. We would have predicted a loss

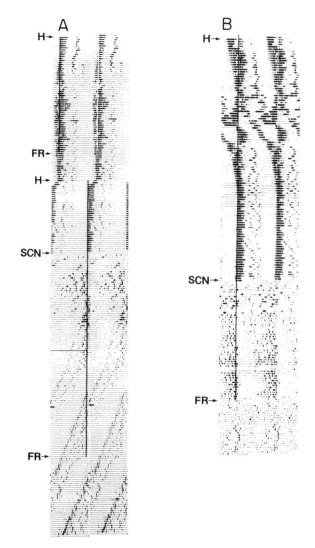

Figure 2-3 Wheel-running activity records of two hamsters housed in continuous dim illumination and exposed to a daily 30 min opportunity to leave their home cages and hoard seeds from a larger box. The availability of hoarding opportunities is indicated by a vertical line and the symbol H. Animals were released to freerun (FR) and received lesions aimed at their suprachiasmatic nuclei (SCN) at the times indicated. (A) This hamster entrains to the daily hoarding opportunity and follows a phase shift in its timing. It received a partial SCN lesion and failed subsequently to re-entrain, freerunning instead with a period shorter than 24 hr. (B) This hamster's activity crosses through the hoarding time without entraining once, then entrains successfully. It received a complete SCN lesion and then began to anticipate the hoarding opportunity. When the hoarding time was discontinued, it failed to generate a freerunning rhythm. [From Rusak et al. (35).]

of circadian rhythmicity and an absence of entrainment to the hoarding opportunity, since the apparent entrainment target, the SCN, were gone. We were surprised again, because after some weeks, a ragged but unambiguous anticipatory rhythm developed (Fig. 2-3B). This was the first clear instance of an anticipatory rhythm we had seen in hamsters, and the first indication that a circadian system susceptible to entrainment by the stimuli associated with the hoarding opportunity existed outside the SCN.

The interpretation of this finding is complex. It appears that in hamsters an oscillator susceptible to nonphotic entrainment exists outside the SCN but is never expressed in the presence of the SCN. The contrast between this finding and the responses of rats to food restrictions might imply, for example, that the SCN in hamsters suppresses the output of the extra-SCN oscillator, while in rats it does not. This is possible, but it does not explain another critical difference between hamsters and rats. Among those hamsters that do show entrainment to the hoarding cue, it is the SCN pacemaker that is entrained, while rats are resistant to pacemaker entrainment by feeding schedules.

The simplest explanation is that the SCN and the FEO in rats are measurably but very weakly coupled, as others have already suggested (43, cf. 3). The FEO in rats can then be readily separated from the SCN and entrained to a different period or phase by an appropriate stimulus that acts on it and not on the SCN. We observe this separated and entrained oscillator as a food-anticipatory activity bout. When the periods of the SCN and the extra-SCN oscillators are very similar, however, even their weak coupling might allow the food-entrained oscillator to synchronize the SCN pacemaker. This suggestion is consistent with the idea that weak coupling permits interactions over only a narrow range of period differences. The result is that one sees rare cases of entrainment of the SCN pacemaker by food-restriction schedules (43).

By contrast, the analogous oscillator in the hamster may be very tightly coupled to the SCN. The consequence would be that nonphotic cues acting on that oscillator must either entrain the entire oscillator complex, including the SCN, or fail to entrain any portion of it. The extra-SCN oscillator cannot be separately entrained and expressed while it remains tightly coupled to the SCN. When the SCN are removed, however, as in our hoarding study, environmental entrainment effects on the extra-SCN oscillator system can be observed.

OTHER CUES: THE ROLE OF AROUSAL

A number of other nonphotic cues have been reported to entrain some animals at some times. Bird song has a weak entraining action on sparrows (19), beavers may entrain socially (6), humans probably do (1), and temperature cycles may entrain some squirrel monkeys (2). Recently, Mrosovsky has demonstrated some striking examples of nonphotic effects on the hamster circadian system. He has shown phase shifts and entrainment to social cues and cage-changing (25), and acceleration of reentrainment as a consequence of activity increases caused by confinement to a novel cage (26). Mrosovsky (25) proposed that all of these cues might operate by increasing the animal's arousal, and that arousal effects are mediated through an oscillator separate from the light-sensitive pacemaker. In his view, phase shifts (and sometimes entrainment) in response to a variety of cues are secondary to the behavioral consequences of these cues that arouse and activate the hamster.

The economy of this hypothesis is attractive, and the idea that these cues act on an oscillator separate from the SCN may be consistent with our lesion data related to entrainment to hoarding opportunities (35). It is also consistent with neurophysiological recordings in rats indicating that meal schedules do not alter the rhythm of neural activity in the SCN (14). If one invokes the hypothesis of tight coupling between the SCN and an arousal-sensitive, extra-SCN oscillator in hamsters, one can generalize the earlier explanation to account for how hoarding opportunities, cage changing, and social cues indirectly phase shift and entrain the SCN-based pacemaker. Presumably the effects of these cues on arousal entrain the extra-SCN oscillator, which in turn synchronizes the SCN to which it is tightly coupled. The relative periods of these oscillators and the entraining cycles may also be critical. Although the appropriate studies have not yet been reported, it could be predicted that rats, with their relatively loose coupling of SCN to extra-SCN oscillators, would show little sign of pacemaker entrainment when exposed daily to cues such as these.

FEEDBACK AND THE PACEMAKER SYSTEM

One implication of this analysis is that the animal's state of arousal can affect the central pacemaker, directly or indirectly. Since one function of the pacemaker is to regulate the animal's arousal, this conclusion implies the existence of feedback in the circadian system, making it a closed- rather than open-loop type of control system, even if the loop is closed indirectly.

Another important implication is for our view of the role of the SCN in the circadian system. The SCN may have achieved their role as a driving pacemaker in mammals because they have privileged access to the most reliable of environmental time cues—lighting information. The importance of this cue may, however, have been overemphasized because of the ease with which lighting can be manipulated in the laboratory. The real world outside the laboratory is filled with periodic stimuli other than lighting cues, and organisms appear to have mechanisms that are sensitive to these as well. The relative difficulty of manipulating and controlling these stimuli in the laboratory may account for our lack of information about their influence on circadian rhythms and the general view that this influence is not very great.

Components of the circadian system other than the SCN may be responsible for mediating the effects of nonphotic environmental factors on rhythms, but the analysis of these factors is so far quite rudimentary. Depending on their functional relations to the SCN, these oscillators may be more or less likely to influence SCN-driven rhythms in various species. This mechanism would create inherent flexibility in the operations of the circadian system. For some species (e.g., hamsters) it might permit some cues other than light to affect the entire circadian system. For others (e.g., rats or bees), it might ensure an ability to anticipate time-constrained opportunities, while preserving photic entrainment of the pacemaker intact.

It is instructive to consider humans from this perspective. Several reports suggest that humans may be susceptible to entrainment by social cues (1), but recent studies have also demonstrated that photic cues are effective (8,13,47). Knowledge that light can affect the human circadian system does not rule out a role for other factors in entraining humans, any more than photic sensitivity rules out sensitivity to other cues in nonhuman species. Nor does evidence of sensitivity to light ensure that other environmental cues are necessarily subordinate to lighting cues in their effects on rhythms. The mammalian circadian system has the capacity to respond to a number of environmental cues. Depending on a variety of factors, including the internal coupling relations among different oscillators, their relative period lengths, and the individual's motivational state, one or another cue may effectively dominate the system. We do not know which cues are most effective in humans, nor what roles motivational factors might play in shifting the balance of control among these cues.

One implication of the findings on nonphotic cues in rodents is that stimuli that affect the behavior of organisms can indirectly affect the light-sensitive pacemaker for the circadian system. This conclusion has implications for the analysis of photic effects on humans. One issue in the literature on photic effects related to seasonal affective disorders has been whether light treatment has its therapeutic effect by changing the entrainment of an abnormally phased oscillator, or by exerting a placebo or nonspecific energizing effect (e.g., 17). The alternatives can be restated in terms of whether light re-entrains the SCN pacemaker or more directly alters the individual's motivational state and activity. If humans resemble hamsters in this regard, this sharp dichotomy may be misleading. Behavioral and motivational changes may act on a component of

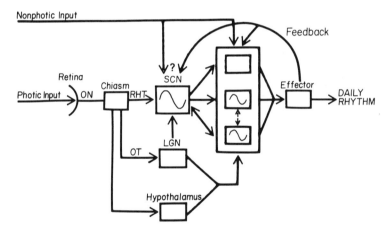

Figure 2-4 A model showing the components of the mammalian circadian system and their possible relations to each other. Photic input impinges on the retina and is conveyed via the optic nerve (ON) to the chiasm from which projections reach the SCN [via the retinohypothalamic tract (RHT)], the lateral geniculate nuclei (LGN), and other parts of the hypothalamus. The LGN projects to the SCN and perhaps to other oscillators in the circadian system. The SCN may affect behavior through their influence on other oscillators, which may also influence each other and the SCN, as well as through nonoscillatory mechanisms. Nonphotic cues reach extra-SCN oscillators but may also affect the SCN directly. The output of effector systems also reaches the extra-SCN oscillators and may directly or indirectly affect the SCN. Other elements for which there is evidence, but which are not shown, include an oscillator in the retina (or other part of the visual system) that is reciprocally connected to the SCN. This model has a closed-loop structure including several avenues for feedback on the central pacemaker. [Modified from Rusak (33).]

the circadian system that, in turn, affects the entrainment of the SCN, regardless of whether the photic cue directly phase shifts the SCN or not. These apparently different proposed effects of light therapy might then converge in causing phase shifts in the SCN pacemaker, either directly, or indirectly as a consequence of induced changes in the individual's behavior.

SUMMARY

Diagrams representing the linear, open-loop control of behavior by a central circadian pacemaker (Fig. 2-1) may be appropriate for some organisms, but are inadequate in describing the complexity of the mammalian circadian system, which might better be modeled as a complex hierarchical structure including a role for feedback (Fig. 2-4). The mammalian pacemaker appears to operate by entraining or gating the expression of a population of circadian oscillators. These and/or other parallel pacemaker systems reside outside the SCN and survive its destruction. Some oscillators in the system are sensitive to a variety of nonphotic cues. These oscillators may in turn entrain the light-sensitive pacemaker in the SCN through their direct coupling to it. Among the stimuli that may affect the extra-SCN oscillator system are the consequences of increased arousal or activity of the organism. These stimuli may, therefore, alter the function of the SCN in a manner that resembles the effects of feedback in a closed-loop control system.

ACKNOWLEDGMENTS

Research reported in this chapter was supported by grants from NSERC and MRC of Canada and the Dalhousie Research Development Fund in the Sciences.

REFERENCES

1. Aschoff J, Fatranská M, Giedke H, Doerr P, Stamm D, Wisser H. Human circadian rhythms in continuous darkness: Entrainment by social cues. *Science* 1971; 171:213–315.
2. Aschoff J, Tokura H. Circadian activity rhythms in squirrel monkeys: Entrainment by temperature cycles. *J Biol Rhythms* 1986; 1:91–99.
3. Aschoff J, von Goetz C. Effects of feeding cycles on circadian rhythms in squirrel monkeys. *J Biol Rhythms* 1986; 1:267–276.
4. Bolles RC, Stokes LW. Rat's anticipation of diurnal and adiurnal feeding. *J Comp Physiol Psychol* 1965; 60:290–294.
5. Boulos Z, Rosenwasser AM, Terman M. Feeding schedules and the circadian organization of behavior in the rat. *Behav Brain Res* 1980; 1:39–65.
6. Bovet J, Oertli E. Free-running circadian activity rhythms in free-living beaver (*Castor canadensis*). *J Comp Physiol* 1974; 92:1–10.
7. Coleman GJ, Harper S, Clarke JD, Armstrong S. Evidence for a separate meal-associated oscillator in the rat. *Physiol Behav* 1982; 29:107–115.
8. Czeisler CA, Allan JS, Strogatz SH, Ronda JC, Sanchez R, Rios CD, Freitag WO, Richardson GS. Bright light resets the human circadian pacemaker independent of the timing of the sleep-wake cycle. *Science* 1986; 233:667–671.

9. Daan S, Berde C. Two coupled oscillators: Simulations of the circadian pacemaker in mammalian activity rhythms. *J Theor Biol* 1978; 70:297–313.

10. Davis FC, Menaker M. Hamsters through time's window: Temporal structure of hamster locomotor rhythmicity. *Am J Physiol* 1980; 239:R149–R155.

11. Eastman CI, Mistlberger RE, Rechtschaffen A. Suprachiasmatic nuclei lesions eliminate circadian temperature and sleep rhythms in the rat. *Physiol Behav* 1984; 32:357–368.

12. Gaston S, Menaker M. Pineal function: The biological clock in the sparrow? *Science* 1968; 160:1125–1127.

13. Honma K, Honma S, Wada T. Phase-dependent shift of free-running human circadian rhythms in response to a single bright light pulse. *Experientia* 1987; 43:1205–1207.

14. Inouye ST. Restricted daily feeding does not entrain circadian rhythms of the suprachiasmatic nucleus in the rat. *Brain Res* 1982; 232:194–199.

15. Krieger DT. Ventromedial hypothalamic lesions abolish food-shifted circadian adrenal and temperature rhythmicity. *Endocrinology* 1980; 106:649–650.

16. Lehman MN, Silver R, Gladstone WR, Kahn RM, Gibson M, Bittman EL. Circadian rhythmicity restored by neural transplant. Immunocytochemical characterization of the graft and its integration with the host brain. *J Neurosci* 1987; 7:1626–1638.

17. Lewy AJ, Sack RL, Singer CM, White DM, Hoban TM. Winter depression and the phase shift hypothesis for bright light's therapeutic effects: History, theory and experimental evidence. *J Biol Rhythms* 1988; 3:121–133.

18. Lolordo VM. Selective associations. In A Dickinson and RA Boakes (eds.), *Mechanisms of Learning and Motivation*. Lawrence Erlbaum, Hillsdale, NJ, 1979: 367–398.

19. Menaker M, Eskin A. Entrainment of circadian rhythms by sound in *Passer domesticus. Science* 1969; 154:1579–1581.

20. Mistlberger RE, Rechtschaffen A. Periodic water availability is not a potent zeitgeber for entrainment of circadian locomotor rhythms in rats. *Physiol Behav* 1985; 34:17–22.

21. Mistlberger RE, Rechtschaffen A. Recovery of anticipatory activity to restricted feeding in rats with ventromedial hypothalamic lesions. *Physiol Behav* 1984; 33:227–235.

22. Mistlberger RE, Rusak B. Palatable daily meals entrain anticipatory activity rhythms in free-feeding rats: Dependence on meal size and nutrient content. *Physiol Behav* 1987; 41:219–226.

23. Mistlberger RE, Rusak B. Food anticipatory circadian rhythms in paraventricular and lateral hypothalamic ablated rats. *J Biol Rhythms* 1988; 3:277–291.

24. Moore RY, Eichler VB. Loss of a circadian adrenal corticosterone rhythm following suprachiasmatic lesions in the rat. *Brain Res* 1972; 2:201–206.

25. Mrosovsky N. Phase response curves for social entrainment. *J Comp Physiol A* 1988; 162:35–46.

26. Mrosovsky N, Salmon PA. A behavioural method for accelerating re-entrainment of rhythms to new light-dark cycles. *Nature (London)* 1987; 330:372–373.

27. Pickard GE, Turek FW. The suprachiasmatic nuclei: Two circadian clocks? *Brain Res* 1983; 268:201–210.

28. Pittendrigh CS. Circadian rhythms and the circadian organization of living systems. *Cold Spring Harbor Symp Quant Biol* 1960; 25:159–184.

29. Pittendrigh CS. Circadian oscillations in cells and the circadian organization of multicellular systems. In FO Schmitt and FG Worden (eds.), *The Neurosciences: Third Study Program*. The MIT Press, Cambridge, MA, 1974: 437–458.

30. Richter CP. *Biological Clocks in Medicine and Psychiatry*. Thomas, Springfield: 1967: 20.

31. Ruis JF, Rietveld WJ, Buys PJ. Effects of suprachiasmatic nuclei lesions on circadian and ultradian rhythms in body temperature in ocular enucleated rats. *J Interdiscipl Cycle Res* 1987; 18:259–273.

32. Rusak B. The role of the suprachiasmatic nuclei in the generation of circadian rhythms in the golden hamster. *J Comp Physiol A* 1977; 118:145–64.

33. Rusak B. Physiological models of the rodent circadian system. In J Aschoff, S Daan, and GA Groos (eds.), *Vertebrate Circadian Systems: Structure and Physiology*. Springer, New York, 1982: 62–74.

34. Rusak B, Groos G. Suprachiasmatic stimulation phase shifts rodent circadian rhythms. *Science* 1982; 215:1407–1409.

35. Rusak B, Mistlberger RE, Losier B, Jones CH. Daily hoarding opportunity entrains the pacemaker for hamster activity rhythms. *J Comp Physiol A* 1988; 164:165–171.

36. Rusak B, Zucker I. Neural regulation of circadian rhythms. *Physiol Rev* 1979; 59:449–526.

37. Satinoff E, Prosser R. Suprachiasmatic nuclear lesions eliminate circadian rhythms of drinking and activity, but not of body temperature, in male rats. *J Biol Rhythms* 1988; 3:1–22.

38. Schulz H, Dirlich G, Zulley J. Phase shift of REM sleep rhythm. *Pflugers Arch* 1975; 358:203–212.

39. Schwartz WJ, Gross RA, Morton MT. The suprachiasmatic nuclei contain a tetrodotoxin-resistant circadian pacemaker. *Proc Natl Acad Sci USA* 1987; 84:1694–1698.

40. Shettleworth SJ. Reinforcement and the organization of behavior in golden hamsters: hunger, environment, and food reinforcement. *J Exp Psychol* 1975; 104:56–87.

41. Stephan FK. Limits of entrainment to periodic feeding of rats with suprachiasmatic lesions. *J Comp Physiol A* 1981; 143:401–410.

42. Stephan FK. Phase shifts of circadian rhythms of activity entrained to food access. *Physiol Behav* 1984; 32:663–671.

43. Stephan FK. The role of period and phase in interactions between feeding- and light-entrainable circadian rhythms. *Physiol Behav* 1986; 36:151–158.

44. Stephan FK, Swann JM, Sisk CL. Anticipation of 24-hr feeding schedules in rats with lesions of the suprachiasmatic nucleus. *Behav Biol* 1979; 25:346–363.

45. Stephan FK, Zucker I. Circadian rhythms in drinking behavior and locomotor activity in rats are eliminated by hypothalamic lesions. *Proc Natl Acad Sci USA* 1972; 69:1583–1586.

46. Terman T, Terman J. A circadian pacemaker for visual sensitivity? *Ann NY Acad Sci* 1985; 453:147–161.

47. Wever R, Polasek J, Wildgruber CM. Bright light affects human circadian rhythms. *Pflugers Arch* 1983; 396:85–87.

3

Sleep–Wake Biorhythms
and Extended Sleep in Man

ROGER BROUGHTON, JOSEPH DE KONINCK,
PiERRE GAGNON, WAYNE DUNHAM, AND CLAUDIO STAMPI

It has been evident for a number of decades that sleep has both homeostatic and biorhythmic properties. The concept of sleep homeostasis goes back at least to the experiments of Piéron (63) in which "une substance hypnotoxique" was believed to accumulate during wakefulness and to be dissipated during sleep. Total sleep deprivation has long been known to increase pressure for sleep and lead to recuperative sleep that is increased in duration and exhibits an initial rebound of slow wave sleep (SWS), followed by one of REM sleep (75). More recently, it has shown to also increase the spectral power in individual lower frequency bands of the sleep EEG (9). Moreover, both SWS and REM sleep show individual homeostasis with increases in SWS occurring after SWS deprivation (1) and increases in REM sleep after REM sleep deprivation (2,23).

The homeostatic features of sleep occur superimposed on powerful underlying biorhythmic fluctuations. The latter include rhythms that, according to their periodicity, have come to be known as circadian, circasemidian, and ultradian. Slower circa-weekly, monthly (menstrual, lunar), and annual (seasonal) infradian rhythms also exist, but will not be considered further.

This chapter provides a brief critical summary of aspects of the chronobiology of human sleep and related models, topics that are more extensively reviewed elsewhere (14), and also presents new data on the use of the extended sleep paradigm for their elucidation.

SLEEP–WAKE BIORHYTHMS IN MAN

Circadian

The term circadian was coined by Franz Halberg to describe those rhythms with a period of about a day (Latin *circa*, around; *dies*, a day), more specifically between 20 and 28 hr. The daily appearance of a major sleep period occurring typically during the nighttime is, of course, the most self-evident rhythmic feature of human sleep. "Free running" studies in environments totally lacking in time cues show both that the daily occurrence of sleep is an endogenous rhythm and that its true period is some 24.5–25.5 hr (72,73). The more or less regular hours of sleep are due to so-called entraining factors or Zeitgebers (German *Zeit,* time; *Geber,* giver), particularly causes of regularity in morning awakening either natural (sunlight, environmental noises) or artificial (alarm clock). The timing of sleep in the entrained state shows more or less consistent phase relationships with other circadian biorhythms, of which the most completely studied is that of body core temperature.

Body core temperature most commonly peaks in the evening, begins to decrease 1–2 hr prior to sleep onset, reaches its lowest point (nadir) in the latter third of night sleep, starts to increase prior to sleep onset, and then increases progressively across the day (20,39). This overall pattern contains both endogenous and superimposed "masking" exogenous (e.g., from activity, meals, environmental temperature) components (27,74). Closely parallel to the body core temperature rhythm are changes in virtually all performance tasks (38) other than those heavily loaded for memory, which peak in the morning (4,29,45). Because these relationships of the circadian body core temperature rhythm and the sleep rhythm are so consistent, and because changes in temperature tend to precede the sleep–wake changes, some authors have suggested that body core temperature is the major determinant of sleep–wake states. However, under "free running" conditions the body core temperature rhythm is highly stable with a period of 24.5–25.5 hr, but may show complex phase relationships with sleep whose period can increase to 48 hr or more (this drifting apart under time isolation conditions of two normally coupled biorhythms has been called "internal desynchronization"— 3). Moreover, when napping is permitted, sleep episodes occur near both temperature peaks and troughs (77). For these and for other reasons it seems unlikely that body core temperature is more than a modulator of sleep probability.

The fact that in the entrained state the major sleep period shows quite consistent recurrence in sidereal time means, of course, that so do all of its main internally consistent features. These include the times of maximum probability (circadian acrophases) of sleep onset, slow wave sleep, REM sleep, and morning awakening. The factors that determine the moment of sleep onset are not fully defined. They include the existing state of entrainment of the underlying circadian sleep–wake oscillator, the amount of prior wakefulness, a decrease in body core temperature (which relates to prior entrainment of the circadian temperature oscillator), degree of subjective sleepiness, voluntary decision to go to sleep, presence of a comfortable and quiet sleep environment, and conditioning of sleep to environmental bedroom cues.

Study of the characteristics of the endogenous sleep–wake and body core temperature rhythms has led to testable theoretical models. A two-process single oscillator model was proposed in 1982 by Borbély (8). It consists of a "process S" similar to the classical hypnogenic substance plus a single endogenous circadian oscillator, process C. The latter is a rhythmic fluctuation in sleep propensity that closely parallels body core temperature. Process S builds up in wakefulness, declines exponentially in sleep, and is believed indexed by the spectral power of EEG slow wave activity. The model, further refined by Daan et al. (21), makes numerous predictions concerning the effects of a number of sleep manipulations, and it has been applied with some success to sleep in depression (44). Folkard and Akerstedt (28) have recently added a sleep inertia (or awakening) factor, "process W," to Borbély's processes C and S, which provides a more accurate prediction of subjective alertness during abnormal sleep–wake schedules.

A two-oscillator model was proposed in the same year by Kronauer et al. (43) that involves a strong X oscillator (governing body core temperature and REM sleep) and a weak Y oscillator (governing sleep–wake state). These oscillators are equivalent to the earlier types I and II oscillators of Wever (72,73). Despite not accommodating the homeostatic properties of sleep, the model predicts sleep under a variety of conditions (33).

A three-oscillator model was proposed by Kawato et al. (35) with separate oscillators for body core temperature, wake onset, and sleep onset. Oscillator states are described only by phase, unlike the differential equations of Kronauer et al. in which both state and amplitude are stipulated. Again, reasonable predictions of major circadian aspects were verified.

Circadian sleep–wake and temperature rhythms are generally treated as more or less sinusoidal events both in data analysis and in models. This methodological assumption is hardly supported by the raw data. First, the sleep–wake state is essentially a binary process. Second, attempts to fit body core temperature into a single sine wave significantly distort the original shape, which is much more complex, quite asymmetrical, and shows superimposed evoked and other "masking" changes related to activity (increases), sleep onset (decrease), and other factors. Other approaches, such as polynomial regression analysis, might give a much more precise description of the shape and timing of the recorded temperature curve. Recording body core temperature under the three conditions of normal sleep–activity patterns, sleep deprivation with constant activity over the 24-hr period, and continuous bedrest with a normal sleep–wake cycle but minimal activity can provide data that, with appropriate subtractive manipulation, can better estimate the endogenous circadian temperature rhythm and reveal a more sinusoidal waveform (27). Finally, correlations of body core temperature with sleep–wake status might be considerably higher using *rate of change* of temperature (indexed by the first derivative) rather than the (probably) biologically less meaningful absolute levels that are currently employed.

Circasemidian

Over the last few years it has become evident that sleep also shows a propensity for an approximately 2/day appearance consisting of a major sleep period (usually nocturnal) and a secondary period of sleepiness or an actual nap (usually mid-afternoon). This bimodal sleep rhythm therefore has a period of about half a day and so can be described as circasemidian or, as Kronauer (42) prefers, as hemicircadian.

The existence of an endogenous 2/day sleep rhythm was first proposed by Broughton (11) and then Webb (70). It was also postulated (11) that there was a related circa 12-hr rhythm of SWS, and that numerous harmonics of the fundamental circadian rhythm could occur at circa 48, 12, 6, 4, 3, and 1.5 hr.

The afternoon period of sleepiness or sleep is, of course, seen as the last nap given up in growth and development, usually when the child has to remain in school for the entire day, and as the usual time of voluntary naps (38) and of daytime sleep in siesta cultures. The latter are generally tropical or subtropical and typically restrict their hours of night sleep by eating and going to bed late (12,14). An afternoon increase in sleepiness is reflected in Blake's (7) so-called "post-lunch dip" in performance and in sleep latency measures by MSLT (65). In pathology, an increase in daytime sleep at this time is seen for narcoleptics in both laboratory studies (6) and in ambulant home monitoring (16,17). It is a robust phenomenon preserved even in the ultrashort sleep schedule of 20 min "days" (7 min for sleep, 13 for wake) of Lavie and Scherson (49). Lavie (48) has called the consistent periods of wakefulness between the circasemidian sleep peaks "forbidden zones for sleep" and Strogatz (67) has called them "wake-maintenance zones." The endogenous nature of the 2/day sleep rhythm is proven by time isolation studies with permitted naps, which show the regular appearance of two sleep periods, a major one usually near the minimum of body core temperature and a minor one near the temperature peak (77).

Evidence also exists that a 12-hr SWS rhythm may be involved in the circasemidian appearance of sleep. It has long been known that the amount of SWS reflects prior wakefulness (71). Indeed studies such as those of Maron et al. (53) and Dijk et al. (25) indicate that evening naps (with longer prior wakefulness) have more slow wave sleep than do mid-afternoon ones. Separation of circadian from state (i.e., sleep) dependent aspects is not easy. Yet it is now well documented in the studies of Gagnon and De Koninck (31) that extended sleep leads to a delayed appearance some 12.5–13.5 hr later of a second major SWS pulse. And in extended sleep that is acutely delayed by 4 hr (from 2400 to 0400 hr), the first night contains three major SWS pulses, the first shortly after sleep onset, the second around 1300 hr (i.e., at about the same time as the second SWS pulse prior to delay, suggesting a circadian time-of-day effect), and a third one some 13 hr after the initial peak (i.e., as part of a sleep-dependent circa 12-hr rhythm). By the fourth night of delayed extended sleep only the 12-hr rhythm persists (32). These features of extended sleep are further examined below. Finally, Campbell and Zulley (19) have recently described a circa 12-hr SWS rhythm in the disentrained time free state.

Limited modeling of the circa 12-hr sleep rhythm has been done. Broughton (11) and Lavie (47) published schematic representations. Recently, Kronauer (42) split his weak Y oscillator into two reciprocal weak Y1 and Y2 oscillators to incorporate this striking feature of sleep biorhythmicity. It has been proposed by Broughton (14) that the fundamental rhythm is probably not one of sleep per se but rather of *wakefulness* with permissive "gates" for sleep occurring between the waking peaks.

Intermediate Ultradian Rhythms

There is considerable evidence for circa 3- to 4-hr rhythms involving sleep. Infants show waking and feeding behaviors at this periodicity (38). Sleep-related 3- to 4-hr periodicity has been documented in EEG signs of drowsiness by automatic analysis (51,52). Such a rhythm appears quite prominently in normals during both continuous bedrest conditions (58) and in the ultrashort sleep paradigm (50). Bedrest studies with *ad libitum* sleep in narcoleptics of Billiard and De Koninck (recent unpublished data) show a prominent 4-hr SWS rhythm. And sleep episodes at this periodicity can occur in time isolation studies (76). The phenomenon needs further study and is not currently incorporated into any model.

Ultradian Rhythms

Night sleep contains rhythmic alternation of NREM and REM sleep states with a period of some 90–120 min in adults (24). Kleitman (37,38) later proposed the existence of a basic rest–activity cycle (BRAC) that would continue around the 24 hr being expressed within sleep as the NREM/REM sleep cycle and within wakefulness as equivalent oscillations in drowsiness–alertness and quiescence–activity. No compelling evidence for waking rhythms of motor rest and activity at this rate has been published; but there is solid evidence for such daytime fluctuations in alertness. These have been documented by studies of EEG (40,51,52,59), vigilance-type performance tasks (18,60), pupillometry (46), and "sleepability" in ultrashort sleep studies (49). The ultradian fluctuations in alertness are accentuated by drowsiness (13) and, at least for the performance aspects, are suppressed by sustained intense motivation (41). In patients, daytime sleep episodes of narcoleptics may show ultradian reappearance whether involving REM sleep (61) or NREM sleep (5), even when such patients are trying to sustain vigilance during prolonged performance testing (69).

The NREM–REM sleep cycle has been modeled by McCarley and Hobson (54) with further refinements including addition of physiological limits on neuronal firing rates by McCarley and Massaquoi (55). This model involves reciprocal interaction between REM-on and REM-off neuronal populations that are expressed as Lotka–Volterra equations. It is quite predictive of the timing of REM periods in both entrained and free-running human data. It does not, however, predict waking ultradian rhythms.

Our knowledge base remains insufficient for more comprehensive modeling of BRAC-related events. It is still not certain, for instance, whether the NREM–REM sleep cycle is sleep dependent or not. Studies that collapse wake time, such as those in the cat of Ursin et al. (68) and in man of Moses et al. (56,57), suggest that REM periodicity is sleep dependent. However, studies in humans sleeping much of the day, such as narcoleptics, indicate that the timing of nocturnal REM periods can be predicted from prior daytime ones (22). It is also not yet known whether the daytime oscillations of sleepiness–alertness are in phase with the nocturnal NREM–REM cycle, which would be an essential prediction of the BRAC hypothesis. Studies of Lavie and Zomer (50) using the ultrashort sleep paradigm showed a nonsignificant trend for greater sleepiness in phase with prior NREM periods. However, children showing ultradian fluctuations in vigilance tended to have more omissions and false positives (suggesting greater sleepiness) in phase with prior REM periods (13). Finally, authors have largely conceptualized REM sleep as a rhythm. Yet even our raw histogram data questions this interpretation. It shows a slow decline through NREM stages and much more abrupt arousals toward REM sleep, creating an asymmetrical "saw-toothed" pattern rather than a sinusoidal event. Considering REM sleep as an all or none *periodic* event, rather than a rhythmic event, would therefore be more realistic (14).

Analysis of the biorhythmic aspects of sleep–wake behavior has employed data from a number of approaches. These include traditional polysomnography, nap studies, bedrest and constant routine studies, extended sleep, ambulatory monitoring, ultrashort sleep schedules, and time isolation studies. The utility of the extended sleep paradigm to document the circadian, circasemidian, and ultradian aspects of sleep will be examined by more detailed analysis of the data in Gagnon and De Koninck (31) and Gagnon et al. (32). A preliminary report (15) has been published.

EXTENDED SLEEP PARADIGM

The extended sleep paradigm was introduced by Gagnon and De Koninck (31) to test the hypothesis (11) of a circa 12-hr SWS rhythm. The reappearance of SWS some 13.5 hr after sleep onset with lights out at 2400 hr in normal subjects chosen for their ability to significantly extend sleep was supportive evidence: but it also could have been due to sleep-dependent or circadian time-of-day factors. To distinguish the latter, the effects of delaying sleep onset of extended sleep were tested both in acute and adapted states. Baseline extended sleep involved simple sleep extension from usual sleep patterns. Acute delayed extended sleep involved both delayed sleep onset *and* sleep extension from usual sleep patterns. And adapted delayed extended sleep involved prior adaptation to delayed sleep onset with normal sleep duration followed by sleep extension. The precise protocols are provided below. As already mentioned, evidence for both transient circadian time-of-day (on night 1) and constant sleep-dependent features was found (32). Other details are given in Gagnon (30).

Further analysis of the data in these studies was indicated for several reasons. It was soon proposed by Horne (34) that the delayed second SWS pulse might be a secondary effect of the increased wakefulness after sleep onset found mainly in the last 3 hr of extended sleep. This possibility had not been excluded by the initial analysis. Second, the acute delay of extended sleep increased prior wakefulness, and the latter's possible role in altering SWS content had not been analyzed. Third, greatly extended sleep provides an excellent paradigm with which to analyze the within sleep circadian, circasemidian, and ultradian features by techniques such as formal time series analysis and curve fitting procedures. It was therefore decided to enter the raw data into a computer data matrix and analyze these other features of extended sleep.

Methods

Subjects

Subjects were chosen from a questionnaire survey of over 450 undergraduates for having a usual habit of 7–9 hr of night sleep combined with an ability to occasionally remain asleep for 12 hr or more. Those with a history of difficulty of falling asleep, remaining asleep, having excessive daytime sleepiness or other signs of hypersomnia, or taking CNS active medication were excluded. All participating subjects were healthy 17- to 22-year-old students. Female subjects were studied outside of the perimenstrual period.

Design. Data in these analyses came from both the reports of Gagnon and De Koninck (31) and Gagnon et al. (32) and were divided into three parts.

1. *Baseline extended sleep:*   15 subjects (12 female, 3 male) had two adaptation nights of 7–8 hr sleep followed by a single night of extended sleep exceeding 14.4 hr, all 3 nights having lights out at 2400 hr.
2. *Acute delayed extended sleep:*   8 of the above subjects (7 female, 1 male) had a readaptation night of 7–8 hr sleep beginning at 2400 hr followed by acute delay of bedtime to 0400 hr and successful extension of sleep for 14.4 hr or more.
3. *Adapted delayed extended sleep:*   6 of 10 other subjects (4 female, 2 male)

had three baseline nights of delayed 7–8 hr duration sleep with bedtime at 0400 hr and then were able to extend their sleep on a fourth night for 14.4 hr or more.

Physiological recordings and staging. Recordings included C3-A1 EEG, EOG, and submental EMG leads and were made using a Tektronix EEG apparatus with paper writeout of 10 mm/sec. Sleep staging was done visually following the criteria of Rechtschaffen and Kales (64) using 1-min epochs. Scoring reliability was checked by independent blind scoring of two judges, and the correlation coefficients for all stages were over 0.85. In all statistical analyses, stages 3 and 4 were combined into SWS.

Data analysis. Visually scored data for the extended nights to be analyzed were entered into a computer matrix. These data involved the 15 nights of extended sleep from midnight, 8 with acute delay to 0400 hr, and 6 with adapted delayed sleep onset at 0400 hr. The procedure therefore involved 25,056 data entries (29 nights × 14.4 hr × 60 min).

Mean raw data plots were made for each of the three conditions using 10-min bins to obtain a visual representation of group evolution across time and to guide subsequent analyses.

Correlation analyses were performed for the baseline extended sleep condition (15 subjects) to ascertain whether the delayed SWS reappearance might be explicable by prior sleep state—in particular by prior within-sleep wakefulness. Correlations were made with the magnitude (min) of SWS occurring after 12 hr and the prior within-sleep amounts of wakefulness after sleep onset (WASO), stage 1, 2, SWS, REM, and WASO + REM.

Ultradian aspects were investigated in the 15 nights of baseline extended sleep using autocorrelational analyses from Box and Jenkins (10). Individual sleep–wake states were averaged into 5-min bins and autocorrelations generated for up to 43 lags. The program provided detection of all peaks exceeding 1 and 2 standard errors and gave their r values. Analyses were also done using 10-min bins. These confirmed the results with 5-min bins, but gave less precision for the mean period, and so are not reported here.

Circadian, circasemidian, and intermediate ultradian features were analyzed by multiple polynomial regression analyses using the algorithms of Pedhazur (62) on averaged data using 10-min bins, that is, equivalent to the mean raw data plots. Such curve fitting employs the least-squares method. In essence, it searches the raw data for a particular sleep–wake state with consecutive stepwise increases in the power of the differential equation until a satisfactory fit is made. The available program goes up to the fifteenth power and the r^2 value indicates the amount of variance expressed in the fitted curve. The program also plots the fitted curve across the raw data.

Sleep stage comparisons were done on the three conditions directly on the data matrix using the two-tailed Student's t test.

Results

Mean Raw Data

The plot of the mean raw data for sleep across 14.4 hr of baseline extended sleep revealed a number of features of interest. They included an evident ultradian dampening of SWS across the first few sleep cycles, a second major SWS peak appearing some 13 hr after sleep onset, apparent ultradian rhythmicity of REM sleep (which was well maintained in amount until around 11–12 hr after sleep onset) and of stage 2 sleep, lack of apparent ultradian rhythmicity of stage 1 and WASO, and an increase in WASO in the last 3 hr of sleep.

Correlational analyses of the magnitude of the delayed SWS peak and prior sleep structure were significant for three variables, but in the direction opposite to that predicted by Horne (34). Negative significant correlations occurred for WASO ($r = -.51, p = .025$), WASO and REM ($r = -.65, p = .002$), and stage 1 ($r = -.48, p = .035$). Moreover, there was a strong trend toward a positive correlation with prior SWS ($r = .38, p = .08$).

Ultradian rhythms were found by autocorrelation time series analysis to be significant for REM sleep with a period of 90 min (18 lags, $r^2 = .44$), SWS at 95 min (19 lags, $r^2 = .37$), and stage 2 at 105 min (21 lags, $r^2 = .25$). Lack of significant rhythmicity of stages 1 and WASO was confirmed.

Circadian, circasemidian, and intermediate ultradian features were clarified by the polynomial regression analysis. The power to which each polynomial was taken and the equivalent r^2 value are provided in Table 3-1.

Wakefulness after sleep onset was minimal until 10 hr after sleep onset, whereafter it comprised about 45% of time with a transient decrease at around 13 hr, when SWS reappearance was maximum. Stage 1 showed a peak with sleep onset drowsiness, then became minimal and increased progressively across the night. Stage 2 was low for the first 2 hr, being out of phase with SWS, essentially flat from 2 to 10 hr, and thereafter showed two decreases at the times of maximum wakefulness (11 hr) and of the second SWS peak (14 hr). SWS had its maximum peak 30 min after sleep onset, decreased with ultradian dampening until 4 hr, then stayed low until after 13 hr, and showed the delayed peak at 14.0 hr. Thus, the interpeak interval was 13.5 hr, essentially identical to that obtained without curve fitting by Gagnon and De Koninck (31). Superimposed on this semicircadian distribution were tertiary level lower amplitude ultradian peaks seen in the fitted data around 2.5, 5.5, 8.5, and 11.5 hr, that is, around every 3 hr. In post hoc analyses, substituting the physiological data between 4 and 13 hr after sleep onset with both random numbers (ranging between 0 and 1 min) and with constant 0 min data and repeating the polynomial regression analysis gave similar circa 3-hr intermediate peaks, implying an artifactual origin. The raw data and fitted curves are shown for baseline extended sleep in Figure 3-1.

Table 3-1 Fitted Curves by Polynomial Regression Analysis

	Baseline extended		Acute delayed		Adapted delayed	
	Power	r^2	Power	r^2	Power	r^2
WASO	14	.97	15	.91	15	.93
1	15[a]	.79	15	.61	15[a]	.63
2	13	.68	12	.50	1	.00
SWS	14	.91	14	.80	15	.79
REM	3	.59	4	.24	4	.24

[a]In these instances the fit was not complete at the fifteenth power and would have been pursued to higher powers had the program permitted.

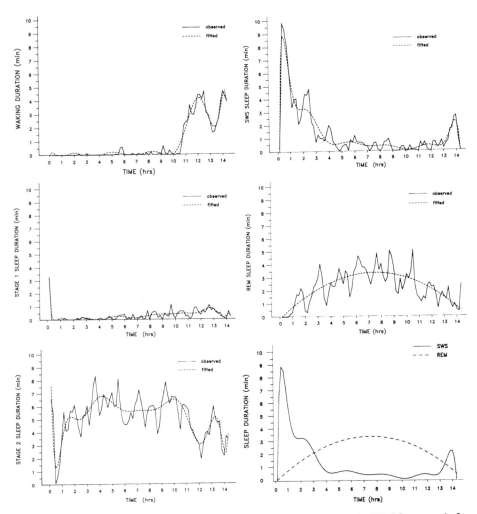

Figure 3-1 Baseline extended sleep showing raw data and fitted curves for WASO, stages 1, 2, SWS, and REM, plus superimposed fitted curves for SWS and REM.

The circadian placement of REM sleep was maximum between the two SWS peaks. The circadian REM acrophase was at 7.5 hr, that is, near the subjects' usual time of awakening. But high amounts of REM sleep were also seen well into the mid-morning period. REM sleep was at 95% of the circadian maximum between 6.5 and 9.0 hr and at 90% between 5.3 and 10.8 hr.

Comparison with Acute Delayed Extended Sleep

The fitted curves for individual sleep–wake states in the acutely delayed condition are provided in Figure 3-2, and statistical comparisons with baseline extended sleep in Table 3-2. The two most striking features are the three peaks in SWS present at 0.5, 8.5, and 13.5 hr after sleep onset. The second peak is close to the clock time of the initial predelay second peak. Secondly, acute delay (but not adapted delay) adds 4 hr of presleep wakefulness and a significant increase in SWS occurred in the acute delay

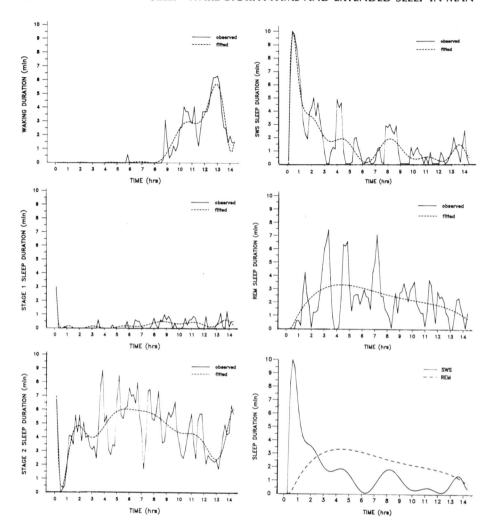

Figure 3-2 Acute delayed extended sleep (as for baseline extended sleep).

condition (Table 3-2). Data were also separated into thirds of the night between conditions and are presented in Table 3-3. Concerning the acute delay condition, two further predictions (other than an anticipated increase in total SWS) were made. The first was that an increase in SWS would occur particularly in the middle third of the night as a circadian effect. The second one was that, due to the relatively slow responsiveness to sleep displacement of the circadian distribution of REM sleep (determined by the Kronauer X oscillator), there would be a greater amount of REM sleep in the first third of the night. These two a priori predictions were tested by the Dunn–Sidak pairways comparisons procedure (36). Both held true at the $p = .05$ level.

Comparison with Adapted Delayed Extended Sleep

The results of the polynomial regression analysis are shown in Figure 3-3. The sleep statistics compared to the other two states are presented in Table 3-2 and by thirds of

Table 3-2 Comparison of All-Night Sleep–Wake Patterns in Extended Sleep in Baseline, Acute Delayed, and Adapted Delayed Conditions

		A Baseline		B Acute delay		C Adapted delay		Significance		
		Mean	SD	Mean	SD	Mean	SD	A vs B	A vs C	B vs C
Sleep period	(min)	850.5	19.2	845.8	41.2	848.5	26.0	NS	NS	NS
Sleep time	(min)	778.7	44.4	757.9	53.8	755.8	71.5	NS	NS	NS
Sleep efficiency	(%)	92.6	5.0	89.7	5.7	89.1	7.9	NS	NS	NS
Sleep latency	(min)	15.9	9.1	9.8	4.7	11.7	7.8	NS	NS	NS
SWS latency	(min)	15.3	3.2	12.9	3.0	15.3	4.3	NS	NS	NS
REM latency	(min)	79.2	24.7	83.9	29.2	63.7	20.6	NS	NS	NS
REMPs	(no.)	8.5	1.3	7.5	1.4	8.2	1.7	NS	NS	NS
REMP efficiency	(%)	94.3	7.3	95.9	4.9	90.8	7.4	NS	NS	NS
REMP duration	(min)	25.8	5.4	27.4	4.6	27.6	5.8	NS	NS	NS
REM cycle duration	(min)	98.8	11.8	102.6	12.0	106.1	23.7	NS	NS	NS
Ws >1 min	(no.)	3.7	2.4	2.5	1.2	3.3	1.8	NS	NS	NS
Stage shifts	(no.)	53.5	8.8	51.2	6.5	57.5	8.1	NS	NS	NS
WASO	(min)	77.3	43.3	106.1	53.8	108.2	71.5	NS	NS	NS
Stage 1	(min)	24.1	8.6	21.2	11.2	41.7	15.1	NS	.01	.01
Stage 2	(min)	447.9	45.3	393.9	58.8	390.8	75.2	.01	.05	NS
Stage SWS	(min)	115.3	27.2	147.0	28.4	125.2	19.3	.01	NS	.05
REM sleep	(min)	199.4	25.9	195.8	37.6	198.2	47.6	NS	NS	NS

Table 3-3 Sleep–Wake Stages (min) by Thirds of Extended Nights in Baseline, Acute Delayed, and Adapted Delayed Conditions

	A Baseline		B Acute delay		C Adapted delay	
	Mean	SD	Mean	SD	Mean	SD
First third						
WASO	0.2	0.8	0.0	0.0	0.0	0.0
1	4.5	3.0	4.0	3.0	8.3	4.8
2	148.8	27.7	113.0	20.2	120.2	7.6
SWS	86.1	18.2	101.8	13.0	93.2	10.8
REM[a]	48.4	16.1	69.2	11.4	66.3	9.3
Second third						
WASO	3.3	5.8	7.8	6.9	18.0	36.0
1	6.4	5.5	7.9	9.4	15.2	9.7
2	170.0	20.4	169.4	22.8	153.7	15.0
SWS[a]	12.4	12.5	26.8	10.6	14.0	13.6
REM	95.9	15.1	76.2	22.0	87.2	32.5
Third third						
WASO	73.9	44.5	98.4	52.3	90.2	56.0
1	13.3	4.4	9.4	2.6	18.2	5.6
2	129.1	32.7	111.5	41.1	117.0	17.0
SWS	16.7	11.5	18.5	15.4	18.0	10.2
REM	55.1	19.4	50.2	19.5	44.7	17.7

[a]A priori Dunn–Sidak pairwise comparisons were done on these variables (see text).

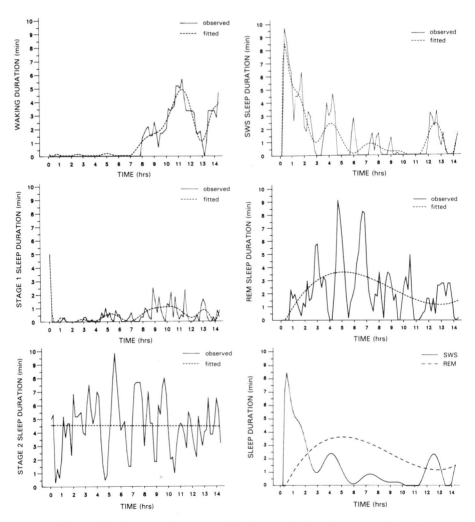

Figure 3-3 Adapted delayed extended sleep (as for baseline extended sleep).

night in Table 3-3. It is evident that the pattern is quite similar to the baseline condition insofar as SWS and REM sleep are concerned: but there is significantly more stage 1 than in both of the other two conditions and significantly less SWS than in the acutely delayed condition with its greater prior wakefulness.

Discussion

The analyses completed in this study further clarify aspects of the chronobiology of sleep. The delayed SWS peak some 13.5 hr after sleep onset could not be explained by greater prior within-sleep wakefulness or wakefulness + REM (or stage 1), as suggested by Horne (34). Indeed, the correlation was the inverse. The less the amount of prior wakefulness or light sleep (and the greater the prior SWS) the larger the magnitude of the delayed SWS peak. Thus unfragmented deep sleep predisposes to greater delayed SWS reappearance.

Coexistent effects of circadian factors and presleep wakefulness were seen in the acute delayed data. In this condition, the underlying sleep–wake and body core temperature (unrecorded) rhythms had been entrained for sleep onset shortly after 2400 hr and 7–8 hr of subsequent sleep. Acute delay of 4 hr involves both an increase in prior wakefulness by this amount and a similar realignment of sleep placement within the context of the prior entrained biorhythms. The resultant effects included changes in sleep–wake amounts and time of occurrence within sleep. The increase in total SWS of some 35 min no doubt reflects the higher amounts of prior wakefulness. The latter would not, however, explain the temporal distribution of SWS within the sleep period. This consisted of three main SWS peaks. The first was in the classical location shortly after sleep onset. The second was around 1300 hr, that is, close to the clock time of the second peak in the baseline extended condition. As previously discussed (32), this is most easily explained by a circadian time-of-day factor, there being essentially no wakefulness between the two peaks. And the third SWS pulse occurred 13.5 hr after the first, and so indicated the coexistence of the previously described sleep-dependent circa 12-hr SWS rhythm. By the fourth night of delayed sleep onset, only the circa 12-hr rhythm was present.

Autocorrelation with 5-min lags supported significant ultradian rhythmicity of stages REM, SWS, and stage 2, but not of stage 1 drowsiness or wakefulness. The somewhat different periods are of interest. The REM sleep period was 90 min, stage 2 period was 95 min, and SWS period was 105 min. The slower periodicities of the NREM sleep stages can be explained by their progressively later appearance on average within the individual NREM/REM cycles.

Curve fitting of slower events by polynomial regression analysis was of interest for several reasons. The SWS interval could be measured more precisely, and in the baseline state was 13.5 hr. A superimposed circa 3-hr SWS rhythm was found which appeared equivalent to the 3- to 4-hr SWS rhythm seen in narcoleptics under continuous bedrest conditions found by Billiard and De Koninck (unpublished data). Unfortunately, post hoc tests suggested that our intermediate range ultradian peaks were probably an artifact of the data processing technique.

The interactions between SWS and other sleep stages were clarified by this form of data processing. Displacement of stage 2 by SWS was evident both in the first 2 hr and in hours 13 and 14 of sleep. Moreover, the circadian REM acrophase was clearly placed between the two SWS pulses, probably reflecting their reciprocal inhibitory nature. And REM sleep was found to continue in high amounts up to 11 hr after sleep onset. This facilitation of REM sleep mechanisms across the morning hours may explain why SOREMPs are much more common when naps are taken at that time in both normals (53) and patients (2). It may also explain the curious and previously mentioned finding that performance tasks with high memory loads are best performed in the morning, the role of REM sleep in memory and learning functions being well documented (26,66).

SUMMARY

Human sleep–wake rhythms show main periodicities around 24, 12, 3–4, and 1.5–2 hr. These periodicities are seen in multiple types of experimental manipulations in normals and occur in sleep pathologies such as narcolepsy. A single approach, such as that of extended sleep, may evidence these periodicities. No comprehensive model yet exists incorporating the many documented periodicities of sleep-related biorhythms (14).

ACKNOWLEDGMENTS

We thank Joel Ginsburg for entering the extended sleep data into computer (which took 6 weeks), the Medical Research Council of Canada and the Natural Sciences and Engineering Research Council of Canada for financial support, and Barbara Reynolds for typing the manuscript.

REFERENCES

1. Agnew HW, Webb WB, Williams RL. Comparison of stage 4 and 1-REM sleep deprivation. *Percept Motor Skills* 1967; 24:851–858.
2. Aguirre M, Broughton R. Complex event-related potentials (P300 and CNV) and MSLT in the assessment of excessive daytime sleepiness in narcolepsy-cataplexy. *Electroenceph Clin Neurophysiol* 1987; 67:298–316.
3. Aschoff J, Wever R. Spontanperiodik des Menschen dei Ausschluss aller Zeitgeber. *Dei Naturwissenschaften* 1962; 49:337–342.
4. Baddeley AD, Hatter J, Scott D, Snashall A. Memory and time of day. *Br J Psychol* 1970; 22:605–609.
5. Baldy-Moulinier M, Arguner A, Besset A. Ultradian and circadian rhythms in sleep and wakefulness. In C Guilleminault and WC Dement (eds.), *Narcolepsy*. Spectrum, New York, 1976: 485–98.
6. Billiard M, Quera Salva M, De Koninck J, Besset A, Touchon J, Cadilhac J. Daytime characteristics and their relationships with night sleep in the narcoleptic patient. *Sleep* 1986; 9:167–174.
7. Blake MFJ. Time of day effects on performance in a range of tasks. *Psychonom Sci* 1967; 9:349–350.
8. Borbély AA. A two process model of sleep regulation. *Hum Neurobiol* 1982; 1:195–204.
9. Borbély AA, Baumann F, Brandeis D, Stauch I, Lehmann D. Sleep deprivation effect on sleep stages and EEG power density in man. *Electroenceph Clin Neurophysiol* 1981; 51:483–493.
10. Box G, Jenkins G. *Time Series Analysis*. Holden-Day, San Francisco, 1976.
11. Broughton RJ. Biorhythmic variations in consciousness and psychological functions. *Can Psychol Rev* 1975; 16:217–230.
12. Broughton RJ. The siesta: Social or biological phenomenon? *Sleep Res* 1983; 12:28.
13. Broughton RJ. Three central issues concerning ultradian rhythms. In *Ultradian Rhythms in Physiology and Behavior*. H Schulz and P Lavie (eds.), Springer-Verlag, Berlin, 1985: 217–233.
14. Broughton R. Chronobiological aspects of models of sleep and napping. In D Dinges and R Broughton (eds.), *Sleep and Alertness: Chronobiological, Behavioral and Medical Aspects of Napping*. Raven, New York 1989: 71–98.
15. Broughton RJ, De Koninck J, Gagnon P, Dunham W, Stampi C. Chronobiological aspect of SWS and REM sleep in extended night sleep of normals. *Sleep Res* 1988; 17:150.
16. Broughton RJ, Dunham W, Suwalski W, Lutley K, Roberts J. Ambulant 24-hour sleep-wake recordings in narcolepsy-cataplexy. *Sleep Res* 1986; 15:109.
17. Broughton RJ, Dunham W, Newman J, Lutley K, Duchesne P, Rivers M. Ambulatory 24-hour sleep-wake monitoring in narcolepsy-cataplexy compared to matched controls. *Electroenceph Clin Neurophysiol* 1988; 70:473–481.

BIOLOGICAL RHYTHMS   39

18. Busby K, Broughton RJ. Waking ultradian rhythms in hyperkinetic and normal children. *J Abnorm Child Psychol* 1983; 11:431–442.
19. Campbell SS, Zulley J. Napping in time-free environments. In DF Dinges and RJ Broughton (eds.), *Sleep and Alertness: Chronobiological Behavioural and Medical Aspects of Napping.* Raven, New York 1989: 121–138.
20. Colquhoun WP, Blake MJF, Edwards RS. Experimental studies of shift work: A comparison of 'rotating' and 'stabilized' 4-hour shift systems. *Ergonomics* 1968; 11:437–453.
21. Daan S, Beersma DGM, Borbely AA. The timing of human sleep: A recovery process gated by a circadian pacemaker. *Am J Physiol* 1984: (Reg Integrative Comp Physiol 12): R161–178.
22. De Koninck J, Quera Salva M, Besset A, Billiard M. Are REM cycle narcoleptic patients governed by an ultradian rhythm? *Sleep* 1986; 9:162–166.
23. Dement WC. The effect of dream deprivation. *Science* 1980; 131:1705–1707.
24. Dement WC, Kleitman N. Cyclic variations in EEG during sleep and their relation to eye movements, body motility and dreaming. *Electroenceph Clin Neurophysiol* 1956; 9:673–690.
25. Dijk DJ, Beersma DGM, Daan S. EEG power density during naps; reflections of an hourglass measuring the duration of prior wakefulness. *J Biol Rhythms* 1987; 3:207–219.
26. Fishbein W, Gutwein BM. Paradoxical sleep and memory storage processes. *Behav Res* 1977; 19:425–464.
27. Folkard S. The pragmatic approach to masking. *Chronobiol Int* 1989; 6:55–64.
28. Folkard S, Akerstedt T. Towards the prediction of alertness on abnormal sleep-wake schedules. In A Coblenz (ed.), *Vigilance and Performance in Automatized Systems.* Kluwer, Dordrecht, 1989: 287–296.
29. Folkard S, Knauth P, Monk TH, Rutenfranz J. The effect of memory load on the circadian variation in performance efficiency under a rapidly rotating shift system. *Ergonomics* 1976; 19:479–548.
30. Gagnon P. Le cycle du sommeil dans des conditions de sommeil prolongé chez les gens adults. Doctoral thesis, University of Ottawa, 1982.
31. Gagnon P, De Koninck J. Reappearance of EEG slow waves in extended sleep. *Electroenceph Clin Neurophysiol* 1984; 58:155–157.
32. Gagnon P, De Koninck J, Broughton J. Reappearance of electroencephalographic slow waves in extended sleep with delayed bedtime. *Sleep* 1985; 8:118–128.
33. Gander PH, Kronauer RE, Czeisler CA, Moore-Ede MC. Modelling the action of Zeitgebers on the human circadian system: Comparisons of simulations and data. *Am J Physiol* 1984; 247 (Reg Integrative Comp Physiol 16): R427–444.
34. Horne J. Presented to the symposium (Koella WP, chairperson) "Organization and regulation of sleep: Various models," at 8th European Congress of Sleep Research, Szeged, Hungary, Sept 1–5, 1986.
35. Kawato M. Fujita K, Suzuki R, Winfree AT. A three-oscillator model of the human circadian system controlling core temperature rhythm and the sleep-wake cycle. *J Theor Biol* 1982; 98:369–392.
36. Kirk RE. *Experimental Design: Procedures for the Behavioral Sciences,* 2nd ed. Brooks/Coles, Belmont, CA: 1982.
37. Kleitman N. The nature of dreaming. In GEW Wolstenholme and MO O'Connor (eds.), *The Nature of Sleep.* Churchill, London, 1961: 349–364.
38. Kleitman N. *Sleep and Wakefulness.* University of Chicago Press, Chicago, 1963: 364.
39. Kleitman N, Jackson DP. Body temperature and performance under different routines. *Am J Appl Physiol* 1950; 3:309–328.
40. Kripke DF. An ultradian biological rhythm associated with perceptual deprivation and REM sleep. *Psychosom Med* 1972; 34:221–234.

41. Kripke DF, Mullaney DJ, Fleck PA. Ultradian rhythms during sustained performance. In H Schulz and P Lavie (eds.), *Ultradian Rhythms in Physiology and Behavior*. Springer-Verlag, Berlin, 1985: 200–216.
42. Kronauer RE. Temporal subdivision of the circadian cycle. *Lect Math Life Sci* 1987; 19:63–120.
43. Kronauer RE, Czeisler CA, Pilato SF, Moore-Ede MC, Weitzman ED. Mathematical model of the human circadian system with two interacting oscillators. *Am J Physiol* 1982; 242 (Reg Integrative Comp Physiol 11): R3–17.
44. Kupfer DG, Ulrich RF, Coble PA, Jarrett DB, Grochocinski V, Doman J, Mathews G, Borbely AA. Application of automated REM and slow wave sleep analysis. II. Testing the assumption of the two-process model of sleep regulation in normal and depressed subjects. *Psychiatr Res* 1984; 13:335–343.
45. Laird DA. Relative performance of college students as conditioned by time of day and day of week. *J Exp Psychol* 1925; 8:50–63.
46. Lavie P. Ultradian rhythms in alertness—a pupillometric study. *Biol Psychol* 1979; 9:49–62.
47. Lavie P. Ultradian rhythms: Gates of sleep and wakefulness. In H Schulz and P Lavie (eds.), *Ultradian Rhythms in Physiology and Behavior*. Springer-Verlag, Berlin, 1985: 148–164.
48. Lavie P. Ultrashort sleep-waking schedule. III. Gates and "forbidden zones" for sleep. *Electroenceph Clin Neurophysiol* 1986; 63:414–425.
49. Lavie P, Scherson A. Ultrashort sleep-waking cycle. I. Evidence of ultradian rhythmicity in "sleepability." *Electroenceph Clin Neurophysiol* 1981; 52:163–174.
50. Lavie P, Zomer J. Ultrashort sleep-waking schedule. II. Relationship between ultradian rhythms in sleepability and the REM-NREM cycles and effects of the circadian phase. *Electroenceph Clin Neurophysiol* 1984; 57:35–42.
51. Manseau C, Broughton RJ. Ultradian variations in human daytime EEGs: A preliminary report. In W Koella (ed.), *Sleep 1982*. Karger, Basel, 1983: 196–198.
52. Manseau C, Broughton RJ. Bilaterally synchronous ultradian EEG rhythms in adult humans. *Psychophysiology* 1984; 21:265–273.
53. Maron L, Rechtschaffen A, Wolpert EA. Sleep cycling during napping. *Arch Gen Psychiat* 1964; 11:503–508.
54. McCarley RW, Hobson JS. Neuronal excitability modulation over the sleep cycle: A structural and mathematical model. *Science* 1975; 189:58–60.
55. McCarley RW, Massaquoi SG. A limit cycle mathematical model of the REM sleep oscillator system. *Am J Physiol* 1986; 251 (Reg Integrative Comp Physiol 20): R1011–1029.
56. Moses J, Lubin A, Johnson LC, Naitoh P. Rapid eye movement cycle is a sleep dependent rhythm. *Nature (London)* 1977; 265:360–361.
57. Moses J, Naitoh P, Johnson LC. The REM cycle in altered sleep-wake schedules. *Psychophysiology* 1978; 15:207–211.
58. Nakagawa Y. Continuous observations of EEG patterns at night and in daytime of normal subjects under restrained conditions. I. Quiescent state when lying down. *Electroenceph Clin Neurophysiol* 1980; 49:524–537.
59. Okawa M, Matousek M, Petersen I. Spontaneous vigilance fluctuations in the daytime. *Psychophysiology* 1984; 21:207–211.
60. Orr WC, Hoffman HG, Hegge FW. Ultradian rhythms in extended peformance. *Aerospace Med* 1974; 45:995–1000.
61. Passouant P, Halberg F, Genicot R, Popoviciu L, Baldy-Moulinier M. La périodicité des accès narcoleptiques et le rythme ultradien du sommeil rapide. *Rev Neurol (Paris)* 1969; 121:155–164.
62. Pedhazur E. *Multiple Regression in Behavioral Research*. Holt, New York, 1982.
63. Piéron H. *Le Problème Physiologique du Sommeil*. Masson, Paris, 1913.

64. Rechtschaffen A, Kales A (eds.). *A Manual of Standardized Terminology, Techniques and Scoring System for Sleep Studies of Human Subjects.* US Government Printing Office, Washington, DC, 1968.

65. Richardson GS, Carskadon MA, Orav WC, Dement WC. Circadian variations of sleep tendency in elderly and young adult subjects. *Sleep* 1982; 5 (Suppl. 2): 82–94.

66. Smith CT. Sleep states and learning: A review of the animal literature. *Neurosci Biobehav Res* 1985; 9:157–168.

67. Strogatz SH. *The Mathematical Structure of the Human Sleep-Wake Cycle.* Springer-Verlag, Berlin, 1986.

68. Ursin R, Moses J, Naitoh P, Johnson LC. REM-NREM cycle in the cat may be sleep dependent. *Sleep* 1983; 6:1–9.

69. Volk S, Simon O, Schulz H, Hansert E, Wilde-Frenz J. The structure of wakefulness and its relationship to daytime sleep in narcoleptic patients. *Electroenceph Clin Neurophysiol* 1984; 57:119–128.

70. Webb W. Sleep and naps. *Spec Sci Technol* 1978; 1:313–318.

71. Webb WB, Agnew HW. Stage 4 sleep: Influence of time course variables. *Science* 1971; 174:1354–1356.

72. Wever RA. The circadian multi-oscillator system in man. *Int J Chronobiol* 1975; 3:19–55.

73. Wever RA. *The Circadian System in Man.* Springer-Verlag, Berlin, 1979.

74. Wever RA. Internal interactions within the human circadian system: The masking effect. *Experientia* 1985; 41:332–342.

75. Williams HL, Hammack JT, Daly RL, Dement WC, Lubin A. Responses to auditory stimulation, sleep loss and EEG stages of sleep. *Electroenceph Clin Neurophysiol* 1964; 16:269–279.

76. Zulley J. The four-hour sleep-wake cycle. *Sleep Res* 1988; 17:403.

77. Zulley J, Campbell S. Napping behavior during "spontaneous internal desynchronization": sleep remains in synchrony with temperature. *Hum Neurobiol* 1985; 4:123–126.

4

Effects of Wakefulness and Sleep on Depression and Mania

THOMAS A. WEHR

"Je schlaflosen die Nacht, um so besser der folgende Tag!"
[The more sleepless the night, the better the following day!]
W. SCHULTE (1966)

Episodes of affective illness are often accompanied by marked changes in sleep. Insomnia frequently occurs in mania, and insomnia or hypersomnia often occurs in depression. At the same time, manipulations of sleep can modify depression and mania. Sleep deprivation improves depression, and it can also induce mania. Conversely, recovery sleep after sleep deprivation can reinduce depression. Thus, sleep appears to have a depressant effect and wakefulness an activating or mood-elevating effect. Since these interactions between affective state and sleep and wakefulness are bidirectional, they appear to constitute a closed-loop feedback system (Fig. 4-1).

In principle, any factor originating in the organism or its environment that impinges on sleep and wakefulness could open this loop and alter affective state. In this way, the sleep–wake cycle could be a medium through which many factors might affect the course of affective illness. Such influences might trigger or terminate episodes of depression or mania, either adventitiously, if they occur spontaneously, or intentionally, if they are employed as treatments (Fig. 4-1).

The biological mechanism(s) of sleep's depressant effect and wakefulness' antidepressant and mania-inducing effects are unknown. A better understanding of mechanisms almost certainly would lead to a better understanding of the pathogenesis of depression and mania; it would undoubtedly also lead to new types of treatment for these states. In writing this chapter, the author's aim is to facilitate an understanding of these mechanisms by reviewing what is known about the effects of sleep–wake manipulations on affective illness, by discussing current hypotheses, and by presenting a new hypothesis that equates sleep, physiologically, with heat, and sleep deprivation with heat deprivation.

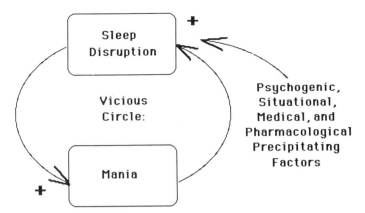

Figure 4-1 Closed-loop positive feedback relationship between mania and sleep duration. Disrupted sleep appears to trigger and intensify mania, and mania in turn causes insomnia. This "vicious circle" suggests a way in which mania, once initiated, might be self-reinforcing, and it could help to explain the tendency of mania to escalate out of control. In principle, the vicious circle of sleep disruption and mania could be set in motion by any psychogenic, situational, medical, or pharmacological factor that disrupts sleep, as indicated in the diagram.

BRIEF DESCRIPTION OF DEPRESSION AND MANIA

Affective illness is a recurrent illness characterized by episodes of depression—and in some cases, mania—that recur and remit repeatedly during the course of a patient's life. During the intervals between episodes patients can recover completely (to the extent that it is possible to recover from any traumatic experience). Most patients have a "unipolar" form of the illness with depression only. Some patients have a "bipolar" form with both depression and mania. The lifetime prevalence of affective illness in the general population is approximately 8%; for the bipolar form of affective illness it is approximately 1% (127). The propensity to develop affective illness is inherited, as is shown by the nearly 70% concordance rate in identical twins of probands with bipolar illness. However, since this rate is substantially less than 100%, factors other than heredity must also be important. The fact that the prevalence of depression in genetically predisposed individuals appears to be increasing in those born after 1940 suggests that nonhereditary factors are becoming increasingly important (85).

Depression is a complex syndrome that includes changes in behavior, cognition, mood, and vegetative functions. When depressed, patients feel sad, anxious, irritable, or angry. They are hopeless, have an unrealistically negative view of themselves, are troubled by feelings of guilt, and ruminate obsessively about real or imagined misdeeds and deficiencies. They tend to withdraw from social activities and relationships; they lose initiative and have difficulty making decisions, even about trivial matters, such as choosing what clothes to wear; and they lose interest in sex and are no longer able to enjoy things that are ordinarily pleasurable. Their appetite, weight, and sleep are disturbed in one of two opposite ways. In "endogenous" depression patients have difficulty sleeping and they lose appetite and weight. In "atypical" depression patients oversleep, crave carbohydrates, overeat, and gain weight (see 198 for review of these differences).

In many respects mania is opposite to depression. It is an excited state. Patients are emotionally unstable and feel elated, angry, or irritable. They are optimistic and often have an unrealistically positive view of themselves. Their thinking moves quickly from one idea to another, sometimes in a superficial or tangential way that has been characterized as a "flight of ideas." They are intrusive and do not like to be interrupted. They make decisions impulsively, spend money recklessly, and alienate friends, colleagues, and family members. Their need for sleep is often markedly reduced.

Drugs are usually used to treat or prevent depression and mania. Tricyclic compounds, such as imipramine, and monoamine-oxidase inhibitors (MAOIs), such as phenelzine, are employed as antidepressants. Lithium carbonate, phenothiazines, such as chlorpromazine, and butyrophenones, such as haloperidol, are employed as anti-manic agents. Lithium carbonate and other drugs are also prescribed as maintenance medications to prevent affective recurrences.

Depression can recur regularly on an annual basis (see 197 for review). There are two principal forms of seasonal affective disorder (SAD) characterized by either recurrent winter depression or recurrent summer depression. Winter depression appears to be triggered by light deficiency, and it responds to treatment with bright artificial light. Factor(s) that trigger summer depression have not been conclusively identified, but heat has been implicated.

EFFECTS OF AFFECTIVE ILLNESS ON SLEEP

Two opposite types of sleep disturbance have been described in connection with depression. Some patients, especially if older, agitated, and/or psychotic, have insomnia, notably early morning awakening. Other patients, especially if younger, lethargic, and/or bipolar, sleep excessively (91).

The composition of a night's sleep and the evolution of sleep stages through the night are often modified in depression (52). Patients frequently exhibit reduced REM sleep latency, increased REM sleep density, especially in the first REM sleep episode, and variably long first REM sleep episodes. Although the total amount of REM sleep is usually normal, these changes cause the temporal distribution of REM sleep to be shifted earlier or advanced, so that relatively more REM sleep occurs in the first part of the sleep period and relatively less in later parts. The total amount of slow wave sleep is usually significantly reduced.

None of these changes appears to be pathognomonic of depression. For instance, reduced REM sleep latency, which once was promoted as a diagnostic marker of depression, has now been described in more than 10 other psychiatric disturbances (see Table 4-1) (11,44,64,69,71,77,93,101,111,129,130,136,145,155,156), and normal REM sleep latencies have been reported in more than 10 studies of depressed patients (see Table 4-2) (5,12,19,72,76,95,105,126,160,161). Decreased slow wave sleep also occurs in many psychiatric and medical conditions (40–42,48).

Most patients appear to require less sleep when they are manic. In fact, some have

Table 4-1 Reduced REM Latency in Disorders Other Than Depression

Disorder	Author(s) (year)	Subjects	N	Latency
Mania	Hudson et al. (1988)	Manic patients	9	46.8
		Normal controls	18	73.9
Schizophrenia	Stern et al. (1969)	Schizophrenic patients	8	53.3
		Normal controls	6	93.7
	Jus et al. (1973)	Schizophrenic patients	11	52.8
		Normal controls	10	93.0
	Hiatt et al. (1985)	Schizophrenic patients	5	47.9
		Normal controls	18	70.4
	Benson et al. (1985)	Schizophrenic patients	12	60.3
		Schizoaffective patients	8	78.3
		Depressed patients	12	60.5
		Normal controls	18	95.9
Borderline personality disorder	Lahmeyer et al. (1985)	Borderline patients	16	68.0
		Depressed patients	16	66.9
	Reynolds et al. (1985)	Borderline patients (I)	10	62.2
		Borderline patients (II)	10	55.0
		Depressed patients	10	44.5
		Normal controls	10	77.8
Anxiety disorder	Foster et al. (1977)	Anxiety patients	10	60.6
		Depressed patients	10	62.3
Anorexia nervosa	Neil et al. (1980)	Anorexic patients	10	62.1
		Normal controls	10	90.8
Panic disorder	Roy-Byrne et al. (1986)	Panic disorder patients	9	74.0
		Normal controls	9	106.0
Dementia	Martin et al. (1986)	Korsakoff patients	7	47.2
		Alzheimer patients	8	57.6
		Normal controls	9	73.5
Alcoholism	Spiker et al. (1977)	Alcoholic patients	10	43.7
		Depressed patients	10	44.9
Obsessive–compulsive disorder	Insel et al. (1982)	Obsessive–compulsive patients	14	48.4
		Depressed patients	14	47.3
		Normal controls	14	80.8
Impotence	Schmidt et al. (1986)	Impotent patients	25	42.1
Insomnia	Schmidt et al. (1986)	Insomnia patients	8	54.4
Sleep apnea	Reynolds et al. (1984)	Apnea patients	12	55.3

total insomnia for one or more nights. Total insomnia can occur on alternate nights at the beginning of manic episodes, giving rise to a distinctive pattern of 48-hr sleep–wake cycles (187) (see Fig. 4-2). Like depression, mania is often accompanied by shortened REM sleep latencies (69).

The association of changes in sleep duration with changes in affective state is most clearly seen in longitudinal recordings of sleep EEG or wrist motor activity in patients with frequent recurrences of mania and depression (see Fig. 4-2). This type of patient often sleeps excessively when depressed and hardly at all when manic. The changes in sleep duration can be extreme. For example, when one patient was allowed to sleep *ad libitum* in a temporal isolation chamber, she slept 12 hr/day (50%) when depressed and 3 hr/day (12%) when manic (190).

Table 4-2 Normal REM Latency in Depression

Author(s) (year)	Subjects	N	Diagnosis	REM latency
Jovanovic (1977)	Depressed patients	60	(20 BP, 40 UP)	77.3
	Normal controls	>200		81.4
Taub et al. (1978)	Depressed young adults	20	(UP)	112.4
	Normal controls	20		108.3
Puig-Anich et al. (1982)	Depressed children	27	(endogenous)	149.6
	Depressed children	27	(nonendogenous)	157.1
	Normal controls	11		150.2
Linkowski et al. (1985)	Depressed patients	9	(BP)	72.9
	Normal controls	7		72.9
Ansseau et al. (1985)	Depressed patients	13		83.3
Jernajczyk (1986)	Depressed patients	10	(BP)	71.3
	Normal controls	10		67.1
Mendelson et al. (1986)	Depressed patients	7	(6 BP, 1 UP)	72.9
	Normal controls	7		70.8
Sack et al. (1986)	Depressed patients	6	(BP)	75.0
	Normal controls	6		88.0
Thase et al. (1986)	Depressed patients	26	(BP)	71.8
	Normal controls	26		72.8
Cashman et al. (1986)	Depressed adolescents	15		—
	Normal controls	15		—
Berger et al. (1988)	Depressed patients	16	(4 BP, 12 UP)	65.5
	Normal controls	16		74.1
	Psychiatric controls	20		73.6

EFFECTS OF SLEEP AND SLEEP MANIPULATIONS ON AFFECTIVE ILLNESS

Improvement of Depression after Total Sleep Deprivation (TSD)

Research on the effects of sleep deprivation on psychiatric illness was carried out in two distinct eras. In the 1950s and 1960s schizophrenia was the focus of research; in the 1970s and 1980s affective illness was the focus. It is remarkable how independent these two phases of investigation were, considering their proximity in time and the underlying unity of their findings. Apparently this situation occurred because the work was carried out by different investigators, with different diagnostic groups, on different continents, in different languages, and from different theoretical perspectives.

Psychoanalytic theories about dreams and psychosis inspired the investigations of sleep deprivation in schizophrenia. Psychoanalytically oriented investigators believed that dreams served as an escape valve through which instinctual drives could be regularly discharged; psychosis was thought to be caused by an intrusion of drives and other unconscious processes into waking life. Similarities between psychotic symptoms and dreams suggested to some that schizophrenia was an intrusion of dreams into wakefulness (43,51). These abstract ideas were reified by the discovery of REM sleep in 1952, and by the subsequent demonstration that sleep deprivation leads to a cumulative REM sleep debt that is discharged during recovery sleep. These observations inspired a series of EEG sleep studies and sleep deprivation experiments in schizophrenic patients and normal individuals (Table 4-3). According to the psychoanalytic

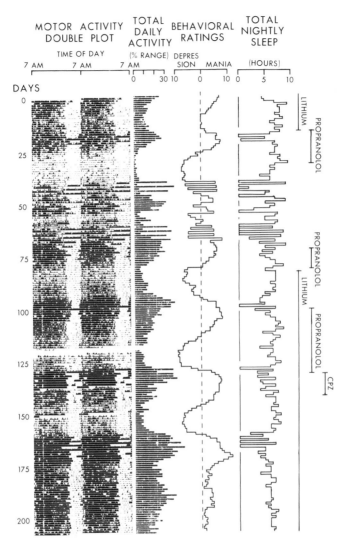

Figure 4-2 Longitudinal recording of wrist motor activity and nurses' observations of sleep show state-dependent changes in levels of activity and duration of sleep during long-term cycles of mania and depression in an 18-year-old woman. Motor activity is shown in a raster format, in which 24-hr segments of 15-min bins of activity counts are plotted consecutively beneath one another. The rasters are doubled plotted to the right to facilitate visual inspection of the data. Nurses daily ratings of depression and mania and nightly estimates of hours of sleep are also shown. Sleep duration is shorter and activity levels are higher during mania than during depression. Switches out of depression into mania are frequently accompanied by one or more nights of total insomnia, which produce a distinctive pattern of 48-hr sleep–wake cycles. [Reprinted from Wehr et al. (187).]

Table 4-3 Activating Effects of Sleep Deprivation in Schizophrenic Patients

Author(s) (year)	Subjects	N	Results
Total sleep deprivation			
Koranyi and Lehmann (1960)	Chronic schizophrenics	6	1. Improvement of negative symptoms: "brighter," "more talkative," "euphoria," "enthusiasm," "increased motor activity"
	Paranoid	2	
	Catatonic	2	
	Hebephrenic	2	2 Induction of positive symptoms: "suspicious," "laught inappropriately," "hallucinated," "motor automatism"
Luby and Caldwell (1967)	Chronic schizophrenics	4	1. Improvement of negative symptoms: "increasingly tractable . . . articulate . . . expressing feelings"
	Catatonic	4	2. Relapse after recovery sleep
Fähndrich (1982)	Schizophrenics	17	1. Improvement of depressive symptoms in 14 / 21 patients; Hamilton ratings 19.4 → 6.8
	Paranoid	13	
	Defect state	2	
	Acute	1	
	Simple	1	
	Schizoaffectives	4	
Selective REM sleep deprivation			
Azumi et al. (1967)		5	1. One patient improved
Vogel and Traub (1968)	Chronic schizophrenics	5	"Virtually no change"
de Barros-Ferreira et al. (1973)	Chronic schizophrenics	11	1. Improvement of negative symptoms: "hyperactivity, subexcitation, and logorrhoea"
			2. Three remained improved after recovery sleep
			3. No induction of psychosis
Gillin et al. (1974)	Chronic schizophrenics	7	1. Improvement of depressive symptoms: "less depressed and anxious . . . but not statistically significant"
	Undifferentiated	5	
	Paranoid	1	
	Catatonic	1	

theory, it was predicted that sleep deprivation would induce psychotic symptoms because it intensifies instinctual drives by blocking their discharge in dreams.

In the early 1950s Koranyi and Lehman attempted to induce psychotic symptoms in chronic schizophrenic patients by depriving them of sleep for 4 days (87). Unexpectedly, they found that depressive-type symptoms improved during the course of the experiment (Table 4-3). They noted that patients who had been withdrawn and apathetic for years gradually brightened and became convivial as sleep deprivation progressed. Ultimately, some did become psychotic. Similar observations were reported subsequently by Luby and Caldwell in 1967 (Table 4-3) (100).

Ultimately this line of investigation was abandoned. There are several reasons for its disappearance. First, there was no therapeutic intent of sleep deprivation; it was used to provoke psychotic symptoms, not to treat depressive symptoms. Thus, the results were not seen as having practical applications; therefore, they were of little interest to clinicians. Second, levels of REM sleep were found to be normal in schizophrenia, contrary to predictions based on the REM sleep-instinctual drive hypothesis of psychosis. Third, findings in normal individuals were discredited to some extent by the revelation that psychostimulants, which can cause psychosis, had been used to facilitate sleep deprivation in some of the experiments. When some of the key researchers in this area abandoned studies of schizophrenia, they turned to nonpsychiatric problems and, in effect, left the field. An exception was Vogel, a bridging figure who extended this work to affective patients and found that selective REM sleep deprivation improved depression, as will be discussed.

The era of sleep deprivation research in affective illness began in 1966 when Schulte described a patient who discovered that he felt better when he slept poorly, and improved dramatically when he stayed awake all night riding a bicycle (see quotation at beginning of chapter) (147). Subsequently, Schulte's associates, Pflug and Tölle, systematically investigated the effects of total sleep deprivation in a series of depressed patients and confirmed this finding (120–123). Subsequently, various investigators studied over 1200 depressed patients' responses to total sleep deprivation and found that about 60% improved substantially during the course of the procedure (3,4, 13,14,17,28 – 33,37,39,50,73,83,86,90,92,94,97,99,102,108,110,120,122,125,137, 143,146,149,158,159,162,165,168,169,175,178,190,202,203,205,208) (Tables 4-4 and 4-5).

The typical antidepressant response to sleep deprivation is rapid and dramatic, but it is often reversed by recovery sleep. A small subgroup of patients, "day 2 responders," shows no improvement on the day after the night of sleep deprivation, but improve on the day following recovery sleep (102,203).

To those who have not witnessed it, it is difficult to describe adequately the remarkable effect of sleep deprivation on depression. A patient who has been severely depressed, withdrawn, hopeless, and suicidal for months or years, can be transformed overnight into someone who is elated, enthusiastic, engaged, and hopeful about the future.

Improvement of Depression after Partial Sleep Deprivation (PSD)

Schilgen and Tölle reported that partial sleep deprivation in the second half of the night, allowing as much as 4 hr of sleep prior to 1 or 2 A.M., is as effective an antidepressant as total sleep deprivation (142,143). This finding has been confirmed by several other investigators (123,139) (Table 4-6). It has important clinical implications. First, it is easier for patients to carry out partial sleep deprivation than total sleep deprivation. Second, since partial sleep deprivation can be more easily repeated on

Table 4-4 Drug Status and Antidepressant Response to Total Sleep Deprivation

Drug status	N	% R
Drug-free ≥ 2 weeks	99	56.6
Drug-free < 2 weeks	456	62.1
On drug	318	51.0
Not stated	144	63.2
Total	1017	58.2

Table 4-5 Antidepressant Responses to Total
Sleep Deprivation in Studies That Employed
the Hamilton Depression Rating Scale and
Explicit Response Criteria

Author(s) (year)	Criterion	N	% R
Wirz-Justice et al. (1979)	>33.3%	52	65.4
Amin et al. (1980)	>30%	22	54.5
Zander et al. (1981)	>10 pts	10	70.0
Elsenga et al. (1983)	>6 pts	20	35.0
Kuhs (1985)	>30%	39	41.0
Reynolds et al. (1988)	>30%	15	40.0
Elsenga et al. (1987)	>6 pts	44	45.5
Wiegand et al. (1987)	>30%	12	75.0
Summary:		214	51.9

subsequent nights, relapses after sleep deprivation might be prevented by repeated use
of the procedure.

Goetze and Tölle reported that partial sleep deprivation in the first half of the night
is relatively less effective an antidepressant (54). This observation was confirmed by
Sack et al. and Elsenga et al. in crossover studies in which the same depressed patients
were partially sleep deprived in the first and second halves of the night on two different
occasions (34,140) (Fig. 4-3).

Improvement of Depression after Changing the Timing of Sleep

Wehr et al. noted that a number of circadian rhythms appeared to be shifted earlier, or
phase-advanced relative to sleep in depressed patients compared with normal individuals, and they hypothesized that this phase disturbance might be responsible for the
abnormally early occurrence of REM sleep in depression (183,186,188). They predicted that if a phase advance of circadian rhythms relative to sleep contributed to the
pathogenesis of depression, then a corresponding advance in the timing of the sleep
schedule would correct the internal phase disturbance and improve depressive symptoms. In a series of uncontrolled experiments they found that shifting the timing of the
sleep schedule 6 hr earlier from its usual 11 P.M.–7 A.M. time to a new 5 P.M.–1 A.M.
time was associated with improvement of depression in several depressed patients
(183,188,189). Subsequently, Souetre et al. and Sack et al. reported similar findings
(139,153).

Table 4-6 Drug Status and Antidepressant
Response to Partial Sleep Deprivation

Drug status	N	% R
Drug-free ≥ 2 weeks	53	56.7
Drug-free < 2 weeks	36	50.0
On drug	94	61.7
Total	183	50.8

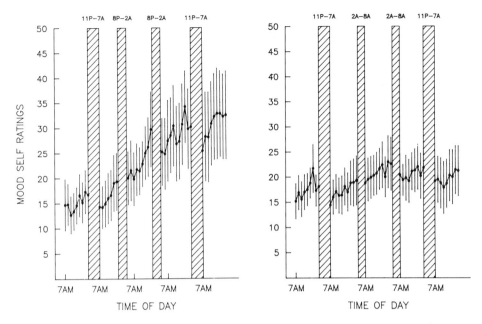

Figure 4-3 Partial sleep deprivation in the second half of the night (left) appears to improve depression more than partial sleep deprivation in the first half of the night (right). Data show self-ratings of mood (mean ± SE) for 16 depressed patients who were treated with each type of partial sleep deprivation in a balanced order cross-over study. [Adapted from a figure published by Sack et al. (140).]

Surridge-David et al. conducted an opposite type of phase shift experiment in 10 normal individuals and found that depressive symptoms were induced by the procedure (157). They shifted the timing of the sleep schedule 6 hr later from its usual 12 P.M.–7:30 A.M. time to a new 6 A.M.–2:00 P.M. time. After the shift, REM sleep measures changed from a normal pattern to one that resembled that seen in depression. For the group as a whole, there was a modest lowering of mood after the shift, and two subjects became markedly depressed. Although it cannot be excluded that the raters were responding to changes in the subject's appearance and behavior that were indicative of fatigue rather than depression, the study raises the possibility that the timing of sleep might also influence mood in normal individuals.

Lewy et al. conducted a similar phase-shift experiment in patients with winter depression whose melatonin circadian rhythm appeared to be shifted later, or phase-delayed relative to sleep. They reported that a corresponding delay in the timing of the sleep schedule, which corrected this internal phase disturbance, improved their depressive symptoms (96).

Improvement of Depression after Selective REM Sleep Deprivation (SRSD)

Most antidepressant drugs suppress REM sleep. In 1968 Vogel and colleagues hypothesized that the capacity of antidepressant effects of drugs to suppress REM sleep was the mechanism of their therapeutic effect. As a corrollary, they predicted that mechanical suppression of REM sleep by forced awakenings might have antidepressant effects similar to the drugs (171,172). To test this hypothesis they conducted a parallel design study in which they assessed endogenous depressives' responses to two treatments carried out for 3 weeks: selective REM sleep deprivation and selective non-REM sleep deprivation. They found that the former was modestly superior to the latter according to observer ratings with the Hamilton Depression Scale (28.4 versus 10.6% reductions in ratings, $p < .03$, one-tailed) (Fig. 4-4). However, they found no significant difference according to patient self ratings with the Zung Depression Scale. Patients who improved were those who showed evidence of REM sleep rebound during recovery night sleep following the REM sleep deprivations. Unfortunately, no one has yet attempted to replicate the results of this interesting, but arduous study.

Onset of Depression or Worsening of Depression after Sleep

Ancient Greek and Roman physicians believed that a lethargic, hypersomnic type of depression could be made worse by sleep. Referring to this belief and to the humoral theory on which it was based, Robert Burton wrote in *The Anatomy of Melancholy* (1621) that "sleep may do more harm than good, in that phlegmatic, swinish, cold, and sluggish melancholy . . . [It] fills the head full of gross humours; causeth distillations, rheums, great store of excrements in the brain" (19).

Consistent with this ancient idea, modern research has shown that patients whose depressions improve after sleep deprivation often relapse after recovery sleep (202). Such relapses can occur after naps as brief as 90 min (202). According to Wiegand et al. such relapses were especially likely to occur when naps included episodes of REM sleep. However, this finding did not reach statistical significance, and it could not be confirmed by Gillin et al. (personal communication). The fact that relapses occur after recovery sleep suggests that sleep may be depressogenic, at least in the special case of patients who have responded to sleep deprivation. Such a depressogenic effect of sleep could be invoked to explain why patients with endogenous depression usually feel worse in the morning, after a period of sleep, and feel best in the evening, after a period of wakefulness. In such patients, the antidepressant effect of total sleep deprivation could be conceptualized as allowing to continue, a process of improvement that is already underway during the course of the day's wakefulness prior to sleep deprivation (167).

On the other hand, some depressed patients have a pattern of diurnal variation in mood that is opposite to that described in endogenous depression: they feel worse in the evening and better in the morning. Interestingly, these patients appear to feel worse after sleep deprivation, according to observations of van den Hoofdakker and Beersma (167). In these patients, it seems, sleep is not depressogenic (it might even be anti-

---

Figure 4-4 Comparison of antidepressant effects of partial sleep deprivation in the second half of the night versus the first half of the night (top) and antidepressant effects of REM sleep deprivation versus non-REM sleep deprivation (bottom). In each case the former treatments were superior to the latter treatments. Left: Sleep EEG data for baseline and treatment conditions for each type of treatment. Sleep during the superior treatments was shorter in duration and contained less REM sleep than the inferior treatments. Middle: Scatter plots showing changes during treatment for each individual for each type of treatment. Right: Patients' mean depression rating scores ($\pm$SD) before and after treatment for each type of treatment. Data from Sack et al. (140) and Vogel et al., (172), respectively.

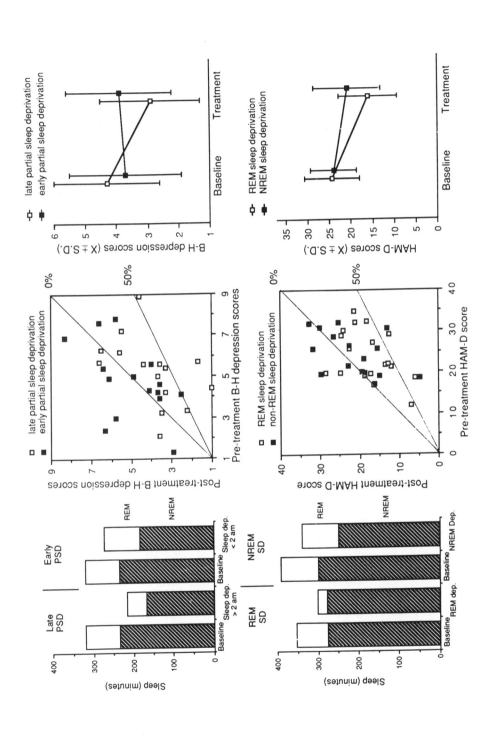

depressant). In light of these patients' paradoxical responses to sleep and sleep deprivation, it would be interesting to know if any of them are "day 2 responders" who
improve after recovery sleep following sleep deprivation.

Onset of Mania after Sleep Deprivation

Like other antidepressant modalities, sleep deprivation appears to be capable of inducing mania or hypomania, at least in depressed bipolar patients, who may be predisposed to develop mania. The idea that sleep has a restorative, calming effect, and
that sleep disruption might aggravate excited states is an intuitive one that appears in
the writings of leading psychiatrists of the nineteenth century. For example, J. C.
Heinroth wrote in 1818 that "morbid excitation is maintained by insomnia to no small
extent" (61).

There is now experimental evidence that sleep deprivation is capable of inducing
mania or hypomania. In 1982, my colleagues and I reported that the majority of a
group of depressed, rapid-cycling, bipolar patients switched into mania or hypomania
the day after they were deprived of sleep for one night (187) (see Table 4-7). Some of
these patients remained manic or hypomanic for days or weeks afterward; others
switched back into depression after recovery sleep. Apparently, ours is the only study
of sleep deprivation in which clinical ratings were employed prospectively to detect
mania or hypomania. However, two other groups prospectively assessed symptoms
that are commonly associated with mania and, consistent with our results, found that
they markedly increased after sleep deprivation. In 1979 Gerner et al. reported that
"ratings of elation and talkativeness (activation) increased dramatically" in a group of
mostly bipolar patients who responded to sleep deprivation (50), and Kasper et al.
reported that self-ratings of elation markedly increased after sleep deprivation in depressed patients, half of whom were bipolar (79).

Switches into mania after sleep deprivation were also described anecdotally by
several other groups of investigators. For example, Kretschmar and Peters reported in
1973 that "in these [bipolar] cases, one has to expect in addition [to the antidepressant
effects] the occurrence of a switch into mania" (89), and Zimanová and Vojtechovsky
stated in 1974 that "the most remarkable effect of deprivation was in our view a shift of
depression into mania in two patients with a bipolar type of depression" (209). Unfortunately, it is difficult to estimate the frequency of switches into mania in most studies
because investigators often did not state the number of bipolar patients who were
investigated, and the studies were not specifically designed to detect mania. There
were no prospective clinical ratings of mania, and no criteria for mania or hypomania
were described. Their focus was on antidepressant effects of sleep deprivation, and
mania was reported incidentally, post hoc. Sleep deprivation studies in which at least a
minimum estimate can be made of the frequency of switches into mania are shown in
Table 4-8 (13,23,26,122,125,158,177,187,203,207).

Occurrence of Mania after Partial Sleep Deprivation,
Selective REM Sleep Deprivation, and Phase-Advance of Sleep

There are almost no systematic studies of mania or hypomania after partial sleep
deprivation, phase-advance of the sleep period, or selective REM sleep deprivation.
My colleagues and I found that some bipolar patients became manic or hypomanic after
phase-advance of the sleep period (183,188,189).

Table 4-7 Responses of Drug-Free Depressed Rapid Cycling Bipolar Patients to One Night's Total Sleep Deprivation[a]

Patient	Age	Sex	Diagnosis	Nurses' ratings before and after TSD[b]								Type of response	Duration of response (days)
				Depression				Mania					
				Day − 1 A.M. / P.M.		Day + 1 A.M. / P.M.		Day − 1 A.M. / P.M.		Day + 1 A.M. / P.M.			
1	34	F	BPI	9	8	8	5	0	0	5	1	Mania	14
2	57	F	BPII	6	6	0	0	0	0	6	1	Mania	50
3	44	F	BPII	9	6	4	0	0	0	0	5	Mania	1
4	36	F	BPI	6	6	0	0	0	0	5	2	Mania	10
5	22	F	BPII	5	5	3	0	0	0	2	7	Mania	1
6	67	F	BPII	4	2	0	0	0	0	1	1	Hypomania	3
7	55	F	BPI	12	8	6	0	0	0	1	1	Hypomania	2
8	49	F	BPII	6	5	3	0	0	0	0	1	Hypomania	1
				7	7	6	0	0	0	0	2	Hypomania	11
				7	7	6	0	0	0	0	1	Hypomania	9
				8	7	6	4	0	0	0	0	Partial	1
9	28	F	BPI	9	9	6	1	0	0	0	2	Hypomania	1
				10	9	9	8	0	0	0	0	None	—
10	56	F	BPII	7	6	5	4	0	0	0	0	Partial	1
11	57	F	BPII	8	6	6	4	0	0	0	0	None	—
				9	3	6	0	0	0	0	0	Euthymia	1
12	21	M	BPII	8	7	6	6	0	0	0	0	None	—

[a]Summary of outcome of 18 sleep deprivations in 12 patients: mania = 5, hypomania = 6, euthymia = 1, partial antidepressant response = 2, no response = 2. Data for patients 1–5, 8, 9, 11, and 12 were previously published in Wehr et al. (187).

[b]TSD, total sleep deprivation.

Table 4-8 Studies Reporting Incidence of Mania or Hypomania after Sleep Deprivation in Depressed Bipolar Patients

Author(s) (year)	Number of Pts.	Mania ratings	Criteria for mania/ hypomania	Manic No. (%)	Hypomanic No. (%)	Total No. (%)
Pflug (1972)	12	None	Not stated	1 (8)	Not stated	1 (8)
Bhanji and Roy (1975)	2	None	Not stated	0	1 (50)	1 (50)
Svendsen (1976)	17	None	Not stated	0	Not stated	0
Post et al. (1976)	9	None	Not stated	0	1 (11)	1 (11)
Wirz-Justice (1975)	7	None	Not stated	0	2 (29)	2 (29)
Cole and Müller (1976)	3	None	Not stated	1 (33)	Not stated	1 (33)
Yamaguchi et al. (1978)	7	None	Not stated	1 (14)	Not stated	1 (14)
Vovin et al. (1982)	7	None	Not stated	1 (14)	Not stated	1 (14)
Wehr et al. (1982)	12	Bunney-Hamburg	Mania >3 Hypomania >0	4 (33)	5 (42)	9 (75)
Dessauer et al. (1985)	4	None	Not stated	1 (25)	1 (25)	2 (50)
Total	80			≥9 (11)	≥10 (13)	≥19 (24)

Problems in the Interpretation of Sleep Manipulation Studies

As we shall see, in a number of the foregoing studies methods were flawed or results were ambiguous. Therefore, in some cases it is difficult to interpret the results.

Medication status and method of clinical assessment of patients do not seem to have affected the results to any significant degree. Although patients who participated in the experiments were often treated simultaneously with various types of medications, the percentages of patients who improved after one night's total or partial sleep deprivation were comparable when the studies were analyzed separately according to whether patients were taking drugs (13,14,17,31,38,54,60,83,99,123,137,142, 143, 146,149,158), withdrawing from drugs (4,32,39,86,94,102,120,125,162,163, 165,175,190), or free of drugs (29,50,73,74,139,207), or where the drug status was not specified (3,97,108,159,190,205) (Tables 4-4 and 4-6). Similarly, although some investigators used standard clinical assessment scales, like the Hamilton Depression Rating Scale, and explicit response criteria (4,30,32,33,90,202,205,206), and others did not, results from the two types of studies were also comparable when they were analyzed separately (Table 4-5).

The natural course of depression is characterized by a tendency to remit spontaneously; therefore, in studies of treatments it is important to control for the influence of spontaneous improvement on the results. Spontaneous improvement is usually gradual, and it is unlikely to occur in a large number of patients on any given day. Thus, it seems unlikely that improvements that occur the day after a single sleep–wake intervention, such as one night's total sleep deprivation, are due to spontaneous remissions (3,4,13,14,17,29,31,32,38,39,50,73,83,86,94,97,99,102,108,120,123,125,137, 143,146,159,163,165,175,190,205,206). However, this is not the case in studies in which multiple sleep–wake interventions were carried out for 1 week or more (28,32, 37,92,94,114,122,125,162,169,180,206). In these studies it seems likely that improvements were due to spontaneous remissions in a larger number of cases. This problem is compounded in studies in which multiple sleep–wake interventions were carried out for one or more weeks while patients were simultaneously treated with antidepressant drugs. In these studies it may be much more likely that patients' improvements were due to spontaneous or drug-induced remissions than to the sleep–wake interventions (31,37,178,180,202). Tables 4-4–4-6 refer only to those studies in which clinical assessments were reported for the day after a single night's total or partial sleep deprivation.

In studies of treatments, it is important to control for the influence of patients' and experimenters' expectations on the results. This is usually done by keeping patients and observers blind to treatment interventions and by comparing active treatments with inactive or less active treatments. Obviously, it is impossible for patients not to be aware that they were deprived of sleep for an entire night or for parts of the night, or that the timing of their sleep schedule was shifted several hours earlier or later than usual. Therefore, in studies of these interventions patients have not been blind to the time of occurrence and to the nature of the intervention. The single exception is selective REM sleep deprivation. Although the patients of Vogel et al. (172) undoubtedly knew when the interventions occurred, it seems quite likely that they did not know whether they were being deprived of REM sleep or non-REM sleep.

In studies of the various types of sleep manipulations it is possible to keep observers blind to the timing and nature of the intervention; however, this has not always been done.

It might seem to be impossible to develop a sham treatment to control for patients' expectations of sleep manipulations. However, any sleep intervention that appears to be inactive could be used as a control treatment, and two such possibilities have emerged from the experiments conducted so far. As Vogel et al. (172) predicted, selective non-REM sleep deprivation appears to be a less effective antidepressant than selective REM sleep deprivation, and the former presumably could be used as a control treatment in future investigations of the latter. Similarly, as Sack et al. (140) and Elsenga et al. (34) predicted, partial sleep deprivation in the first half of the night seems to be a less effective antidepressant than partial sleep deprivation in the second half of the night, and it might also prove useful as a control treatment in future investigations of the latter. In contrast to the situation with REM and non-REM sleep deprivation, patients would be able to discriminate between the two partial sleep deprivation schedules and would therefore not be blind to these differences. However, there is no obvious reason to think that their expectations of the former would be very different from their expectations of the latter.

Difficulties in controlling patients' expectations of antidepressant treatments are not peculiar to studies of sleep interventions. A similar problem exists in studies of phototherapy of winter depression, in which the treatment must be seen to be effective (197), and in studies of antidepressant drugs, in which, because of side effects, patients and observers are usually able to distinguish between active treatments and placebo (68).

In their interventions different investigators have attempted to evaluate the specific effects of manipulations of sleep stages, sleep duration, or the timing of sleep; however, in practice these variables have usually been confounded in their studies. For example, Vogel et al. (172) sought to compare the antidepressant effects of selective REM sleep deprivation and selective non-REM sleep deprivation, but sleep duration was less during the former, which was the superior treatment, than during the latter (Fig. 4-4). Sack et al. (140) and Elsenga et al. (34) sought to compare the antidepressant effects of being awake in the last part of the night and the first part of the night, but

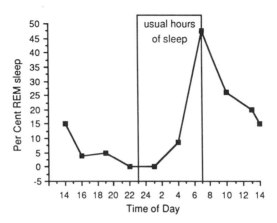

Figure 4-5 REM sleep propensity exhibits a circadian rhythm that reaches a peak at dawn near the end of the usual sleep period and a trough in the evening near the beginning of the usual sleep period. Data show the percentage REM sleep in naps allowed for 1 hr every 3 hr in a group of normal individuals. Most antidepressant sleep–wake manipulations reduce REM sleep because they interfere with sleep in the second half of the night. Data are from Weitzman et al. (200).

in the Sack et al. study, in which sleep EEG recordings were obtained, sleep duration and total minutes of REM sleep were both less during the former, which was the superior treatment, than during the latter (Fig. 4-4). The study of Sack et al. (140) was designed to investigate the possibility, raised by previous uncontrolled studies of the antidepressant effects of phase advance of sleep, that the timing of sleep and wakefulness might be a critical variable in depressed patients' responses to sleep manipulations. In designing the study, we anticipated, on the basis of previous studies of normal individuals, that it would be more difficult for patients to sleep in the evening than in the early morning (210). To increase the likelihood that durations of sleep would be balanced in the two conditions, we decided to restrict sleep to approximately 4 hr in each condition. Therefore, patients were partially deprived of sleep in each condition, but we were not so much interested in studying partial sleep deprivation as we were in controlling the duration of sleep while we studied the importance of its timing. As it turned out, this goal proved difficult to achieve. In designing the study, we also presumed that evening sleep would contain less REM sleep than early morning sleep, as a consequence of the circadian rhythm in REM sleep propensity, which reaches its maximum near dawn (see Fig. 4-5), but there seemed to be no simple way to control for this difference. These technical difficulties will continue to challenge investigators who attempt to conduct controlled studies of the antidepressant effects of sleep–wake manipulations in the future.

CLINICAL IMPLICATIONS

Sleep Manipulations as Treatments for Depression

Many depressed patients improve dramatically after they are deprived of sleep for one night. The rapidity of this response contrasts favorably with the long latency of patients' responses to antidepressant drugs. Unfortunately, most patients who respond to sleep deprivation relapse equally rapidly after returning to sleep. The fact that sleep deprivation's antidepressant effects are often so easily reversed has limited its usefulness as a practical treatment.

There are a few patients for whom one night's total sleep deprivation is an effective approach to treatment. One group that appears to benefit from sleep deprivation consists of depressed bipolar patients who respond to the procedure by definitively switching out of their depressed phase into a sustained hypomanic phase (187). As long as the hypomania is mild, this may be a satisfactory outcome. Another group consists of certain patients with recurrent premenstrual depressions. Such patients appear to respond favorably to total and partial sleep deprivation (119). Since premenstrual depressions can be relatively brief, the short duration and rapid onset of the antidepressant effects of sleep deprivation may actually be preferable to the slower acting antidepressant drugs. In contrast to drugs, which need to be prescribed on a continuing basis, sleep deprivation treatments can be applied only when they are needed during the premenstrual phase.

If sleep deprivation could be administered on an ongoing basis, like drugs, perhaps its beneficial effect might be sustained. Of course, this approach would not be possible with total sleep deprivation, but it could be attempted with partial sleep deprivation in the second half of the night, phase advance of sleep, and selective deprivation of REM sleep. In fact, Vogel et al. treated depressed patients with REM sleep deprivation for several weeks, allowing recovery sleep once every few nights (171). Patients who seemed to respond to the treatments maintained their improvement and many were ultimately discharged from the hospital without medications. However, REM sleep deprivation does not seem to be a very practical approach because it is technically difficult to carry out.

Repeated partial sleep deprivations in the second half of the night might prove to be a practical treatment for patients who are able to comply with the procedure. It can be carried out several times a week, and patients do not seem to relapse after one night of recovery sleep following two consecutive nights of partial sleep deprivation (see Fig. 4-3). Phase advance of sleep can also be used as an ongoing treatment, because it incurs little sleep loss (139,183,188,189).

In contrast to some other types of treatment, patients play a major role in the implementation of sleep interventions. Therefore, their understanding of the procedures and their attitude toward them are critical for their success. Because of the special demands that the treatments place on the patients, they have a unique perspective on their use. For these reasons, patients' observations about their experience with sleep interventions are of particular interest. The following case report includes one of my patients' account of his experience with this type of treatment.

CASE REPORT. A professor with many scholarly and administrative responsibilities, who had had mild mood swings most of his life, became markedly depressed, for the first time, at age 39. Normally he was an energetic and productive person and was highly successful in his field. However, during his depression he found it extremely difficult to think clearly or imaginatively, and to make decisions. He felt paralyzed and ruminated about possible errors in his work. He was overwhelmed by a feeling of insecurity and uncertainty, and no longer felt like the leader and energizer of his department, of which he was the chairman. Sometimes his thoughts turned to suicide as an escape. His energy level decreased markedly, he lost interest in sex and gained weight, and his sleep was disturbed by early awakening and bad dreams. Compared with his former self, he felt like "the ember of a dying flame." These symptoms continued unabated for 10 months, except for a brief remission during a trip to the Far East.

At the time of his first visit, I suggested several treatment options, including sleep manipulations. He decided to try the sleep manipulations, and he recorded the following observations about his experience with them:

"I chose to attempt sleep modification as the initial therapeutic intervention to combat my depression because: 1) it seemed more 'natural' than medications; 2) it gave me a sense of power and control over my mood and being; 3) it was more 'collaborative' in concept than just passively taking medication; 4) I liked being part of 'cutting edge' therapy; 5) the notion of 'sleep as a toxin' resonated with my experience."

"The sleep intervention program consisted of instructions that I was to wake up at 2:00 A.M., that during the early morning hours I should try to spend time outdoors where it was cold, and that I was not under any circumstances to allow myself to nap or doze for even a brief period of time during those early morning hours, for I risked switching back off any therapeutic benefit that I might have obtained. When I asked when I should start, I was told, 'why not tonight?' I was not quite prepared for that; in fact I wanted to procrastinate the intervention much as I had procrastinated my work tasks, but resolving to play the role of patient, I followed instructions and indeed arose at 2:00 A.M. the next morning."

"The first night that I awakened at 2:00 A.M. it was extremely difficult for me to stay awake. I remember that around 5:00 A.M. I fell asleep for 30 minutes or so. During the day that followed, I felt somewhat more energized as if a veil had partially lifted but there was still darkness present; I was better, but nowhere nearly completely recovered. I awoke at 2:00 the next morning and this time had an easier time staying awake, although there were moments when I felt as if there would be nothing sweeter than a nap. At work that day, something had changed. My depression had lifted. I had entered a new world, or more precisely one that I had known in the past but with which I had not been in contact for a long time. Everything around me seemed brighter, crisper, clearer. I was more engaged and more confident in my interactions with colleagues. I had a zest for those little details that before seemed a burden and a bother. The change was palpable and evident. My wife noticed it immediately."

"Over the next week, I was able to solidify these gains. I had been told that I had two choices: either I could gradually arise later each morning, in an attempt to fool my internal time clock, so that I would be able eventually to awaken at a more normal time or I could try arising at 2:00 on a schedule that was compatible with the rest of my life but which maintained the therapeutic gains. I chose the latter for two reasons. I liked getting up at 2:00 in the morning. It gave me private time, something which I ordinarily had very little of between a very demanding wife and a very demanding job."

"Gradually the early morning hours took on a structure. I would be awakened by an alarm clock, walk downstairs, turn on the espresso machine, read the previous day's newspapers for an hour to an hour and a half, and then either read something for pleasure, spend time on a creative work project, or do repetitive tasks such as straightening out a room in the house. The best antidote to feelings of fatigue at 2:00 in the morning is to engage in a repetitive and physically taxing task, e.g., building a piece of furniture."

"I have been utilizing 2:00 A.M. arising for eight months. Usually I schedule it two days per week, although I am able to use the intervention as a drug which I can take more of when necessary. The late morning of a 2:00 A.M. arousal day I am usually quite tired. I find that a 30 minute mixture of a transcendental meditation session and a nap at about 3:00 in the afternoon helps to keep me refreshed and vital. I usually go to bed between 10:00 and 10:30 on weekdays regardless of when I am scheduled to arise, so that on days in which I have a 2:00 A.M. arising I sleep approximately 3½ hours. A 3½ hour sleep period fits in well with what I have found is a natural cycle of sleep for me—3 hours. Anything less than

3 hours of sleep, and I am inordinately tired. Anything very much longer than three hours, and I am drowsy and disoriented."

"During the eight month period that I have been arising at 2:00 in the morning, I have had one serious bout of depression. I pushed myself to arise at 2:00 in the morning for several consecutive days, and found that I could not remain awake. This episode of depression lasted approximately 2 weeks. An observation which I made during this episode and which I found particularly intriguing is the on–off nature of the condition. During the course of a day, I would find myself completely debilitated and paralyzed one minute and energized and bright the next. It was as if a switch were being thrown several times a day."

"I feel that I have been given a life-restoring gift, a tool that I can use to modulate my own moods. For that I am eternally grateful. It has allowed me to maintain close touch with the me that I like. I have become more productive, have a better marriage, and feel that I am master of my own destiny once again."

Manipulations of sleep may be more generally useful in the treatment of depression when they are combined with medications. This has been done in several ways. First, the night after sleep deprivation, patients who have responded to the procedure have been given drugs in an attempt to prevent relapse during recovery sleep. Using this strategy Baxter et al. were able to sustain the antidepressant effect of sleep deprivation with lithium carbonate (9). The known capacity of lithium carbonate to prevent affective recurrences was the rationale for this approach. In a controlled study Elsenga and van den Hoofdakker et al. found that initiation of treatment with the tricyclic antidepressant, clomipramine, seemed to sustain patients' antidepressant responses to total and partial sleep deprivation (33). Initial results with these approaches seem promising, but they need to be supported by further studies.

In the Elsenga and van den Hoofdakker study, sleep deprivations were repeated several times during the first weeks of clomipramine treatment. This approach could also be viewed as an attempt to hasten the response to the drugs, or to ameliorate depressive symptoms during the long latency period of the drug response. A Danish survey of psychiatric hospitals suggests that this approach has been adopted in conventional clinical settings by psychiatrists who treat depression. Christiansen and Hedesmand found that in 1979 18 of 58 psychiatric departments employed sleep deprivation to treat depression (20). A total of 598 treatments were administered in that year in 166 therapeutic series, corresponding to 3.6 sleep deprivation treatments per series. The investigators speculated that clinicians were using sleep deprivation to alleviate depressive symptoms until the effect of coadministered antidepressant drugs became apparent.

Sleep manipulations have also been carried out with patients who have been taking antidepressant drugs for several weeks but have not yet responded. The aim was to provoke a drug response. In uncontrolled studies, Wasik and Puchala and Sack et al. reported some success with this strategy using partial sleep deprivation and phase advance of sleep, respectively (139,180).

In considering possible interactions of sleep deprivation and antidepressant medications, it may be relevant that certain drugs, such as MAOIs and psychostimulants, cause a sustained reduction in sleep duration (29). It is conceivable that the ongoing partial sleep deprivation induced by these drugs contributes to their antidepressant and mania-inducing effects.

Sleep as an Intensifier of Depression

Psychic pain and impaired functioning leads many depressed patients to withdraw from responsibilities and relationships. Sometimes, they seek the oblivion of sleep as an escape. One patient described his sleep behavior as follows:

> I sought solace in sleep. I would stay in bed later than I ought, not wanting to face the day. I would take naps during the day at work. Work, in fact, became one long exercise in getting through the day without getting caught. I would fall asleep at dinner during evenings out with friends. Sleep became an escape from all the responsibilities, mostly work-related, that I could not keep up with.

This was the same patient whose successful treatment with partial sleep deprivation was cited earlier. If, as experiments suggest, sleep is depressogenic, then this sleep-seeking behavior would intensify depressive symptoms. In this way, depression, once induced, could become self-reinforcing. It is also conceivable that depression might begin in this manner in individuals who use sleep to escape from unpleasant emotional responses to life events.

Sleep Disruption as a Preventable Cause of Mania

If disruption of sleep can trigger mania, then any factor that disrupts sleep might trigger mania (Fig. 4-1). Furthermore, avoidance of sleep disruption might help to prevent mania. Knowledge of these facts would obviously be extremely useful to patients, families, and physicians who wish to understand and manage the illness.

A host of factors might trigger mania by disrupting sleep. These factors could be categorized as psychological, situational, medical, and pharmacological (Fig. 4-1). Emotional reactions to life events, such as grief, joy, infatuation, fear, and anger, are psychogenic factors that frequently cause insomnia and might thereby trigger mania. Various types of emergencies, shift-work, travel, and noise are situational factors that can interfere with sleep and sleep schedules and might trigger mania. Medical illness, drugs, and drug withdrawal can also cause insomnia.

The psychiatric literature contains many reports that point to these and other factors as possible causes of manic episodes in patients with bipolar illness (reviewed in 194). In fact, some authors who have written about causes of mania even seem to have recognized the possibility that sleep disruption might be an intervening variable. For example, the noted German psychiatrist, Wilhelm Griesinger, wrote in 1855 that "frequently . . . insanity originates indirectly . . . from the psychical causes . . . A mediator . . . of especial importance and frequency . . . is continued sleeplessness . . . which overexcites the brain . . . It presents, therefore, in the preliminary stages of insanity, a symptom which may be often combatted by therapeutic measures" (58). Schulte, who called attention to the antidepressant effects of sleep deprivation also referred to "a psychosis-provoking effect of unaccustomed sleep deprivation" (148) [see also Gove (56)].

Among the psychogenic causes of mania, a stress factor that is frequently cited is bereavement. In one study, bereavement appeared to precipitate mania in one-third of the episodes in which a stress factor could be identified (2). The euphoria and optimism of mania seem to be paradoxical and inappropriate responses to the loss of a loved one. However, manic reactions to grief are not so surprising when one considers that grief very often causes insomnia (22), and insomnia might in turn trigger mania. According to this interpretation, mania is not so much an inappropriate emotional response to loss as it is an unfortunate complication of an appropriate emotional response. A possible mediating role of insomnia can be inferred in some reports of bereavement mania in the literature, as the following excerpts illustrate:

CASE REPORT. "Mrs. A, a 44-year-old widow, was admitted to a psychiatric hospital 2 days after the death of her 18-year-old son and 4 days after he had been in a one-car accident.

"When Mrs. A. was notified of her son's accident and his serious condition, she went into a 'shock-like' state, showing virtually no emotion as she took her turn at the bedside vigil and performed her usual chores. She was at home when word of his death reached her, and she responded by lying on the floor and screaming incoherently for several minutes. Following this she arose and 'went about her business as if nothing had happened.' "

"For the next 2 days, Mrs. A. ate practically nothing, *slept only 2 or 3 hours a night,* and sat alone in a darkened room staring into space. At the funeral, after the coffin had been lowered into the ground, she had to be restrained from pursuing the hearse as she tearfully cried, 'they're taking my son away!' "

"For the next 2 weeks, Mrs. A.'s behavior was almost entirely manic. With her psychiatrist she was coy, seductive, and manipulative; with others she was happy, bubbly, and even gleeful . . . She ate little, was decidedly hyperactive, and slept hardly at all except when heavily sedated." [italics my own] [From Hollender and Goldin (67)]

CASE REPORT. "A 28-year-old woman was first seen as an outpatient six months after the birth of her second child in a stable de facto marriage. The uncomplicated pregnancy and birth had been followed by a period of subjective well-being, but from three months post-partum, she had suffered from gradually increasing depression of mood . . . The condition did not remit or fluctuate during the following month. At this point, the patient's de facto husband was killed in a recreational flying accident."

"Having received the news in the early evening, *she spent a restless night.* Within 24 hours she was excited, elated, and incessantly active; she talked constantly and would brook no contradiction . . . She did not sleep for more than one hour each night for the following week, claiming that such sleep was adequate. She exhausted her perplexed relatives by her unwonted garrulousness, irritability and euphoria." [italics my own] [From Rosenman and Taylor (133)]

The following account of a patient's reaction to work-related sleep deprivation shows how situational factors that interfere with sleep might also trigger mania:

CASE REPORT. A 33-year-old attorney, who was married, had two children, and held a responsible, high-level position in a major corporation, was, by all accounts, a stable and conservative person who had been in good physical and mental health all of his life. However, several of his relatives had manic-depressive (bipolar) illness. His paternal grandfather had had violent episodes of mania. A paternal aunt had been hospitalized and treated with electroconvulsive therapy (ECT). A paternal cousin had been hospitalized several times for treatment of mania and was taking lithium carbonate as prophylaxis.

The attorney was working on a difficult and important case. A trial date had been set, and as it approached he realized that he did not have enough time to prepare in his usual thorough manner. Therefore, the night before the trial he decided to go without sleep and continue his preparations through the night. The next morning he became increasingly talkative, impulsive and euphoric. He had racing thoughts and was preoccupied with the idea that he could become a negotiator between nations and solve many of the world's problems. When his wife questioned his judgment, he got angry and struck her. He became increasingly manic, the police were called, and he was hospitalized involuntarily. He was treated with tranquilizers and lithium carbonate and gradually improved. Six weeks later he was discharged and returned to work. Four months after the onset of the episode he discontinued his medications, and he did well for the next three years.

At age 36, exactly the same sequence of events occurred. He stayed awake all night preparing for a trial, became manic, and was again treated with lithium carbonate. He has had no other episodes.

This patient's family history suggests that he had a genetic predisposition to develop mania. It is known that many individuals who are genetically predisposed to develop mania never become ill. Apparently, other factors must interact with the genes to cause the illness to become manifest. Sleep disruption could be such a factor. With regard to the attorney, it is conceivable that he might never have become ill if he had not decided to go without sleep. He was told that he might be able to prevent future episodes of mania by avoiding sleep deprivation.

Other examples illustrating the possible role of sleep disruption as an intervening variable in the precipitation of mania are published elsewhere (192,194).

Sleep Disruption as an Intensifier of Mania

Manic patients seem to have a reduced need for sleep. Furthermore, their increased rate of thinking and their tendency to seek out others and to become involved in various types of activities and projects can interfere with their obtaining even the diminished amount of sleep they require. If curtailment of sleep provokes mania, as the experimental data suggest, then the reduction in sleep that accompanies mania might intensify the condition. In this way mania, once induced, might become self-reinforcing and no longer dependent on the factors that triggered it in the first place (Fig. 4-1). Indeed, the course of mania is usually marked by a progressive intensification of symptoms. Once patients become manic, they often rapidly escalate out of control.

In the days before effective treatments were available, mania could follow a malignant course and terminate in death. In 1849 Bell described 40 cases of mania that were characterized by an acute onset and a florid course (10). At least 30 of these episodes ended fatally. In almost every case patients experienced a sustained and nearly total insomnia. Bell commented that the typical patient "makes constant attempts to get out of bed, and if permitted to do so, will stand until exhausted." He went on to say that "the patient will get so little food, so little sleep, and be exercised with such constant restlessness and anxiety, that he will fall off from day to day," will become increasingly emaciated, and "at the expiration of two or three weeks . . . will sink in death." At autopsy, Bell found only a "very meagre and scarcely appreciable amount of changes." For one patient he published data about the nightly duration of sleep during the course of a fatal manic episode. These data are shown graphically in Figure 4-6.

A possible parallel to these fatal cases can be found in animal deaths after long-term experimental sleep deprivation. Rechtschaffen and his colleagues subjected rats to chronic, nearly total sleep deprivation with a special apparatus that was designed to minimize the influence of factors not specifically related to sleep deprivation (36). They found that the animals progressively lost weight and died after 2–5 weeks. Like Bell, they found at necropsy that "there was no observable pathology common to all TSD [totally sleep deprived] rats. Neither was there any observable anatomical abnor-

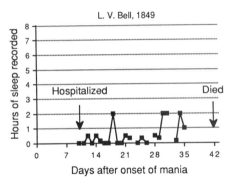

Figure 4-6 Nightly duration of sleep in a 30-year-old manic patient who was admitted to McLean Asylum for the Insane in 1830. After several weeks of nearly total insomnia, the patient died. Animal studies suggest that such deaths, which were not uncommon in the days before effective treatment for mania were available, might be caused by sleep deprivation per se (see text). Data from Bell (10).

mality that could account for imminent or actual death." The factors leading to emaciation and death in these animals are unknown and are the focus of ongoing research.

These animal experiments raise the possibility that chronic sleep loss per se might be partly responsible for the fatal outcome in severe untreated mania.

Sleep as a Treatment for Mania

Sedation is commonly employed to treat acute mania. Furthermore, specific treatments for mania, such as lithium carbonate and major tranquilizers, often have marked sedative effects. There is little question that sedation acutely controls mania, if only because patients cannot exhibit the behavioral symptoms of mania during sleep. Since sleep disruption appears to induce and to intensify mania, it is possible that drug-induced sleep not only masks the symptoms of mania, but also might reverse the underlying process that is responsible for the condition. However, there do not appear to be any systematic studies of the effects of sedation per se on the course of mania.

Wet sheet packs are sometimes used to treat excited, psychotic states, such as mania (134). In this type of treatment, patients are restrained by being wrapped in wet sheets for periods as long as 2 hr. The treatment often has a dramatic calming effect (134). As it progresses, the treatment causes body temperature to rise, sometimes so much so that hyperthermia occurs as a complication of the procedure. Possibly because of this warming effect, patients become drowsy, and they sometimes fall asleep (134). Whether the sedating effect of the treatment plays any role in its antimanic efficacy has not been investigated.

RELEVANCE TO OTHER PSYCHIATRIC DISORDERS

Schizophrenia

"Negative" symptoms in schizophrenia, such as apathy, social withdrawal, and lack of motivation, resemble symptoms of depression. In addition, "positive" symptoms of schizophrenia, such as agitation, hyperactivity, insomnia, emotional lability, delusions, and hallucinations, resemble symptoms of mania. In view of these similarities, it is interesting that total sleep deprivation, partial sleep deprivation in the second half of the night, and possibly selective REM sleep deprivation, appear to improve negative symptoms and to provoke positive symptoms, just as they improve depression and provoke mania (Table 4-3) (7,25,38,87,100,171). For example, Koranyi and Lehmann totally deprived apathetic chronic schizophrenic patients of sleep for 4 consecutive days (87). At first the patients became more lively and enthusiastic; then they became progressively more agitated and, ultimately, psychotic. Luby and Caldwell reported similar improvement of negative symptoms after sleep deprivation, and they found that patients lost this improvement after recovery sleep, just as occurs with depression (100). Using the Hamilton Depression Rating Scale, Fähndrich reported that two-thirds of his schizophrenic patients improved after total sleep deprivation, a response rate that is exactly the same as that of depressed patients (38). Höchli et al. and Holsboer-Trachsler and Ernst, also using the Hamilton Depression Rating Scale, reported that schizophrenics' depressive symptoms improved significantly after repeated partial sleep deprivations in the second half of the night and to a lesser extent worsened after recovery sleep (66,68). In view of this evidence showing similar effects of sleep and wakefulness on comparable symptoms of affective illness and schizophrenia, it might be more accurate to describe the effects of sleep deprivation more generally as improving inhibited states and provoking excited states.

The clinical implications of these findings might be the same for schizophrenia as for affective illness. Sleep might intensify negative or depressive symptoms of schizophrenia, and sleep deprivation might be a useful adjunct in the treatment of these symptoms. On the other hand, disruption of sleep might provoke outbursts of positive symptoms associated with acute schizophreniform psychosis, and avoidance of sleep disruption might prove to be useful in the prevention of psychotic decompensations.

Panic Disorder

Roy-Byrne et al. reported that sleep deprivation provoked panic attacks in 33% of patients who had histories of panic disorder (135). This effect could be viewed as yet another manifestation of the tendency of sleep deprivation to provoke excited states. The implications for prevention are obvious.

BIOLOGICAL MECHANISMS

In view of the growing evidence that affective illness is a medical illness in which genetic and other biological factors play a central role in pathogenesis, it seems likely that the mechanisms of the effects of sleep–wake manipulations on the illness have a biological basis. It also seems likely that elucidation of these mechanisms would substantially increase our understanding of the pathogenesis of the illness and lead to novel types of pharmacological and other treatments. The task of identifying biological mechanisms would be easier if we knew precisely what aspects of the sleep–wake manipulations are responsible for their clinical effects. Sleep deprivation, for example, is a complex procedure in which many factors are manipulated besides sleep. Patients sit, stand, or walk around at a time when they would ordinarily be lying in bed. They are exposed to light instead of darkness. They are engaged in social activities instead of being alone. They may eat or drink instead fasting. They are active instead of resting, and so on. In principle, any or all of these changes might be responsible for the antidepressant effect of the procedure. In fact, sleep deprivation, per se, might not even be responsible for the effect. The situation with sleep–wake manipulations is very similar to that with antidepressant and antimanic drugs. The drugs have many physiological and biochemical effects, but we do not know which of these effects are critical for their clinical effects.

Different groups have investigated the importance of sleep, timing of sleep, sleep stage content of sleep, and environmental light in patients' responses to sleep–wake manipulations, as discussed below.

CRITICAL PARAMETERS OF EFFECTIVE SLEEP–WAKE MANIPULATIONS

Antidepressant Effects of Sleep–Wake Manipulations

To determine what parameters of sleep manipulations are responsible for their effectiveness, we have to be able to discriminate between effective and ineffective manipulations. But, in view of the methological problems that have been discussed previously, how can we be confident that any particular sleep–wake manipulation really affects clinical state? In studies of treatments of depression, improvements can occur spontaneously or nonspecifically as a consequence of patients' expectations of the treatments. It is customary to control for the effect of spontaneous improvements by including a comparison group that receives no treatment. Such a group can also control for effects of patients' expectations if they are given some type of inactive treatment. Of the more than 100 studies of antidepressant sleep interventions published, only three have included these types of controls: the REM sleep versus non-REM sleep deprivation study of Vogel et al. (172) and the late versus early partial sleep deprivation study of Sack et al. (140) and Elsenga et al. (34). It is encouraging that these studies seem to indicate that at least two types of sleep–wake manipulations improve symptoms of depression; however, it is worth noting that the effects observed in each study were relatively modest, and that no one else has tried to replicate the results of either type of study. Also, since the study of Sack et al. (140) confounded timing of sleep and sleep duration and the study of Vogel et al. (172) might be considered to have confounded sleep stage content of sleep with duration of sleep, we cannot be certain what aspect(s) of the interventions were actually responsible for their antidepressant effects (Fig. 4-4). We can conclude only that interventions that include these features are active. Nevertheless, these studies appear to show that the antidepressant effects of sleep–wake manipulations cannot be attributed solely to spontaneous improvements or patients' expectations of the procedures.

It could also be argued that in the uncontrolled studies improvements that occur within 1 day of a sleep–wake intervention, such as total or partial sleep deprivation, are probably not the result of spontaneous improvement, because spontaneous improvement usually occurs gradually and is unlikely to occur in a large number of patients on any given day.

In conclusion, the similar findings in the two controlled studies and in the large

number of uncontrolled studies make it clear that some form(s) of partial sleep deprivation are sufficient to improve depression. Taken together, the results of the studies of
Vogel et al. (172) and Sack et al. (140) show that the effective treatments were those in
which sleep in the second half of the night was disrupted, REM sleep was disrupted,
and sleep was shorter in duration. It is not possible to decide which factor(s) were
critical for the response.

Sleep deprivation is also darkness deprivation, because the sleep deprivation
procedure usually exposes patients to light at a time when they would ordinarily be
asleep in the dark. Since, at least one form of depression, winter depression, improves
when patients are exposed to light and worsens when the light is withdrawn, it is

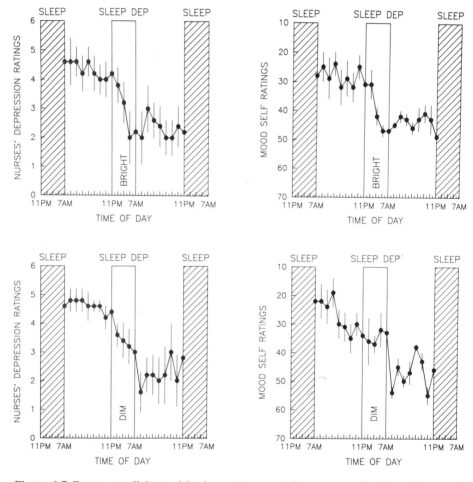

Figure 4-7 Exposure to light at night does not appear to be necessary for the antidepressant
effect of one night's total sleep deprivation. Diagrams show patients' self-ratings of mood (mean
± SD) before, during, and after sleep deprivation. Patients were sleep deprived on two occasions, once in very bright light (top) and once in nearly total darkness (bottom). The degree of
improvement was similar the day after each type of sleep deprivation (however, patients did
appear to improve more rapidly during the bright light condition).

possible that increased exposure to light at night is responsible for the antidepressant effect of sleep deprivation. Furthermore, some studies of winter depression suggest that exposure to light at the end of the night, the time when sleep deprivation appears to be most effective, is also the time when phototherapy appears to be most effective. However, my colleagues and I carried out an experiment that suggests that exposure to light at night is not necessary for the antidepressant effect of total sleep deprivation (190). We deprived five depressed patients of sleep on two different occasions, once in nearly total darkness and once in very bright light. The light manipulations took place between 11 P.M. and 7 A.M. of the sleep deprivation night. All of the patients eventually improved to an equal degree the day after each type of sleep deprivation. However, it is worth noting that the patients appeared to improve more rapidly during the night of sleep deprivation when they were exposed to bright light (Fig. 4-7).

Depressant and Mania-Inducing Effects of Sleep–Wake Manipulations

The idea that sleep might induce or intensify depression seems plausible in view of the finding that sleep deprivation improves depression. Also, the idea that sleep deprivation might induce or intensify mania seems plausible considering that other antidepressant modalities, such as drugs and electroconvulsive therapy, may induce mania (193). Furthermore, the rapidity of the onset of these responses to sleep and sleep deprivation, as with the antidepressant effect of sleep deprivation, makes it unlikely that the responses are the result of spontaneous changes in clinical state. However, the possibility that the changes result from patients' expectations of the procedures cannot be ruled out. Therefore, the growing evidence from uncontrolled studies that sleep induces or intensifies depression and that sleep deprivation induces or intensifies mania needs to be confirmed in controlled studies.

Constraints on Hypotheses

Until the results of future studies make it possible to unconfound the effects on clinical state of duration of sleep, timing of sleep, and sleep stage content of sleep, it seems unreasonable to allow any of these factors to constrain in any decisive way hypotheses about the biological mechanisms of sleep–wake manipulations.

CIRCADIAN RHYTHM (PROCESS C) HYPOTHESES AND THE INTERNAL COINCIDENCE MODEL

A number of years ago Wirz-Justice and I suggested that the depressant effect of sleep might depend on the circadian phase at which sleep occurred (186). According to this "internal coincidence model," depression occurred when sleep coincided with a circadian phase that was sensitive to sleep's depressant effects, and depression might improve if the timing of sleep were shifted to a different circadian phase that was less sensitive to these effects, or, conversely, if the timing of the circadian phase were shifted relative to sleep. The numerous studies of circadian rhythms that had been published at that time suggested that the timing of circadian rhythms in several different physiological and biochemical variables was shifted abnormally early, or phase-advanced in depression

(184,185,188). Since REM sleep is governed by a process that exhibits a circadian rhythm, this apparent advance in circadian rhythms' phases seemed to provide a possible explanation for the advance within sleep of the temporal distribution of REM sleep that had often been observed in depression (Fig. 4-5). Considering these findings, we specifically hypothesized that a circadian phase that was sensitive to the depressant effects of sleep was harmless when it normally coincided with the first hours of wakefulness in the morning, but triggered depression when it was phase-advanced along with other circadian rhythms and coincided with the last hours of sleep. On the basis of this hypothesis we predicted that advancing the timing of the sleep schedule correspondingly earlier would cause the circadian phase that was sensitive to sleep's depressant effect to once again coincide with wakefulness and would thereby improve depression (183). This prediction seemed to be bourne out by observations that phase advance of sleep and sleep deprivation in the second half of the night were effective antidepressants while sleep deprivation in the first half of the night was not (34,54,139,140,142, 153,183,188,189). However, as already discussed, no study was successfully controlled for all other possible influences that might have been responsible for these findings. Also, phase advance of circadian rhythms has not been consistently observed in studies carried out after the hypothesis was published (195). The most consistent finding is that the nadir of the circadian rhythm in plasma levels of cortisol is abnormally phase-advanced in unipolar depression (195).

The most basic postulate of the internal coincidence model is that sleep induces or intensifies depression when sleep coincides with a circadian phase that is sensitive to these effects of sleep, and that wakefulness improves depression (and induces mania) when it coincides with this circadian phase. This postulate of the model can be considered separately from the question of whether or not circadian rhythms are phase-advanced in depression. Several types of experiments suggest that the timing of sleep and wakefulness might be important in patients' responses to sleep–wake manipulations (34,54,139,140,142,153,183,188,189). Until timing has been ruled out as a critical factor in patients' responses, the internal coincidence model remains plausible and merits further investigation. The model does not specify the process whose sensitivity to sleep is modulated by a circadian rhythm. One possibility, to be discussed later, is that this process is REM sleep. REM sleep is sensitive to sleep in the sense that it can occur only during sleep, and it is modulated by a circadian rhythm such that it most likely to occur in the latter half of the night (when sleep deprivation appears to be more effective) and least likely to occur earlier in the night (when sleep deprivation appears to be less effective) (Fig. 4-5).

THE REM SLEEP HYPOTHESIS

Vogel hypothesized that suppression of REM sleep was the therapeutic mechanism of antidepressant drugs, and he found that mechanical deprivation of REM sleep improved depression to a degree and with a time course that, he argued, resembled responses to antidepressant drug treatments (171,173). In further support of his hypothesis, he noted that in his study patients who did not improve after REM sleep deprivation also did not improve after treatment with an antidepressant drug, imipramine, that patients who responded favorably to either modality exhibited REM sleep rebound when the treatment is withdrawn, and that REM sleep deprivation produces several behavioral changes in animals that are in some respects opposite to changes that occur in depression (172,173).

Vogel used Hobson and McCarley's reciprocal interaction, two-oscillator model of the REM–non-REM cycle to conceptualize REM sleep abnormalities in depression, and the antidepressant effects of REM sleep deprivation (65,105,173). According to this model, REM sleep is generated by a group or network of neurons, possibly located in the medial pontine reticular formation, and it is inhibited by another group or network of neurons, possibly the monoaminergic cells in the midbrain, pons, and medulla. In the model, the latter group of cells is stimulated by the former, and their reciprocal interactions are responsible for the cyclicity of REM and non-REM sleep. According to Vogel, an increase in the percentage of REM sleep early in the sleep period in depression is caused by a reduction in strength of the REM sleep inhibiting component of the oscillating system. A decrease in the percentage of REM sleep late in the sleep period in depression is caused by a reduction in strength of the REM generating component. According to Vogel, REM sleep deprivation acts to strengthen both components of the oscillator. He suggested that weakening of the REM–non-REM oscillator might be responsible for symptoms of depression, and that strengthening of the damaged oscillator by REM sleep deprivation might be responsible for the antidepressant effects of that procedure as well as those of drugs used to treat depression.

Vogel had little to say about therapeutic mechanisms of other types of sleep–wake manipulations. However, it should be noted that total and partial sleep deprivation and phase-advance of sleep all reduce REM sleep because the circadian rhythm in REM sleep propensity reaches its peak in the second half of the night (see Fig. 4-5), and all three procedures prevent sleep at that time. In view of these facts, the results of the experiment of Vogel et al. raise the possibility that the antidepressant effect of all these procedures depends on their capacity specifically to reduce REM sleep (as discussed previously, the same argument could be made for reduced sleep duration, which is confounded with REM sleep deprivation in most of the procedures) (see Fig. 4-4). However, it is difficult to reconcile this hypothesis with the fact that the first three types of treatment relieve depression within hours, while selective REM sleep deprivation, according to Vogel et al., requires 3 weeks to achieve its therapeutic effect (172). However, this issue is clouded by Vogel's having stated in an earlier report of a pilot study of REM sleep deprivation that its antidepressant effects were apparent within a few days (171).

Wiegand et al.'s finding that the presence of REM sleep in short naps tended to be associated with relapses after total sleep deprivation would provide another kind of support for the REM sleep hypothesis if it were statistically more robust (202).

Considering the evidence accumulated so far, the hypothesis that effects on REM sleep are specifically responsible for the effects of sleep–wake manipulations on clinical state is still one of the most parsimonious explanations for all the observations, and it appears to merit further investigation.

THE SLOW-WAVE SLEEP (PROCESS S) HYPOTHESIS

In contrast to Vogel, Borbély and Wirz-Justice focused on a process related to slow-wave sleep in their hypothesis about the therapeutic mechanism of sleep deprivation (16). Borbély developed a model of sleep regulation in which sleep propensity and sleep duration were considered to be functions of the level of a homeostatic process, S, that accumulates during wakefulness and is discharged during sleep (15). In this model transitions from sleep to wakefulness and wakefulness to sleep occur when process S crosses thresholds that are modulated by a second process, C. Process S is equated with slow-wave sleep, or, more precisely, with power density in the EEG spectrum during sleep. Borbély and Wirz-Justice hypothesized that in depression process S accumulates abnormally slowly during wakefulness and is therefore abnormally low at the time of sleep onset. According to the model, deficient process S at sleep onset would explain the long sleep latencies, the low levels of slow-wave sleep, and the early morning awakening that are frequently observed in patients with depression. Since process S accumulates during wakefulness, sleep deprivation, by extending wakefulness, would tend to restore process S to more nearly normal levels in depressed patients. If the hypothesized deficiency in process S were responsible for depressive symptoms, then its increase during sleep deprivation would explain the therapeutic effect of the procedure.

So far, evidence concerning the process S deficiency hypothesis of depression and therapeutic sleep deprivation has been inconsistent. A basic problem is that reduced slow-wave sleep is not specifically related to depression; it is found in many other types of psychiatric and medical illness (40,42,48). Furthermore, although Borbély found that power density was abnormally low in depression (16), others have not been able to confirm this observation (167). Finally, a prediction of the hypothesis that augmentation of process S was responsible for the antidepressant effect of sleep deprivation was not supported by van den Hoofdakker and Beersma's finding that improvement after one night's total sleep deprivation was not correlated with increased power density during recovery sleep (167).

SLEEP AS HEAT, WAKEFULNESS AS COOLING

Relative Hyperthermia after Sleep Onset

Physiological responses to sleep resemble responses to heat exposure. Shortly after sleep onset, thermolytic responses, such as vasodilation and sweating, increase dramatically (24,59). At the same time thermogenic processes and resting metabolic rate decrease (59). Apparently, thermolysis increases and thermogenesis decreases because the hypothalamic set point for temperature regulation is reset approximately 0.4°C lower during sleep than during wakefulness (53,62,179). This resetting appears to take place immediately after sleep onset. However, because of the thermal inertia of the body, the regulated lowering of core body temperature caused by this resetting takes place gradually. Because set point resetting is immediate and temperature lowering is gradual, the organism could be considered to be in a state of relative hyperthermia at the beginning of sleep. Thus, the resemblance between sleep and heat exposure is more than superficial; relatively speaking, sleep is a form of heat exposure.

Some of the neuroendocrine changes that accompany sleep onset could also be understood as components of a physiological response to heat. For example, the secretion of thyroid-stimulating hormone (TSH), a pituitary hormone that helps to stimulate thermogenesis, is inhibited by sleep just as it is inhibited by heat exposure

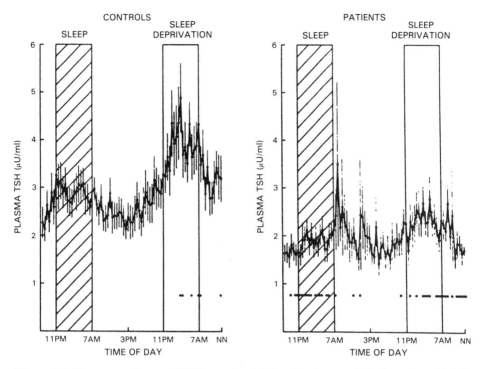

Figure 4-8 The nocturnal surge of TSH secretion is blunted in depressed bipolar patients (right) compared with normal individuals (left). Sleep inhibits TSH secretion, and total sleep deprivation disinhibits or stimulates TSH secretion. Data are from Sack et al. (141).

(Fig. 4-8) (63). Secretion of prolactin, a pituitary hormone that is thermolytic insofar as it helps to regulate sweating (106,116,132), is stimulated by sleep just as it is stimulated by heat exposure.

This heat-like property of sleep might be important in the mechanisms of clinical responses to sleep–wake manipulations in patients with affective illness. Specifically, "heat deprivation" might be responsible for the antidepressant effect of sleep deprivation. In this connection, it is interesting that preliminary evidence suggests that a seasonal form of affective illness characterized by recurrent summer depression might be triggered by seasonal changes in temperature (196,197). In one experiment, depressive symptoms appeared to be induced in patients with a history of recurrent summer depression by exposing them to heat for 2 days (196). The relatively rapid time course of these clinical responses to heat is similar to the time course of changes observed after sleep–wake manipulations.

Measurements of body temperature and of TSH levels suggest that depressed patients might be abnormally warm during sleep. A number of studies have shown that rectal temperature is abnormally high during sleep in depression, and that it returns to normal levels during remission (see Figs. 4-9 and 4-10) (6,150,154,184). Several studies have also revealed that the nocturnal surge in TSH secretion is blunted in depression and returns to normal levels after remission (see Table 4-9 and Figs. 4-8 and 4-11) (55,80,82,84,141,152,181,182). Blunting of nocturnal TSH secretion could be

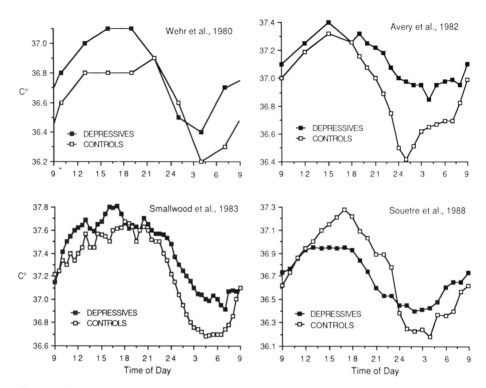

Figure 4-9 Several studies show that nocturnal temperature is elevated in depressed patients compared with normal individuals. Data are from Wehr et al. (184), Avery et al. (6), Smallwood et al. (150), and Souêtre et al. (154).

interpreted as a physiological response to elevated body temperatures during depression. In fact, Souetre et al. measured rectal temperature and TSH levels in the same patients before and after recovery and found an inverse relationship between the two variables (Fig. 4-11) (154).In depression, nocturnal rectal temperature was elevated and nocturnal TSH secretion was blunted; after remission nocturnal temperature decreased and nocturnal TSH secretion increased. These changes are very similar to reciprocal changes in rectal temperature and TSH secretion that O'Malley et al. induced by heating normal individuals with thermal blankets (see Fig. 4-11) (112).

Since sleep deprivation prevents the relative hyperthermia that is associated with sleep onset, it could be conceptualized as a kind of heat deprivation. The heat deprivation is relative. Body temperature is actually higher during sleep deprivation than during sleep, but the temperature controller responds as though the body were cooler because its set point is higher. The "cooling" effect of sleep deprivation might also be further enhanced by a decrease in the efficiency of heat-conserving mechanisms that seems to be caused by sleep deprivation (47,200).

Like cold exposure, sleep deprivation dramatically stimulates the nocturnal surge of TSH secretion (113,117). In depressed bipolar patients Sack et al. found that nocturnal TSH secretion was blunted during sleep and that it was partially normalized by one night's total sleep deprivation (Fig. 4-8) (141). Sleep deprivation also improved these patients' depressions.

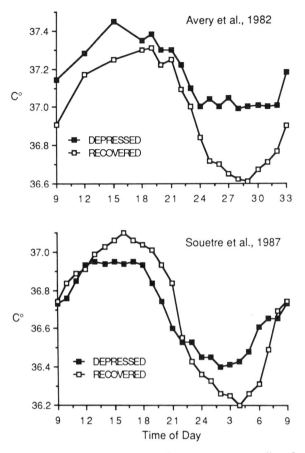

Figure 4-10 Depressed patients' elevated nocturnal temperatures normalize after recovery. Data are from Smallwood et al. (150) and Souêtre et al. (154).

Table 4-9 Blunted Nocturnal TSH Secretion in Depression

	Blunted		Normal	
Author(s) (year)	N	Subjects	N	Subjects
Weeke et al. (1978)	19	Depressed, Endog.		
Golstein et al. (1980)	8	Depressed UP	5	Depressed BP
			6	Normal
Weeke et al. (1980)			2	Depressed BP
			2	Depressed UP
			13	Normal
Kijne et al. (1982)			9	Depressed, endog.
			9	Remitted, endog.
Kjellman et al. (1984)	32	Depressed MDD	24	Remitted MDD
			9	Remitted UP
			8	Remitted BP
			32	Normal
Souêtre et al. (1986)	12	Depressed UP/BP	12	Remitted UP/BP
			13	Normal
Sack et al. (1988)	8	Depressed BP	8	Normal
Kasper et al. (1988)	46	Depressed UP/BP	13	Normal

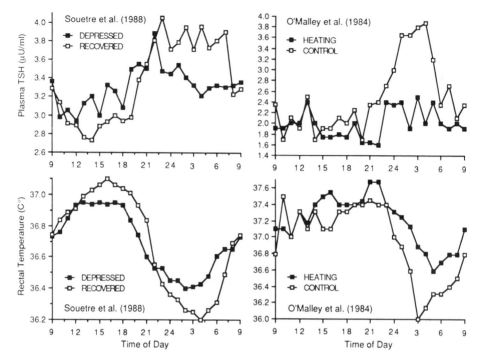

Figure 4-11 Elevated nocturnal temperature in depression may cause blunting of the nocturnal surge of TSH secretion. Reciprocal changes in temperature and TSH are seen after recovery in depressed patients studied by Souêtre et al. (154). Similar reciprocal changes were induced by external heating with a thermal blanket by O'Malley et al. (112). In the latter study heating produced changes in rectal temperature and TSH levels that are similar to those seen in depression.

Brain Heating during REM Sleep

Processes that occur in the central nervous system during REM sleep heat the brain. Neuronal firing rates, CNS oxygen consumption, and CNS glucose utilization all increase diffusely and dramatically during REM sleep (35,45,75). These changes produce heat and raise brain temperature (57,81,118,202). Changes in structures adjacent to the CNS during REM sleep also produce heat. Increased resting tone and rapid movements of eye muscles generate heat during REM sleep. In addition, during REM sleep brown adipose tissue (BAT) along the spine appears to produce heat, which is conveyed into the vertebral venous plexus surrounding the spinal cord (46,151). As a result, CNS temperature increases dramatically during REM sleep, and it can reach levels higher than those observed during wakefulness (81).

I have hypothesized elsewhere that thermogenesis may be an important function of REM sleep (199). REM sleep may represent a mode of homeothermic temperature regulation characterized by thermogenesis in a thermal core that is reduced in size and confined mainly to the CNS during sleep. According to this interpretation, the peculiar features of REM sleep can be understood as mechanisms by which structures lying within this core produce heat. According to this model, the cyclicity of REM sleep results from the behavior of an on–off type of thermostat control mechanism whose thermosensitive and thermoeffector elements are situated in rhombencephalic structures that have been implicated in the generation and inhibition of REM sleep.

REM sleep deprivation presumably prevents the dramatic brain heating that occurs during REM sleep. Therefore, REM sleep deprivation, like total sleep deprivation, may be equivalent physiologically to heat deprivation, or cooling. Thus, relative or absolute cooling may be a common feature of all the antidepressant types of sleep–wake manipulations. Conversely, relative or absolute heating occurs during sleep, which appears to be depressant. Thermoregulatory effects of sleep and wakefulness appear to account for many of the physiological and neuroendocrine effects of the two states. These thermoregulatory effects might also explain the clinical effects of sleep and wakefulness. Results of an experiment in progress support this hypothesis (T. A. Wehr, unpublished data). Eleven patients were sleep deprived for one night on two occasions, once in an ambient temperature of 18°C, and once in an ambient temperature of 33°C. External heating markedly attentuated both the clinical and neuroendocrine effects of sleep deprivation. Depressive symptoms and nocturnal prolactin secretion were augmented by the heating, while nocturnal TSH secretion was blunted by the heating. These results suggest that many of the observations about the effects of sleep–wake manipulations on affective illness might be understood within the framework of thermoregulatory physiology. These results also raise the possibility that heating and cooling maneuvers might be used to treat or prevent episodes of affective illness.

REFERENCES

1. Abrams RM, Hutchison AA, Jay TM. Local cerebral glucose utilization non-selectively elevated in rapid-eye movement sleep of the fetus. *Dev Brain Res* 1988; 40:65–70.
2. Ambelas A. Psychologically stressful events in the precipitation of manic episodes. *Br J Psychiat* 1979; 135:15–21.
3. Amin M. Response to sleep deprivation and therapeutic results with antidepressants. *Lancet* 1978; 2(8081):165.
4. Amin M, Khalid R, Khan P. Relationship between sleep deprivation and urinary MHPG levels. *Int Pharmacopsychiat* 1980; 15:81–85.
5. Ansseau M, Machowski R, Franck G, Timsit-Berthier M. REM sleep latency and contingent negative variation in endogenous depression. Suggestion for a common cholinergic mechanism. *Biol Psychiat* 1985; 20:1303–1307.
6. Avery DH, Wildschiodtz G, Rafaelsen OJ. Nocturnal temperature in affective disorder. *J Affect Disord* 1982; 4:61–71.
7. Azumi K, Takahashi S, Takahashi K, Maruyama N, Kikuti S. The effects of dream deprivation on chronic schizophrenics and normal adults: A comparative study. *Folia Psychiatr Neurol Jpn* 1967; 21:205–225.
8. Barcia D, Ruiz E, Soler V. Sleep deprivation: Treatment for depression. *Rev Psiquiatr Psicol Med* 1979; 14(3):201–208.
9. Baxter LR. Can lithium carbonate prolong the antidepressant effect of sleep deprivation? *Arch Gen Psychiat* 1985; 42:635.
10. Bell LV. On a form of disease resembling some advanced stages of mania and fever. *Am J Insan* 1849; 6:97–127.

11. Benson KL, Zarcone VP. Testing the REM sleep phasic event intrusion hypothesis of schizophrenia. *Psychiat Res* 1985; 15:163–173.
12. Berger M, Riemann D, Wiegand M, Joy D, Höchli D, Zulley J. Are REM sleep abnormalities in depression more than an epiphenomenon? In WP Koella, F Obál, H Schulz, and P Visser (eds.), *Sleep 1986,* Gustav Fisher Verlag, Stuttgart, New York, 1988: 218–222.
13. Bhanji S, Roy GA. The treatment of psychotic depression by sleep deprivation: A replication study. *Br J Psychiatr* 1975; 127:222–226.
14. Bhanji S, Roy GA, Baulieu C. Analysis of mood change during and following sleep deprivation therapy. *Acta Psychiatr Scand* 1978; 58:379–383.
15. Borbély AA. A two process model of sleep regulation. *Hum Neurobiol* 1982; 1(3):195–204.
16. Borbély AA, Wirz-Justice A. Sleep, sleep deprivation, and depression. *Hum Neurobiol* 1982; 1(3):205–210.
17. Buddeberg C, Dittrich A. Psychological aspects of sleep deprivation: A controlled study on depressives and normals. *Arch Psychiatr Nervenkr* 1978; 225:249–261.
18. Burton R. *The Anatomy of Melancholy,* 1621, edited by F Dell and P Jordan-Smith. Tudor Publishing, New York, 1927:216.
19. Cashman MA, Coble P, McCann BS, Taska L, Reynolds CF III, Kupfer DJ. Sleep markers for major depressive disorder in adolescent patients. *Sleep Res* 1986; 15:91.
20. Christensen PH, Hedemand E. Sleep deprivation treatment in Denmark. *Ugeskr Laeger* 1981; 143:1727–1729.
21. Christodoulou GN, Malliaras DE, Lykouras EP, Papadimitriou GN, Stefanis CN. Possible prophylactic effect of sleep deprivation. *Am J Psychiat* 1978; 135:375–376.
22. Clayton PJ. Bereavement. In ES Paykel (ed.), *Handbook of Affective Disorders,* Guilford, New York, 1982:403–415.
23. Cole MG, Müller HF. Sleep deprivation in the treatment of elderly depressed patients. *J Am Geriatr Soc* 1976; 24(7):308–313.
24. Day R. Regulation of body temperature during sleep. *Am J Dis Child* 1941; 61:734–746.
25. De Barros-Ferreira, Goldsteinas L, Lairy GC. REM sleep deprivation in chronic schizophrenics: Effects on the dynamics of fast sleep. *Electroencephalogr Clin Neurophysiol* 1973; 34:561–569.
26. Dessauer M, Goetze U, Tölle R. Periodic sleep deprivation in drug-refractory depression. *Neuropsychiatry* 1985; 13:111–116.
27. Doongaji DR, Vahia VN, Lakdawala PD, Parikh MD, Singh AR, Thatte SS, Lotlikar KD. Sleep deprivation in depression (a preliminary study). *Postgrad J Med* 1979; 25(1):4–11.
28. Dourdil-Pérez F, Sala Ayma JM. Sleep deprivation in the treatment of depression and urinary amines. *Actas Luso-Esp Neurol Psiquiatr Ciencias Afines* 1980; 8:491–496.
29. Duncan WC, Gillin JC, Post RM, Gerner RH, Wehr TA. Relationship between EEG sleep patterns and clinical improvement in depressed patients treated with sleep deprivation. *Biol Psychiat* 1980; 15(6):879–890.
30. Duncan WD, Tamarkin L, Sokolove P, Wehr TA. Chronic clorgyline treatment of the Syrian Hamster: An analysis of circadian effects. *J Biol Rhythms* 1988; 3:305–322.
31. Elsenga S, Van den Hoofdakker RH. Clinical effects of sleep deprivation and clomipramine in endogenous depression. *J Psychiatr Res* 1983; 17(4):361–374.
32. Elsenga S, van den Hoofdakker RH. Clinical effects of several sleep/wake manipulations on endogenous depression. *Sleep Res* 1983; 12:326.
33. Elsenga S, van den Hoofdakker RH. Response to total sleep deprivation and clomipramine in endogenous depression. *J Psychiat Res* 1987; 21:157–161.
34. Elsenga A, van den Hoofdakker RH, Dols LCW. Clinical effects of early and late partial sleep deprivation in endogenous depression. In WP Koella, F Obál, H Schulz and P Visser (eds.), *Sleep 1986.* Gustav Fischer Verlag, Stuttgart, 1988:448–450.

35. Evarts EV, Bental E, Bihari B, Huttenlocher PR. Spontaneous discharge of single neurons during sleep and waking. *Science* 1962; 135:726–728.
36. Everson CA, Bergmann BM, Rechtschaffen A. Sleep deprivation in the rat. III. Total sleep deprivation. *Sleep* 1989; 12(1):13–21.
37. Fähndrich E. Effects of sleep deprivation on depressed patients of different nosologic groups. *Psychiatr Res* 1981; 5:277–285.
37a. Fähndrich E. Schlafentzugs-Behandlung depressiver syndrome bei schizophrener grunderkrankung. *Nervenarzt* 1982; 53:279–283.
38. Fähndrich E. Effect of sleep deprivation as a predictor of treatment response to antidepressant medication. *Acta Psychiatr Scand* 1983; 68:341–344.
39. Feinberg I. Changes in sleep cycle patterns with age. *Psychiat Res* 1974; 10:283–306.
40. Feinberg I, Floyd TC. Systematic trends across the night in human sleep cycles. *Psychophysiology* 1979; 16:283–291.
41. Feinberg I, Hiatt JF. Sleep patterns in schizophrenia: A selective review. In RL Williams, I Karacan and C Moore (eds.), *Sleep Disorders, Diagnosis and Treatment*. Wiley, New York, 1988:205–231.
42. Fisher C, Dement WC. Studies on the psychopathology of sleep and dreams. *Am J Psychiat* 1963; 119:1160–1168.
43. Foster FG, Grau T, Spiker DG. EEG sleep in generalized anxiety disorder. *Sleep Res* 1977; 6:145.
44. Franck G, Salmon E, Poirier R, Sadzot B, Franco G. Etude du métabolisme glucidique cérébral chez l'homme, au cours de l'éveil et du sommeil, par tomographie à émission de positrons. *Rev Electroencephalogr Neurophysiol Clin* 1987; 17:71–77.
45. Franzini C, Ciance T, Lenzi P, Libert JP, Horne JA, Parmeggiani PL. Influence of brown adipose tissue on deep cervial temperature during sleep in the young rabbit. *Experientia* 1986; 42:604–606.
46. Fuller CA, Sulzman FM, Moore-Ede MC. Thermoregulation is impaired in an environment without circadian time cues. *Science* 1978; 199:794–795.
47. Gaillard J. Chronic primary insomnia: Possible physiopathological involvement of slow wave sleep deficiency. *Sleep* 1978; 1:133–147.
48. Gay C, Loo H, Olie JP, Benhadj AB, Tabeze JP, Caire M, Susini-Delucas H, Kameleddine F, Askienaty R. Sleep deprivation and dexamethasone suppression test in healthy volunteers. *Encephale* 1983; 9:273–277.
49. Gerner RH, Post RM, Gillin JC, Bunney WE Jr. Biological and behavioral effects of one night's sleep deprivation in depressed patients and normals. *J Psychiatr Res* 1979; 15:21–40.
50. Gillin JC, Wyatt R. Schizophrenia: Perchance a dream? *Int Rev Neurobiol* 1975; 17:297–342.
51. Gillin JC. The sleep therapies of depression. *Prog in Neuro-Psychopharmacol Biol Psychiat* 1983; 7:351.
52. Glotzback SF, Heller HC. Central regulation of body temperature during sleep. *Science* 1976; 194:537–539.
53. Goetze V, Tölle R. Antidepressant effect of partial sleep deprivation during the first half of the night. *Psychiatr Clin (Basel)* 1981; 14:129–149.
54. Golstein J, Van Cauter E, Linkowski P, Vanhaelst L, Mendlewicz J. Thyrotropin nyctohemeral pattern in primary depression: differences between unipolar and bipolar women. *Life Sci* 1980; 27:1695–1703.
55. Gove WR. Sleep deprivation: A cause of psychotic disorganization. *Am J Sociol* 1970; 75:782–799.
56. Greenberg JH. Sleep and the cerebral circulation. In J Orem and CD Barnes (eds.), *Physiology in Sleep*, Vol. 3. Academic Press, New York, 1980.

57. Griesinger W. *Mental Pathology and Therapeutics,* 1882, CL Robertson (trans.). William Wood, New York, 1855:163.
58. Hammel HT, Jackson DC, Stotwijk JAJ, Hardy JD, Stromme SB. Temperature regulation by hypothalamic proportional control with an adjustable set point. *J Appl Physiol* 1963; 18:1146–1154.
59. Hâsto J. Sleep deprivation in the treatment of endogenous depressions. *Ceskoslovenska Psychiatr* 1978; 74:357–358.
60. Heinroth JC. *Textbook of Disturbances of Mental Life* (1818), J Schmorale (trans.). Johns Hopkins University Press, Baltimore, 1975.
61. Heller HC, Grof R, Rautenberg W. Circadian and arousal state influences on thermoregulation in the pigeon. *Am J Physiol* 1983; 245:R321–R328.
62. Hersham JM, Read DG, Bailey AL. Effect of cold exposure on serum thyrotropin. *J Clin Endocrinol* 1970; 30:430–434.
63. Hiatt FJ, Floyd TC, Katz PH, Feinberg I. Further evidence of abnormal non-rapid-eye-movement sleep in schizophrenia. *Arch Gen Psychiat* 1985; 42:797–802.
64. Hobson JA, McCarley R, Wyzinski PW. Sleep cycle oscillation: Reciprocal discharge by two brainstem neuronal groups. *Science* 1975; 189:55–58.
65. Höchli D, Trachsler E, v. Luckner N, Woggon B. Partial sleep deprivation therapy of depressive syndromes in schizophrenic disorders. *Pharmacopsychiatry* 1985; 18:134–135.
66. Hollender MH, Goldin ML. Funeral mania. *J Nerv Ment Dis* 1978; 166:890–892.
67. Holsboer-Trachsler E, Ernst K. Sustained antidepressive effect of repeated partial sleep deprivation. *Psychopathology* 1986; 19(2):172–176.
68. Hudson JI, Lipinski JF, Frankenburg FR, Grochocinski VJ, Kupfer DJ. Electroencephalographic sleep in mania. *Arch Gen Psychiat* 1988; 45:267–273.
69. Hughs JR, Krahn D. Blindness and the validity of the double-bind procedure. *J Clin Psychopharmacol* 1985; 5:138–142.
70. Insel TR, Gillin JC, Moore A, Mendelson WB, Loewenstein RJ, Murphy DL. The sleep of patients with obsessive-compulsive disorder. *Arch Gen Psychiat* 1982; 39:1372–1377.
71. Jernajczyk W. Latency of eye movement and other REM sleep parameters in bipolar depression. *Biol Psychiat* 1986; 21:465–472.
72. Jimerson DS, Lynch HJ, Post RM, Wurtman RJ, Bunney WE Jr. Urinary melatonin rhythms during sleep deprivation in depressed patients and normals. *Life Sci* 1977; 20:1501–1508.
73. Joffe RT, Brown P, Dienenstock A, Mitton J. Neuroendocrine predictors of the antidepressant effects of partial sleep depression. *Biol Psychiat* 1984; 19(3):347–352.
74. Jouvet M. Neurophysiology of the states of sleep. *Physiol Rev* 1967; 47:117–177.
75. Jovanovic UJ. The sleep profile in manic-depressive patients in the depressive phase. *Waking Sleeping* 1977; 1:199–210.
76. Jus K, Bouchard M, Jus AK, Villeneuve A, Lachance R. Sleep EEG studies in untreated longterm schizophrenic patients. *Arch Gen Psychiat* 1973; 29:386–390.
77. Kasper S, Moises HW, Beckmann H. Dexamethasone suppression test combined with total sleep deprivation in depressed patients. *Psychiatr Clin* 1983; 16:17–25.
78. Kasper S, Katzinski L, Lenarz T, Richter R. Early and late auditory evoked potentials in depressed patients and therapeutic sleep deprivation. *Psychiat Res* 1988; 25:91–100.
79. Kasper S, Sack DA, Wehr TA, Kick H, Voll G, Viera A. Nocturnal TSH and prolactin secretion during sleep deprivation and prediction of antidepressant response in patients with major depression. *Biol Psychiat* 1988; 24:631–641.
80. Kawamura H, Sawyer CH. Elevation in brain temperature during paradoxical sleep. *Science* 1965; 150:912–913.
81. Kijne B, Aggermaes H, Fog-Muller FF. Circadian variation of serum thyrotropin in endogenous depression. *Psychiat Res* 1982; 6:277–282.

82. King D, Dowdy S, Jack R, Gardner R, Edwards P. The dexamethasone suppression test as a predictor of sleep deprivation antidepressant effect. *Psychiat Res* 1982; 7:93–99.
83. Kjellman BF, Beck-Friis J, Ljunggren JG, Wetterberg L. Twenty-four-hour serum levels of TSH in affective disorders. *Acta Psychiatr Scand* 1984; 69:491–502.
84. Klerman GL. The current age of youthful melancholia: Evidence for increase in depression among adolescents and young adults. *Br J Psychiat* 1988; 152:4–14.
85. Knowles JB, Southmayd SE, Delva N, Prowse A, MacLean AW, Cairns J, Letemendia FJ, Waldron J. Sleep deprivation: Outcome of controlled single case studies of depressed patients. *Can J Psychiat* 1981; 26:330–333.
86. Koranyi EK, Lehmann HE. Experimental sleep deprivation in schizophrenic patients. *Arch Gen Psychiat* 1960; 2:534–544.
87. Kraft AM, Willner P, Gillin CG, Janowsky D, Neborsky R. Changes in thought content following sleep deprivation in depression. *Compr Psychiat* 1984; 25:283–289.
88. Kretschmar JH, Peters UH. Sleep deprivation as a treatment of endogenous depression. In UJ Jovanovich (ed.), *The Nature of Sleep*. Gustav Fischer Verlag, Stuttgart, 1973.
89. Kuhs H. Dexamethasone suppression test and sleep deprivation in endogenous depression. *J Affect Disord* 1985; 9:121–126.
90. Kupfer DJ, Reynolds CF III, Grochocinski VJ, Ulrich RF, McEachran A. Aspects of short REM latency in affective states: A revisit. *Psychiat Res* 1986; 17:49–59.
91. Kvist J, Kirkegaard C. Effects of repeated sleep deprivation on clinical symptoms and the TRH test in endogenous depression. *Acta Psychiatr Scand* 1980; 62:494–502.
92. Lahmeyer HW, Val E, Moises Gaviria F, Prasad BR. EEG sleep in borderline personality disorder. *Sleep Res* 1985; 14:133.
93. Larsen JK, Lindberg ML, Skovgaard B. Sleep deprivation as treatment for endogenous depression. *Acta Psychiatr Scand* 1976; 54:167–173.
94. Linkowski P, Mendlewicz J, Leclercq R, Brasseur M, Hubain P, Golstein J, Copinschi G, Van Cauter E. The 24-hour profile of adrenocorticotropin and cortisol in major depressive illness. *J Clin Endocrinol Metab* 1985; 61:429–438.
95. Lewy AJ, Sack R, Singer CM, White DM, Hoban TM. Winter depression and the phase-shift hypothesis for bright light's therapeutic effects. History, theory, and experimental evidence. *J Biol Rhythms* 1988; 3:121–134.
96. Loosen PT, Ackenheil M, Athen D, Beckman H, Benkert O, Dittmer T, Hippius H, Matussek N, Rüther E, Scheller M. Therapy of endogenous depression by sleep deprivation, 2nd communication: Comparison of psychopathological and biochemical parameters. *Drug Res* 1974; 24(8):1075–1077.
97. Loosen PT, Merkel U, Amelung U. Combined sleep deprivation and clomipramine in primary depression. *Lancet* 1976; 2:156–157.
98. Loosen PT, Merkel U, Amelung U. Combined sleep deprivation/chlormipramine therapy of endogenous depressions. *Drug Res* 1976; 26:1177–1178.
99. Luby ED, Caldwell DF. Sleep deprivation and EEG slow wave activity in chronic schizophrenia. *Arch Gen Psychiat* 1967; 17:361–364.
100. Martin PR, Loewenstein RJ, Kaye WH, Ebert MH, Weingartner H, Gillin JC. Sleep EEG in Korsakoff's psychosis and Alzheimer's disease. *Neurology* 1986; 36:411–414.
101. Matussek N, Ackenheil M, Athen D, Beckman H, Benkert O, Dittmer T, Hippius H, Loosen P, Rüther E, Scheller M. Catecholamine metabolism under sleep deprivation therapy of improved and not improved depressed patients. *Neuropsychopharmakology* 1974; 2:108–114.
102. Matussek N, Römisch P, Ackenheil M. MHGP excretion during sleep in endogenous depression. *Neuropsychobiology* 1977; 3:23–29.
103. McCarley R, Hobson JA. Neuronal excitability modulation over the sleep cycle. A structural and mathematical model. *Science* 1977; 196:678–680.

104. Mendelson WB, James SP, Martin JV, Wagner R, Sack DA, Garnett D, Milton J, Wehr TA. Frequency analysis of the sleep EEG in depression. *Psychiat Res* 1987; 21:89–94.
105. Mills DE, Robertshaw D. Response of plasma prolactin to changes in ambient temperature and humidity in man. *J Clin Endocrin Metab* 1981; 52:279–283.
106. Müllen PE, Linsell CR. Sleep deprivation, dieting, and depression markers. *Lancet* 1987; 7(8538):323.
107. Müller C, Fialho O. L'Agrypnie un nouveau traitement antidepressif. *L'Evol Psychiatr* 1982; 663–670.
108. Nasrallah HA, Kuperman S, Coryell WH. Reversal of dexamethasone nonsuppression with sleep deprivation in primary depression. *Am J Psychiat* 1980; 137(11):1463–1464.
109. Nasrallah HA, Coryell WH. Dexamethasone nonsuppression predicts the antidepressant effects of sleep deprivation. *Psychiat Res* 1982; 6:61–64.
110. Neil JF, Merikanges JR, Foster FG, Merikanges KR, Spiker DG, Kupfer DJ. Waking and all-night sleep EEG's in anorexia nervosa. *Clin Electroencephalogr* 1980; 11:9–15.
111. O'Malley BP, Richardson A, Cook N, Swart S, Rosenthal FD. Circadian rhythms of serum thyrotropin and body temperature in euthyroid individuals and their responses to warming. *Clin Sci* 1984; 67:433–437.
112. O'Malley BP, Cook N, Richardson A, Barnett DB, Rosenthal FD. Circulating catecholamine, thyrotrophin, thyroid hormone and prolactin responses of normal subjects to acute cold exposure. *Clin Endocrinol* 1984; 21:285–291.
113. Papadimitriou GN, Christodoulou GN, Trikkas GM, Malliaras DE, Lykouras EP, Stefanis CN. Sleep deprivation psychoprophylaxis in recurrent affective disorders. *Bibl Psychiatr* 1980; 160:56–61.
114. Papousek M, Frank HP, Stohr H. Sleep deprivation: Effects on circadian rhythms. In P Levin and WP Koella (eds.), *Sleep 1974*. Karger, Basel, 1975:474–477.
115. Parker DC, Rossman LG, Vanderlan EF. Relation of sleep-entrained human prolactin release to REM-non-REM cycles. *J Clin Endocrinol Metab* 1974; 38:646–651.
116. Parker DC, Pekary AE, Hershman JM. Effect of normal and reversed sleep-wake cycles upon nyctohemeral rhythmicity of plasma thyrotropin: Evidence suggestive of an inhibitory influence in sleep. *J Clin Endocrinol Metab* 1976; 43:318–329.
117. Parmeggiani PL, Zamboni G, Perez E, Lenzi P. Hypothalamic temperature during desynchronized sleep. *Exp Brain Res* 1984; 54:315–320.
118. Parry BL, Wehr TA. Therapeutic effect of sleep deprivation in patients with premenstrual syndrome. *Am J Psychiat* 1987; 144:808–810.
119. Pflug B, Tölle R. Disturbance of the 24-hour rhythm in endogenous depression and the treatment of endogenous depression by sleep deprivation. *Int Pharmacopsychiat* 1971; 6:187–196.
120. Pflug B, Tölle R. Therapy of endogenous depression by sleep deprivation: Practical and theoretical consequences. *Nervenartz* 1971; 42:117–124.
121. Pflug B. Sleep deprivation as an ambulant therapy for endogenous depression. *Nervenartz* 1972; 12:614–622.
122. Pflug B. The effect of sleep deprivation on depressed patients. *Acta Psychiatr Scand* 1976; 53:148–158.
123. Philipp M. The course of depression after sleep deprivation. *Nervenarzt* 1978; 49:120–123.
124. Post RM, Kotin J, Goodwin FK. Effects of sleep deprivation on mood and central amine metabolism in depressed patients. *Arch Gen Psychiat* 1976; 33:627–632.
125. Puig-Antich J, Goetz R, Hanlon C. Sleep architecture measures in prepubertal children with major depression. *Arch Gen Psychiat* 1982; 39:932–939.
126. Regier DA, Boyd JH, Burke JD, Rae DS, Myers JK, Kramer M, Robin LN, George LK,

Karno M, Locke BA. one-month prevalence of mental disorders in the United States. *Arch Gen Psychiat* 1988; 45:977–986.

127. Reyero F, Müller C. Repeated sleep deprivation in the treatment of depression. *Encephale* 1977; III:55–61.

128. Reynolds CF, Kupfer DJ, McEachran AB, Taska LS, Sewitch DE, Coble PA. Depressive psychopathology in male sleep apneics. *J Clin Psychiat* 1984; 45:287–290.

129. Reynolds CF, Soloff PH, Kupfer DJ, Taska LS, Restifo K, Coble PA, McNamara ME. Depression in borderline patients: A prospective EEG sleep study. *Psychiat Res* 1985; 14:1–15.

130. Reynolds CF, Kupfer DJ, Hoch CC, Stack JA, Houck PA, Berman SR. Sleep deprivation effects in older endogenous depressed patients. *Psychiat Res* 1988; 21:95–109.

131. Robertson MT, Boyajian MJ, Patterson K, Robertson WVB. Modulation of the chloride concentration of human sweat by prolactin. *Endocrinology* 1986; 119:2439–2444.

132. Rosenman SJ, Tayler H. Mania following bereavement: A case report. *Br J Psychiat* 1986; 148:468–470.

133. Ross DR, Lewin R, Gold K, Ghuman HS, Rosenblum B, Salzberg S, Brooks AM. The psychiatric uses of cold wet sheet packs. *Am J Psychiat* 1988; 145:242–245.

134. Roy-Byrne P, Uhde TW, Post RM, Joffe RT. Relationship of response to sleep deprivation and carbamazepine in depressed patients. *Acta Psychiatr Scand* 1984; 69:379–382.

135. Roy-Byrne P, Uhde TW, Post RM. Effects of one night's sleep deprivation on mood and behavior in patients with panic disorder. Comparison with depressed patients and normal controls. *Arch Gen Psychiat* 1986; 43:895–899.

136. Rudolf GA, Tölle R. The course of the night with total sleep deprivation as antidepressant therapy. *Waking Sleeping* 1978; 2:83–91.

137. Rudolf GA, Tölle R. Sleep deprivation and circadian rhythms in depression. *Psychiatr Clin* 1978; 11:198–212.

138. Sack DA, Nurnburger J, Rosenthal NE, Wehr TA. The potentiation of antidepressant medications by phase-advance of the sleep-wake cycle. *Am J Psychiat* 1985; 142:606–608.

139. Sack DA, Duncan W, Rosenthal NE, Mendelson WE, Wehr TA. The timing and duration of sleep in partial sleep deprivation therapy of depression. *Acta Psychiatr Scand* 1988; 77:219–224.

140. Sack DA, James SP, Rosenthal NE, Wehr TA. Deficient nocturnal surge of TSH secretion during sleep and sleep deprivation in rapid-cycling bipolar illness. *Psychiat Res* 1988; 23:179–191.

141. Schilgen B, Tölle R. Partial sleep deprivation as therapy for depression. *Arch Gen Psychiat* 1980; 37:267–271.

142. Schilgen B, Bischofs W, Blaszkiewicz F, Bremer W, Rudolf GA, Tölle R. Totaler und partieller schlafentzug in der behandlung von depressionen. *Drug Res* 1976; 26:1171–1173.

143. Schmidt H. Short REM latency and dream interruption insomnia. Presented at the Society of Biological Psychiatry Annual Meeting, May 7–11, 1986, Washington, DC.

144. Schmidt H. Short REM latencies and repetitive REM awakenings in impotence without depression. *Sleep Res* 1986; 15:203.

145. Schmocker W. Der schlafentzug. Eine klinische, psychophysiologische und biochemische untersuchung. *Arch Psychiatr Nervenkr* 1975; 221:111–122.

146. Schulte W. Kombinerte psycho- und pharmakotherapie bei melancholikern. In H Kranz (ed.), *Probleme pharmakopsychiatrischer kombinations und langzeithandlungen.* Karger, Basel, 1966:150–169.

147. Schulte W. Über die bedeutung des klinischen details: Protrahiertes herausgeraten aus

melancholischen phasen. In H Hippius and H Selbach (eds.), *Das Depressive Syndrom.* Karger, Basel, 1969:415–420.

148. Sidorowicz W. Sleep deprivation in treatment of depression, summary. *Psychiatr Pol* 1976; 10(5):507.

149. Smallwood RG, Avery DH, Pascualy RA, Prinz PN. Circadian temperature rhythms in primary depression. *Sleep Res* 1983; 12:215.

150. Smith RE, Horwitz BA. Brown fat and thermogenesis. *Physiol Rev* 1969; 49:330–425.

151. Souêtre E, Salvati E, Pringuey D. The circadian rhythm of plasma thyrotropin in depression and recovery. *Chronobiol Int* 1986; 3:197–205.

152. Souêtre E, Salvati E, Pringuey D, Plasse Y, Savelli M, Darcourt G. Antidepressant effects of the sleep/wake cycle phase advance. *J Affect Disord* 1987; 12:41–46.

153. Souêtre E, Wehr TA, Sack DA, Krebs B, Darcourt G. 24-hour profiles of body temperature and plasma TSH in bipolar patients during depression and during remission and in normal control subjects. *Am J Psychiat* 1988; 145:1133–1137.

154. Spiker DG, Foster FG, Coble PA, Love D, Kupfer DJ. The sleep disorder in depressed alcoholics. *Sleep Res* 1977; 6:161.

155. Stern M, Fram D, Wyatt RJ, Grinspoon L, Tursky B. All night sleep studies of acute schizophrenics. *Arch Gen Psychiat* 1969; 20:470–477.

156. Surridge-David M, MacLean A, Coulter ME, Knowles JB. Mood change following an acute delay of sleep. *Psychiat Res* 1987; 22:149–158.

157. Svendson K. Sleep deprivation therapy in depression. *Acta Psychiatr Scand* 1976; 54:184–192.

158. Sydor L. Sleep deprivation in the treatment of depressive syndromes. *Psychiatr Pol* 1978; 12(1):71–77.

159. Taub JM, Hawkins DR, Van de Castle R. Electroencephalographic analysis of the sleep cycle in young depressed patients. *Biol Psychiat* 1978; 7:203–214.

160. Thase ME, Kupfer DJ, Ulrich RF. Electroencephalographic sleep in psychotic depression. *Arch Gen Psychiat* 1986; 43:886–893.

161. Tringer L. Depressios betegek kezelese alvasmegvonassal. *Ideggyogyaszati Szemle* 1977; 30:112–126.

162. Uhde TW, Post RM, Ballenger JC, Cutler NR, Jimmerson DC, Weizman ED, Bunney WE Jr. Circadian rhythm and sleep deprivation in depression. In *Sleep 1980.* Karger, Basel, 1981:23–26.

163. van Bemmel AL, van den Hoofdakker RH. Maintenance of therapeutic effects of total sleep deprivation by limitation of subsequent sleep. *Acta Psychiatr Scand* 1981; 63:453–462.

164. van den Burg W, van den Hoofdakker RH. Total sleep deprivation in endogenous depression. *Arch Gen Psychiat* 1975; 32:1121–1125.

165. van den Hoofdakker RH, Beersma DGM, Dijk DJ, Bouhuys AL, Dols ACW. Effects of total sleep deprivation on mood and chronophysiology in depression. In C Shagass et al. (eds.), *Biological Psychiatry 1985.* Elsevier, Amsterdam, 1986.

166. van den Hoofdakker RH, Beersma DGM. On the contribution of sleep wake physiology to the explanation and the treatment of depression. *Acta Psychiatr Scand* 1988; 77:53–71.

167. van Scheyen JD. Sleep deprivation in the treatment of unipolar (endogenous) depressions. *Ned T Geneesk* 1977; 121(14):564–568.

168. Vein AM, Airapetov RG. Nocturnal polygraphic studies during treatment of depressive patients with sleep deprivation. *Nevropatologiia* 1983; 4:577–583.

169. Vogel GW. REM deprivation: Dreaming and psychosis. *Arch Gen Psychiat* 1968; 18:312–329.

170. Vogel GW, Traub AC, Ben-Horin P, Meyers GM. REM deprivation II. The effects on depressed patients. *Arch Gen Psychiat* 1968; 18:301–311.
171. Vogel GW, Thurmond S, Gibbons R, Sloan K, Walker M. REM sleep reduction effects on depression syndromes. *Arch Gen Psychiat* 1975; 32:765–777.
172. Vogel GW, Vogel F, McAbee R, Thurmond AJ. Improvement of depression by REM sleep deprivation. New findings and a theory. *Arch Gen Psychiat* 1980; 37:247–253.
173. von Waldman KD, Hass S, Greger J. Schlafentzug in der therapie endogener depressionen. *Dt Gesundh-Wesen* 1979; 34:2419–2421.
174. Voss A, Kind H. Outpatient treatment of endogenous depressions by sleep deprivation. *Schweiz Rundsch Med Prax* 1974; 63:564–565.
175. Vovin Ry, Aksenova IO, Sverglov LS. The use of sleep deprivation in the treatment of protracted depressive states. *Zh Nevropat Psikhiatr Korsakov* 1979; 79(4):449–453.
176. Vovin RY, Aksenova IO, Sverdlov LS. Sleep deprivation in the treatment of chronic depressive states. *Neurosci Behav Physiol* 1982; 12:92–96.
177. Vovin RY, Kakturovich. Sleep deprivation as a method of endogenous depression treatment. *Zh Nevropat I Psikhiatr Korsakov* 1985; 560–564.
178. Walker JM, Berger RJ. Sleep as an adaptation for energy conservation functionally related to hibernation and shallow torpor. *Prog Brain Res* 1980; 53:255–278.
179. Wasik A, Puchala G. Analysis of the treatment of depressive states by the method of sleep deprivation. *Psychiat Pol* 1978; XII(4):463–468.
180. Weeke A, Weeke J. Disturbed circadian variation of serum thyrotropin in patients with endogenous depression. *Acta Psychiatr Scand* 1978; 57:281–289.
181. Weeke A, Weeke J. The 24-hour pattern of serum TSH in patients with endogenous depression. *Acta Psychiatr Scand* 1980; 62:69–74.
182. Wehr TA, Wirz-Justice A, Goodwin FK, Duncan W, Gillin JC. Phase advance of the circadian sleep wake cycle as an antidepressant. *Science* 1979; 206:710–713.
183. Wehr TA, Muscettola G, Goodwin FK. Urinary 3-methoxy-4-hydroxyphenylglycol circadian rhythm: Early timing (phase-advance) in manic-depressives compared with normals. *Arch Gen Psychiatry* 1980; 37:257–263.
184. Wehr TA, Goodwin FK. Biological rhythms and psychiatry. In S Arieti and HKH Brodie (eds.), *American Handbook of Psychiatry,* Vol VII, 2nd ed. Basic Books, New York, 1981.
185. Wehr TA, Wirz-Justice A. Internal coincidence model for sleep deprivation and depression. In WP Koella (ed.), *Sleep 1980.* Karger, Basel, 1981:26–33.
186. Wehr TA, Goodwin FK, Wirz-Justice A, Breitmaier J, Craig C. 48 hour sleep-wake cycle in manic-depressive illness: Naturalistic observations and sleep deprivation experiments. *Arch Gen Psychiat* 1982; 39:559–565.
187. Wehr TA, Wirz-Justice A. Circadian rhythm mechanisms in affective illness and in antidepressant drug action. *Pharmacopsychiatry* 1982; 15:31–39.
188. Wehr TA, Goodwin FK. Introduction. In TA Wehr and FK Goodwin (eds.), *Biological Rhythms and Psychiatry.* Boxwood Press, Pacific Grove, CA, 1983.
189. Wehr TA, Rosenthal NE, Sack DA, Gillin JC. Antidepressant effects of sleep deprivation in bright and dim light. *Acta Psychiatr Scand* 1985; 72:161–165.
190. Wehr TA, Sack DA, Duncan W, Rosenthal NE, Mendelson WB, Gillin JC, Goodwin FK. Sleep and circadian rhythms in affective patients isolated from external time cues. *Psychiat Res* 1985; 15:327–339.
191. Wehr TA, Sack DA. Sleep disruption: A treatment for depression and a cause of mania. *Psychiatr Ann* 1987; 17(10):655–663.
192. Wehr TA, Goodwin FK. Can antidepressants cause mania and worsen the course of affective illness? *Am J Psychiat* 1987; 144:1403–1411.

193. Wehr TA, Sack DA, Rosenthal NE. Sleep reduction as a final common pathway in the genesis of mania. *Am J Psychiat* 1987; 144(2):201–203.
194. Wehr TA. Chronobiology of affective illness. In W Hekkens, GA Kerkhof and W Rietveld (eds.), *Trends in Chronobiology*. Pergamon Press, Great Britain, 1988:367–379.
195. Wehr TA, Kasper S, Giesen H. Effects of light and heat on remitted summer depressives. Submitted.
196. Wehr TA, Rosenthal NE. Seasonality and affective illness. *Am J Psychiat* 1989; 146:829–839.
197. Wehr TA, Giesen H, Schulz PM, Joseph-Vanderpool JR, Kelly K, Kasper S, Rosenthal NE. Summer depression: Description of the syndrome and comparison with winter depression. In NE Rosenthal and M Blehar (eds.), *Seasonal Affective Disorders and Phototherapy*. New York, Guilford Press, 1988:55–63.
198. Wehr TA. A brain-heating function for REM sleep. Submitted.
199. Weitzman ED. Effects of a prolonged 3-hour sleep-wake cycle on sleep stage, plasma cortisol, growth hormone and body temperature in man. *J Clin Endocrin Metab* 1974; 38:1018–1070.
200. Wever RA. Internal interactions within the human circadian system: The masking effect. *Experientia* 1985; 41:332–342.
201. Wiegand M, Berger M, Zulley J, Lauer C, von Zerssen D. The influence of daytime naps on the therapeutic effect of sleep deprivation. *Biol Psychiat* 1987; 22:386–389.
202. Wirz-Justice A, Pühringer W, Hole G. Sleep deprivation in depression: Effects on the diurnal rhythm of plasma free tryptophan and relation to clinical response. Presented at the *Second International Sleep Research Congress*, Edinburgh, 1975.
203. Wirz-Justice A, Pühringer W, Hole G. Sleep deprivation and clomipramine in endogenous depression. *Lancet* 1976; 2:912.
204. Wirz-Justice A, Pühringer W, Hole G. Response to sleep deprivation as a predictor of therapeutic results with antidepressant drugs. *Am J Psychiat* 1979; 136:1222–1223.
205. Wurtz RHK. Physiological correlates of steady state potential shifts during sleep and wakefulness. II. Brain temperature, blood pressure, and potential changes across the ependyma. *Electroencephalogr Clin Neurophysiol* 1967; 22:43–53.
206. Yamaguchi N, Maeda K, Kuromura S. The effects of sleep deprivation on the circulation rhythms of plasma cortisol in depressive patients. *Folia Psychiatr Neurol,* Japan 1978; 32:479–487.
207. Zander KJ, Lorenz A, Wahlländer B, Ackenheil M, Rüther E. Biogenesis of the antidepressive effect of sleep deprivation. In *Sleep 1980*. Karger, Basel, 1981:9–15.
208. Zimanová J, Vojtechovsky M. Sleep deprivation as a potentiation of antidepressive pharmacotherapy. *Act Nerv Super (Praha)* 1974; 16(3):188–189.
209. Zulley J, Wever R, Aschoff J. The dependence of onset and duration of sleep on the circadian rhythm of rectal temperature. *Pflügers Arch* 1981; 391:314–318.

5

A Method for Assaying the Effects of Therapeutic Agents on the Period of the Endogenous Circadian Pacemaker in Man

CHARLES A. CZEISLER, JAMES S. ALLAN,
AND RICHARD E. KRONAUER

Abnormalities in the period of the endogenous circadian pacemaker have been implicated in the pathogenesis of certain forms of affective illness and circadian rhythm sleep disorders. Several pharmacologic and nonpharmacologic interventions used successfully in the treatment of these conditions are believed to have an effect on circadian period. However, attempts to evaluate circadian period in these clinical conditions have been methodologically flawed in that the free-running period of the rest–activity cycle—not the intrinsic period of the endogenous circadian pacemaker—has been assessed.

We describe a method for determining the period of the endogenous circadian pacemaker, free from confounding influences from exogenous stimuli and the rest–activity cycle. Because this method utilizes frequent serial phase estimations to determine period, greater accuracy of period determination and its variability over time can be achieved.

Affective Illness

In 1947, Georgi postulated that patients with affective illness have phase misalignments among internal markers of circadian rhythmicity, and between these internal rhythms and the external light–dark cycle (1). Halberg has further proposed that the cyclic mood swings observed in manic-depressive illness may be due to the presence of an internal circadian rhythm with a non-24-hr period that is not synchronized to the 24-hr day (2), a hypothesis that is consistent with data from several clinical case reports (3). Wehr and Goodwin (4) have observed that the early morning wakefulness, diurnal variation in mood, and seasonality and cyclicity of depression have stimulated interest in the relationship between biological rhythms and affective illness. Shorter REM sleep latencies and an increased amount of REM sleep in the early night among depressed patients have led some investigators to propose that an internal phase advance of the circadian pacemaker may play a role in the pathogenesis of this affective disorder (5,6). Circadian rhythms of other markers of the endogenous pacemaker have also been reported to be phase-advanced relative to the timing of the sleep–wake cycle in depression (7,8), although it has also been reported that a subset of depressed patients may have phase-delayed circadian rhythms (9).

Wehr has suggested several potential mechanisms including abnormalities in circadian period that could produce the phase misalignment seen in affective illness (10). Wehr's hypothesis is further supported by the fact that lithium, a drug known to lengthen the circadian period in the rat (11–13), is commonly employed in the treatment of bipolar affective disorders. Several studies of free-running human subjects taking lithium have yielded inconclusive results (14–16). However, all of those studies assessed the free-running period of the rest–activity cycle, rather than the intrinsic period of the endogenous circadian pacemaker.

Circadian Rhythm Sleep Disorders

It has been postulated that certain circadian rhythm sleep disorders (17), such as delayed sleep phase syndrome, advanced sleep phase syndrome, and/or hypernychthemeral sleep–wake syndrome, may result from an abnormality of either endogenous circadian period or phase-resetting capacity (18–21). In delayed sleep phase insomnia, most often seen in younger patients, the preferred bedtimes and wake times are intractably shifted to an abnormally late hour. When the degree of the shift is large, the sleep schedule typically produces significant disruptions of school and/or work requirements, despite attempts to modify sleep and wake times. Sleep attempted at a more conventional hour is disrupted and unsatisfying, leading patients to seek help for a complaint of insomnia. Conversely, individuals with the advanced sleep-phase syndrome have markedly advanced circadian phase and complain of early morning wakefulness with corresponding difficulty in staying awake in the evening. Because the entrained phase relationship of the circadian timing system to the environment is, in part, a function of the endogenous circadian period, a systematic assay of the endogenous periods of these patients may reveal much about the pathophysiology of these disorders.

Research in normal subjects has shown that there is an age-dependent advance of circadian phase that may be responsible for the higher incidence of insomnia seen in the elderly population, and *in extremis* may underlie the early morning wakefulness often seen in elderly patients. Changes in the endogenous circadian period with advancing age have been observed in animals (22). In addition, we have shown that an abnormally advanced circadian phase is associated with an abnormally intrinsic period in an elderly subject (19), consistent with predictions based on oscillator theory.

The hypernychthemeral sleep–wake syndrome (21,23,24) occurs when a patient's maximal capacity to phase advance is insufficient to compensate for the difference between the >24-hr endogenous circadian period and the 24-hr environmental cycle. Patients afflicted with this syndrome are not stably entrained to the 24-hr day. Instead, such patients present with progressive delays in sleep onset and waketimes. Patients are alternately symptomatic or asymptomatic, as their endogenous circadian rhythms move in and out of phase with the geophysical day. It has been hypothesized that a sufficiently aberrant circadian period could cause this disorder. It is evident that the period of the behavioral rest–activity cycle is longer than 24-hrs in such patients, but methods are required to determine whether this syndrome is due to a deficiency in phase-resetting capacity or an abnormality of intrinsic period.

Finally, although the nonparametric effects of bright light on human circadian phase have recently been described (25), less is known about the ability of light to induce parametric changes in the human circadian timing system, such as might be required in the treatment of hypernychthemeral sleep–wake syndrome. Studies in Germany have suggested that differing light intensities do not have a systematic effect on period, yet these studies also measured the period of the free-running rest–activity cycle rather than the intrinsic period of the pacemaker (26).

In this article, we introduce a method of assessing a fundamental property of the human circadian timing system: the intrinsic period of the endogenous circadian pacemaker.

IDENTIFYING THE INTRINSIC PERIOD OF THE CIRCADIAN PACEMAKER

Under conditions of normal entrainment, the light–dark cycle and other environmental time cues are capable of synchronizing the human circadian timing system to the 24-hr geophysical day (25,27). However, in the absence of external time cues, human subjects exhibit a free-running period of the rest–activity cycle that averages about 25 hrs (14).

It is important to realize that this 25-hr period typically observed in short-term time isolation studies represents a compromise between two oscillatory processes: the intrinsic period of the circadian pacemaker and those periodic behavior patterns that constitute the rest–activity cycle (14). Most commonly, these two processes remain synchronized with each other—a condition known as internal synchronization. However, in nearly all long-term free-running studies (and in about one-fourth of the short-term studies), the rest–activity cycle will adopt a period different than that of the circadian pacemaker. This condition is unique to human subjects and is known as internal desynchrony. During this state of desynchrony, the circadian pacemaker has a remarkably stable period, whereas the period of the rest–activity rhythm shows marked day-to-day variation.

Measurement of physiologic and behavioral functions under the condition of internal desynchrony shows that the circadian pacemaker drives daily cycles in a variety of physiologic functions including core body temperature, cortisol release, the duration and organization of sleep and sleep stages, REM sleep propensity, urinary potassium excretion, alertness, and cognitive and psychomotor performance (14,28–31). During internal desynchrony, the observed period of these pacemaker-driven rhythms is either shorter or longer than that observed during conditions of internal synchrony, depending on whether the rest–activity cycle desynchronizes with an average period shorter or longer than that of the intrinsic period of the circadian pacemaker. The condition of internal desynchrony allows the identification of those physiologic rhythms that are merely passive responses to the rest activity cycle, not reflective of the output of the circadian pacemaker.

Several groups have attempted to model mathematically the interaction between

these two oscillators (32). However, only one of these models incorporates the observed influence of the rest–activity cycle on the period of the endogenous circadian
pacemaker, via mutual coupling (33). Simulations using this model confirm that the
free-running period observed during synchrony does not represent the intrinsic period
of the endogenous circadian pacemaker. They further suggest that the intrinsic period
of the endogenous circadian pacemaker, not the average period of the rest–activity
cycle, is the dominant parameter in determining entrained phase relationships (33,34).
Thus, the intrinsic period of the endogenous circadian pacemaker can be measured only
during desynchrony when the period of the rest–activity cycle is substantially different
from the period of the endogenous circadian pacemaker. Because the intrinsic period of
the endogenous circadian pacemaker is the dominant influence on the outputs of the
human circadian timing system, very small perturbations in the intrinsic period of that
oscillator can lead to profound changes in the internal phase relationships between the
many neurohumoral and physiologic functions under circadian control. For example,
as shown in Figures 5-1 and 5-2, a 66-year-old woman with a markedly advanced
endogenous circadian temperature phase exhibited an unusually short endogenous circadian temperature period of 23.7 hrs. Likewise, intrinsic abnormalities of the endogenous pacemaker sufficient to produce significant disruptions of entrained phase relationships may not be reflected in the synchronized free-running period, which may fall
well within the normal range because of the compromise between the intrinsic period
of the endogenous pacemaker and the behavioral influence of the rest–activity cycle.
Therefore, a protocol that characterizes the clinically significant intrinsic period

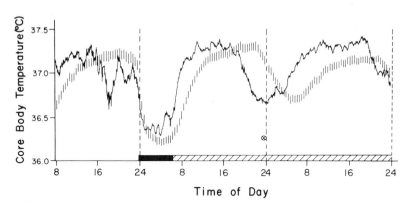

Figure 5-1 The core body temperature rhythm (solid line) of a healthy, 66-year-old woman is
shown under both entrained (first 22 hrs of recording) and constant routine conditions (subsequent 42 hrs depicted). Black bar indicates the time of the sleep period during the entrained day
(scheduled at its habitual time). The hatched bar shows the time of the constant routine, a period
of enforced semirecumbent wakefulness designed to expose the endogenous component of the
daily rhythm. The encircled cross indicates the time of the minimum of a harmonic regression
curve fitted to the constant routine temperature data (ECPmin). This minimum occurred at 23:35
(11:35 P.M.). When this waveform is compared to that of averaged data from 29 normal, young
subjects (vertical bars, mean ± SEM), it can be seen that this elderly subject has a markedly
advanced phase of the endogenous core body temperature rhythm. This phase advance is not
readily seen during measurements made during the entrained day because of masking effects.
Thus, the utility of constant routine assessment is manifest.

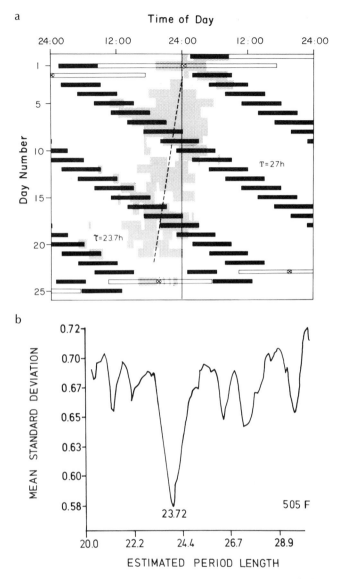

Figure 5-2 (a) During a subsequent study of the subject shown in Fig. 5-1, a 27-hr sleep–wake schedule was imposed to desynchronize sleep–wake behavior from the output of the endogenous circadian pacemaker (as marked by the core body temperature rhythm). The rest–activity pattern is plotted in double raster format, with successive days of study plotted both next to and beneath each other. Solid bars represent episodes of scheduled bed rest. Open bars indicate the times of constant routine assessments of circadian phase. The ECPmin is indicated by encircled crosses. Regression throughout the ECPmin (dashed line) yields a period estimate of 23.79 hrs. A single plot of the times when the body temperature was below the mean entrained body temperature (36.83°C) is depicted with stippling. (b) Spectral analysis using the minimum variance technique is shown for the temperature data collected during the desynchronized portion of the study illustrated in a. The period estimate of 23.72 hrs correlates well with that obtained by regression analysis through the initial and final ECPmin ($p < .01$).

of the endogenous circadian pacemaker, independent of the timing of the rest–activity cycle, is required to diagnose abnormalities in the endogenous circadian period, and to assess the efficacy of therapeutic modalities designed to affect circadian period.

DESIGN OF PERIOD ASSESSMENT PROTOCOL

Characterization of the period of the endogenous circadian pacemaker presents several experimental challenges. First, as indicated above, the effects of the rest–activity cycle on the observed period of the endogenous circadian pacemaker must be minimized and controlled. Second, estimates of phase must be made using a physiologic marker that reliably reflects the output of the endogenous circadian pacemaker under conditions that reduce contamination from the potential masking effects of exogenous stimuli. Third, that marker must be followed for a long enough duration so that regression analysis of frequent serial phase estimates can yield an accurate determination of the period of the endogenous circadian pacemaker. Each of these issues is considered in turn below.

Reduction of the Effects of the Rest–Activity Cycle on the Period of the Endogenous Pacemaker

The rest–activity cycle has its maximum effect on the period of the endogenous pacemaker when it is cycling at periods that are within the range of entrainment of the endogenous pacemaker. Thus, scheduling day lengths 23.5–25.5 hrs long would certainly be expected to cause the intrinsic period of the endogenous circadian pacemaker to adopt the imposed period of the rest–activity cycle. On the other hand, rest–activity cycle periods shorter than 21–22 hrs or longer than 27–28 hrs would be expected to force the rest–activity cycle to desynchronize from the endogenous circadian pacemaker (as illustrated in Fig. 5-2a). Under these conditions of forced internal desynchrony, the intrinsic period of the endogenous circadian pacemaker can be observed (Fig. 5-2b). Analyses of both experimental data and model simulations indicate that both forced and spontaneous internal desynchrony allow the intrinsic period of the endogenous circadian pacemaker to be estimated, although there may be greater residual effects of the rest–activity cycle on the observed period of the temperature cycle in spontaneous desynchrony than in forced desynchrony (34–36).

Estimation of Endogenous Circadian Phase

A number of physiologic parameters have been linked to the endogenous pacemaker during studies of internally desynchronized subjects. These include urinary volume and electrolyte excretion, plasma cortisol levels and urinary free cortisol excretion, computation speed, subjective alertness assessments, rapid eye movement (REM) sleep propensity, and core body temperature (14,29). Other markers, such as melatonin secretion, have been proposed (37), but unfortunately these outputs have never been demonstrated to persist during internal desynchrony. Of those markers known to reflect circadian function, core body temperature can be continuously recorded and readily analyzed (14,28,29,38). Like all other markers, core body temperature is subject to a variety of masking effects that obscure the endogenous component of the observed oscillation. Sleep–wake transitions, exercise, and changes in ambient temperature are known to cause considerable masking of the core body temperature rhythm.

A technique known as the constant routine, first suggested by Mills, has been refined and coupled with methods of phase estimation to yield a reproducible and accurate technique for estimating endogenous circadian phase (28,38,39). We have found that the endogenous circadian temperature rhythm can be reliably observed by instituting a constant routine of enforced semirecumbent wakefulness in constant indoor room light with caloric intake evenly distributed in hourly snacks throughout day and night. The phase of the endogenous circadian temperature minimum can be estimated using the dual harmonic regression method (39). The correlation between this and the traditional method of spectral analysis/waveform education during desynchrony is high [Pearson's correlation coefficient .998 ($p < .01$)] (28). Determination of endogenous circadian period can therefore be made by regression analysis of successive phase estimations using subjects on forced desynchrony protocols by scheduling constant routines during the waking portion of those days when the rest–activity cycle is about 180 degrees out of phase with the endogenous component of the temperature cycle.

Duration of Protocol Required for Precise Period Determination

Presuming an invariate period, the accuracy of the period estimation is determined by the length of the forced desynchrony protocol and the precision of the serial phase estimations. Assuming that phase assessments are accurate within a range of 2 hrs, it should be possible to determine period to within ±9 mins (±.15 hr) in 2 weeks of forced desynchrony. If greater precision is required, the length of the forced desynchrony must be extended. Any error in the period estimate is cumulatively reduced as the number of cycle studies is increased. A 3-week protocol of forced desynchrony should therefore allow determination of period to within ±6 mins (±.1 hr).

METHOD TO ASSAY THE EFFECTS OF THERAPEUTIC AGENTS ON THE PERIOD OF THE ENDOGENOUS CIRCADIAN OSCILLATOR

The protocol illustrated in Figure 5-3 incorporates the above considerations into an experiment designed to assess the effect of a pharmacologic or nonpharmacologic agent on the period of the endogenous pacemaker.

The full 30-day study is divided into three segments, carried out in an environment free of external time cues. Continuous measurements of core body temperature (rectal) is made throughout all segments of the study.

Segment I consists of 2 days when the subject will be scheduled to a 24-hr day. During this time, appropriate measurements and assessments of physiologic and behavioral functions are performed to characterize the subject's entrained state.

Segment II commences on the third day when the subject will be placed on an imposed 28-hr rest–activity schedule. This will force a state of internal desynchrony that will be maintained throughout the remainder of the study.

Because the trough of the core body temperature cycle is the most reliable point

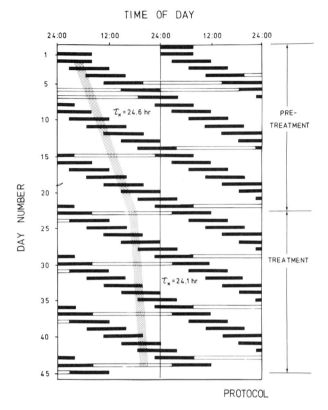

Figure 5-3 A protocol for assessing the effect of a treatment on the endogenous circadian period is shown. Symbols as in Figure 5-2a. The use of frequent constant routines during the waking portion of days when the endogenous circadian phase is approximately 180 degrees out of phase with the rest–activity cycle allows precise estimation of circadian period (via regression analysis) and could indicate the time course over which dynamic changes were occurring. In this hypothetical study, a pretreatment circadian period of 24.6 hrs and a posttreatment circadian period of 24.1 hrs were chosen. The time when the stippled line crosses the open horizontal bars represents the time of the anticipated ECPmin, assuming these periods.

from which to make phase estimations, constant routines will be performed on those days when the temperature cycle is approximately 180 degrees out of phase with the rest–activity cycle. Conveniently, this is also when the residual coupling influence of the rest–activity cycle on the temperature cycle is at a minimum. Ambulatory temperature recordings can be used to schedule the constant routines since the daily variations of the masked temperature rhythm are lowest when the rest–activity and temperature cycles are in phase opposition. The length of Segment II may be modified to accommodate the degree of accuracy desired.

Segment III marks the midpoint of the study. From this point on, the agent to be assayed may be administered. The only restriction on the nature of this therapy is that its administration must not interfere with the subject's sleep–wake schedule or create excessive exogenous stimulation during a time when an endogenous circadian phase estimate is being made. It is important to note at this point that the exact phase of administration of the agent should be carefully chosen. Much research has indicated that the efficacy, and even the nature of the effect of pharmacologic and nonpharmacological agents on the circadian timing system are highly dependent on the timing of their administration. Serial phase estimations are performed as described for Segment II. Likewise, the length of Segment III should be tailored to accommodate the desired degree of accuracy.

Changes in the period of the endogenous circadian pacemaker may be quantified by regression analysis of the endogenous circadian phase assessments.

VALIDATION STUDY

A normal male subject, age 22, was studied for 25 days in an environment free of external time cues (Fig. 5-4a). During the first 4 days of study, baseline measurements of the entrained condition were made and an endogenous circadian phase assessment was performed. From days 5 to 25, the subject was scheduled to a day length of 28 hrs to force a condition of internal desynchronization. During those times when a core body temperature trough was anticipated to coincide with a period of scheduled wakefulness, the subject was placed on a constant routine. Circadian phase was estimated using the method described by Brown (39) from the temperature collected on days 8, 15 and 22. The final constant routine was extended so that two additional

TIME OF DAY

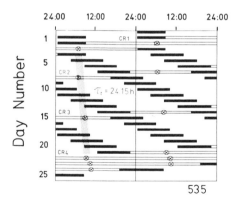
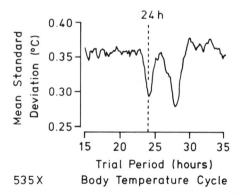

Figure 5-4 (a) Results of a 25-day validation study in a healthy young male are shown. Symbols as in Figure 5-2a. Following baseline measurements, a rest–activity cycle of 28 hrs was imposed. An initial phase assessment (days 2–3) revealed a normal ECPmin, occurring approximately 2 hrs prior to the subject's habitual waketime. During the subsequent period of forced internal desynchronization, circadian phase was reassessed five times (including data collected during a final 70-hr constant routine). Regression analysis (stippled line) of the ECPmin demonstrated an endogenous circadian period of 24.16 hrs. (b) Spectral analysis using the minimum variance technique is shown for the temperature data collected during the desynchronized portion of the study illustrated in a. The period estimate of 24.15 hrs correlates well with that obtained by regression analysis through the multiple ECPmin ($p < .01$).

measurements of circadian phase could be obtained. The intrinsic period of the endogenous circadian pacemaker was determined both by linear regression through the temperature minima, and by the traditional method of nonparametric spectral analysis/
waveform education of continuously monitored core body temperature data.

The imposition of a 28-hr day length successfully induced a state of internal
desynchronization. Linear regression through the ECP minima indicated an intrinsic
period of 24.16 hrs. The period of the temperature cycle [as estimated by the minimum
variance technique (29)] during forced desynchrony was 24.15 hrs (Fig. 5-4b). Similar
methods of comparison applied to three other subjects during desynchrony (both forced
and spontaneous) indicate that correlation between these two forms of measurement
was highly significant (Pearson's correlation coefficient $= .999, p < .01$).

CONCLUSION

This paper has proposed a method of assessing the intrinsic period of the endogenous
circadian pacemaker in human subjects. Through the use of serial phase assessments
during forced desynchrony, the period of the endogenous circadian pacemaker can be
determined with a high degree of accuracy. Additionally, this technique has the advan-
tage of allowing the detection of dynamic changes in the period of the endogenous
circadian pacemaker that are likely to be found in the course of therapeutic intervention.

It has been suggested that modifying the period of the endogenous circadian
pacemaker may be important in the management of a number of disorders of circadian
regulation. The technique we have proposed is a fundamental step in evaluating the
effectiveness of such treatments.

ACKNOWLEDGMENTS

Supported in part by research Grants NIA 1 R01 AG04912-01, AFOSR-83-0309, NIH DRR
BRSG 2S07RR05489, and NIH DRR GCRC 5-M01-RR00888, by the Schering Corporation,
and by fellowships from the Josiah Macy Foundation, the Christopher Walker Fund, and the
Sandoz Corporation (C.A.C.).

REFERENCES

1. Georgi F. Psychophysische korrelationen: psychiatrische probleme im lichte der rhythmus-
   forschung. *Schweiz Med Wochenschrift* 1947; 77:1276–1280.
2. Halberg F. Physiological considerations underlying rhythmometry, with special reference to
   emotional illness. In J de Ajuriaguewa (ed.), *Cycles Biologiques et Psychiatric*. Masson et
   Cie, Geneva, 1968: 73–126.
3. Atkinson M, Kripke DF, Wolf SR. Autorhythmometry in manic-depressives. *Chronobiologia* 1975; 2:325–335.
4. Wehr TA, Goodwin FK. Biological rhythms and psychiatry. In S Arieti and HK Brodie
   (eds.), *American Handbook of Psychiatry*. Basic Books, New York, 1981: 46–74.

5. Kripke DF. Phase advance theories for affective illness. In TA Wehr and FK Goodwin (eds.), *Circadian Rhythms in Psychiatry*. Boxwood Press, Pacific Grove, CA, 1983: 41–69.

6. Wehr TA, Wirz-Justice A, Goodwin FK, Gillin JC, Duncan W. Phase advance of the circadian sleep-wake cycle as an anti-depressant. *Science* 1979; 206:710–713.

7. Doig RJ, Mummenz RV, Wills MR, Elkes A. Plasma cortisol levels in depression. *Br J Psychiat* 1966; 112:1263–1267.

8. Fullerton DT, Wenzel FJ, Lohrenz FN, Falls H, Marshfield W. Circadian rhythm of adrenal cortical activity in depression: A comparison of depressed patients with normal subjects. *Arch Gen Psychiat* 1968; 19:674–681.

9. Lewy AJ, Sack RL, Singer CM. Assessment and treatment of chronobiologic disorders using plasma melatonin levels and bright light exposure: The clock-gate model and the phase response curve. *Psychopharmacol Bull* 1984; 20:561–565.

10. Wehr TA, Goodwin FK. Biological rhythms in manic-depressive illness. In TA Wehr and FK Goodwin (eds.), *Circadian Rhythms in Psychiatry*. Boxwood Press, Pacific Grove, CA, 1983: 129–184.

11. Engelmann W. A slowing down of circadian rhythms by lithium ions. *Z Naturforsch* 1973; 28:733–736.

12. Kripke DF, Wyborney V, McEachron D. Lithium slows rat activity rhythms. *Chronobiologia* 1979; 6:122.

13. Kripke DF, Wyborney VG. Lithium slows rat circadian activity rhythms. *Life Sci* 1980; 26:1319–1321.

14. Wever RA. *The Circadian System of Man*. Springer-Verlag, New York, 1979.

15. Johnsson A, Engelman W, Pflug B. Period lengthening of human circadian rhythms by lithium carbonate, a prophylactic for depressive disorders. *Int J Chronobiol* 1983; 8:129–147.

16. Welsh DK, Nino-Murcia G, Gander PH, Keenan S, Dement WC. Regular 48-hour cycling of sleep duration and mood in a 35-year-old woman: Use of lithium in time isolation. *Biol Psychiat* 1986; 21:527–537.

17. Czeisler CA, Allan JS. Pathologies of the sleep-wake schedule. In RL Williams and I Karacan (eds.), *Sleep Disorders*. Wiley, New York, 1988: 109–129.

18. Dement WC, Guilleminault C, Zarcone V. The pathologies of sleep: A case series approach. In DB Tower (ed.), *The Nervous System: The Clinical Neurosciences*. Raven, New York, 1975: 501–518.

19. Czeisler CA, Allan JS, Strogatz SH, Ronda JM, Sanchez R, Rios CD, Freitag WO, Richardson GS, Kronauer RE. Bright light resets the human circadian pacemaker independent of the timing of the sleep-wake cycle. *Science* 1986; 233:667–671.

20. Czeisler CA, Richardson GS, Coleman RM, Zimmerman JC, Moore-Ede MC, Dement WC, Weitzman ED. Chronotherapy: Resetting the circadian clocks of patients with delayed sleep phase insomnia. *Sleep* 1981; 4:1–21.

21. Kokkoris CP, Weitzman ED, Pollack CP, Spielman AJ, Czeisler CA, Bradlow H. Long-term ambulatory temperature monitoring in a subject with a hypernychthemeral sleep-wake cycle disturbance. *Sleep* 1978; 1(2):177–190.

22. Dement WC, Richardson GS, Prinz P, Carskadon MA, Kripke D, Czeisler CA. Changes of sleep and wakefulness with age. In CE Finch and EL Schneider (eds.), *Handbook of the Biology of Aging*. Van Nostrand Reinhold, New York, 1985: 692–717.

23. Eliott AL, Mills JN, Waterhouse JM. A man with too long a day. *J Physiol* 1971; 212:30–31P.

24. Miles LEM, Raynal DM, Wilson MA. Blind man living in normal society has circadian rhythms of 24.9 hours. *Science* 1977; 198:421–423.

25. Czeisler CA, Kronauer RE, Allan JS, Duffy JF, Jewett ME, Brown EN, Ronda JM. Bright

light induction of strong (Type O) resetting of the human circadian pacemaker. *Science* 1989; 244:1328–1333.

26. Wever R. Autonome circadiane periodik des menschen uter dem einfluss verschiedener beleuchtungs-bedingungen. *Eur J Physiol* 1969; 306:71–91.

27. Czeisler CA, Richardson GS, Zimmerman JC, Moore-Ede MC, Weitzman ED. Entrainment of human circadian rhythms by light-dark cycles: A reassessment. *Photochem Photobiol* 1981; 34:239–247.

28. Czeisler CA, Brown EN, Ronda JM, Kronauer RE, Richardson GS, Freitag WO. A clinical method to assess the endogenous circadian phase (ECP) of the deep circadian oscillator in man. *Sleep Res* 1985; 14:295.

29. Czeisler CA. Internal organization of temperature, sleep-wake, and neuroendocrine rhythms monitored in an environment free of time cues. Ph.D. Thesis, Stanford University, Stanford, 1978.

30. Czeisler CA, Guilleminault C (eds.). *REM Sleep: Its Temporal Distribution*. Raven, New York, 1980.

31. Czeisler CA, Weitzman ED, Moore-Ede MC, Zimmerman JC, Knauer RS. Human sleep: Its duration and organization depend on its circadian phase. *Science* 1980; 210:1264–1267.

32. Moore-Ede MC, Czeisler CA (eds.). *Mathematical Models of the Circadian Sleep-Wake Cycle*. Raven, New York, 1984.

33. Kronauer RE, Czeisler CA, Pilato SF, Moore-Ede MC, Weitzman ED. Mathematical representation of the human circadian system: Two interacting oscillators which affect sleep. In MH Chase (ed.), *Sleep Disorders: Basic and Clinical Research*. Spectrum Publications, New York, 1983: 173–194.

34. Kronauer RE, Fookson JE, Strogatz SH. The period of the deep circadian oscillator observed in desynchrony depends on the desynchronizing conditions. *Sleep Res* 1986; 15:274.

35. Gander PH, Kronauer RE, Czeisler CA, Moore-Ede MC. Modeling the action of zeitgebers on the human circadian system: Comparisons of simulations and data. *Am J Physiol* 1984; 247:R427–R444.

36. Gander PH, Kronauer RE, Czeisler CA, Moore-Ede MC. Simulating the action of zeitgebers on a coupled two-oscillator model of the human circadian system. *Am J Physiol* 1984; 247:R418–R426.

37. Lewy AJ. Human melatonin secretion (II): A marker for the circadian system and the effects of light. In RM Post and JC Ballenger (eds.), *Frontiers of Neuroscience: Neurobiology of Mood Disorders*. Williams & Wilkins, Baltimore, 1984: 215–226.

38. Mills JN, Minors DS, Waterhouse JM. The circadian rhythms of human subjects without timepieces or indication of the alternation of day and night. *J Physiol (London)* 1974; 240:567–594.

39. Brown EN, Czeisler CA. A method for quantifying phase position of the deep circadian oscillator and determining a confidence interval. *Sleep Res* 1985; 14:290.

6

Bright Light, Melatonin, and Biological Rhythms in Humans

ALFRED J. LEWY, ROBERT L. SACK, AND CLIFFORD M. SINGER

In the past few years, the field of chronobiology, particularly its clinical subdiscipline, has changed greatly. This has come about, in part, because of the discovery that bright light has chronobiologic effects in humans (25,27,28,33,52). Previously, it was thought that humans were not affected by light: social cues were considered to be stronger zeitgebers (51). Research over the last decade on light has also provided support for the one-pacemaker model proposed by Eastman (10) and by Daan and co-workers (7).

We have tended to agree with the one-pacemaker model. Our thinking has grown out of our studies on light. In our view, a master pacemaker is distinguished from a slave oscillator, in that the former is sensitive to environmental time cues, whereas slave oscillators receive information about environmental time cues from the master pacemaker. In other words, we think that there may be several slave oscillators for the various circadian rhythms, but that there is only one master pacemaker that is entrained to environmental time cues; the master pacemaker, in turn, entrains the other (slave) oscillators.

Wever's group (51) holds that zeitgebers act equally on two master pacemakers. Another group in Boston (19) has proposed that these zeitgebers act primarily on one pacemaker (the one for the activity–rest cycle) that in turn entrains a second pacemaker for the other endogenous circadian rhythms such as temperature and cortisol. However, recently, the Boston group has apparently abandoned their idea that the activity–rest oscillator is the primary interpreter of environmental time cues (4). When the Boston group assured themselves that light could directly shift the phase of endogenous circadian rhythms independent of the sleep–wake cycle, they changed this component of their two-pacemaker theory (4). It is not clear, however, if this group now considers there to be one or two master pacemakers.

Actually, the Boston group did not need to wait until they had confirmed the direct phase-shifting effect of light on circadian rhythms to abandon their theory. There were already several demonstrations for this effect in humans. The turning point seemed to be in 1980 when we published (33) our finding that bright light suppresses nighttime melatonin production in humans but that ordinary-intensity room light is ineffective

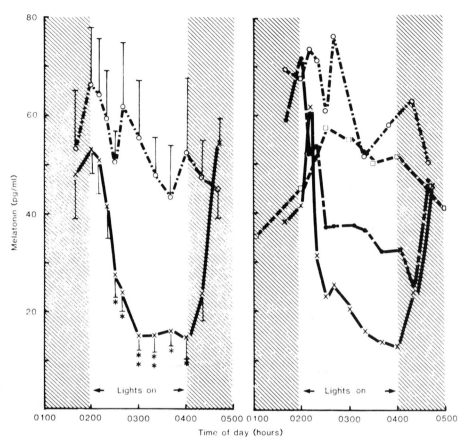

Figure 6-1 (Left) Effect of light on melatonin secretion. Each point represents the mean concentration of melatonin ($\pm$SEM) for six normal control subjects. Time is given in military time. Subjects were awakened and exposed to light between 2 and 4 A.M. A paired t test, comparing exposure to 500 lux with exposure to 2500 lux, was performed for each data point. A two-way analysis of variance with repeated measures and the Newman–Keuls statistic for the comparison of means showed significant differences between 2:30 and 4 A.M. ($*p < .05$; $**p < .01$). [From Lewy et al. (33), with permission.] (Right) Effect of different light intensities on melatonin secretion. The averaged values for two of the subjects studied in the same protocol as described above are shown. Exposure to the intermediate light intensity of 1500 lux appeared to have an intermediate effect on suppression of melatonin production, suggesting a dose–response or fluence–response relationship. (○) 500 lux; (×) 2500 lux; (●) 1500 lux; and (□) asleep in the dark. [From Lewy et al. (33), with permission.]

(Fig. 6-1). Melatonin production occurs only at night in both diurnal and nocturnal species (37). Similar to previous human chronobiology studies, attempts to suppress human nighttime melatonin with light were uniformly negative (1,2,15,34,45,46, 49,50). These negative results caused both clinical chronobiologists and pineal physiologists to conclude that humans were uniquely unaffected by light. Some investigators (16) went so far as to state that perhaps the neural pathways found in mammals that relayed photic information from the retina to the hypothalamus were lacking in humans.

When we published our findings in 1980 that bright light suppressed human nighttime melatonin production, we suggested that bright light might have other chronobiologic effects as well in humans (33). Many investigators immediately realized that this was probably true. But it was in 1983 that Wever first showed that bright light could increase the range of entrainment of the human temperature and sleep–wake rhythms (31). In the same year (25), we published our hypothesized phase response curve (PRC) (Fig. 6-2) for humans with some preliminary data indicating that patients with advanced and delayed circadian rhythms could be treated using bright light to provide corrective shifts (for a discussion of PRCs, see p. 104). However, no research group held the sleep–wake cycle constant in these early studies: it could be argued that bright light was working through the activity–rest (sleep–wake) pacemaker.

Then in 1984 we showed that the human melatonin circadian rhythm could be shifted by shifting the (bright) light–dark cycle while holding the sleep–wake cycle constant (27,28). Four normal volunteers were studied for 15 days. They slept between 11 P.M. and 6 A.M. After measuring their melatonin pattern on day 1 when dusk was between 7:30 and 9 P.M. and dawn was between 6 and 7:30 A.M., we advanced "dusk" by keeping them in a dimly lit room after 4 P.M. each day for 1 week. On the first day, there was an advance in the melatonin onset of 1.5 hr and no change in the offset. There was very little change in the melatonin onset or offset on the second or third day. The immediate advance of the melatonin onset (and not the offset) observed on the first day was probably due to an acute unmasking (removal of the suppressant effect of evening light) on the signal that initiates nighttime melatonin production. By the end of the week, there was an additional advance of one more hour, which is consistent with the removal of bright light from the delay portion of our hypothesized PRC for humans (phase-shifting effects often occur over several days). For the second week of the study, we delayed "dawn" by keeping the subjects in the dimly room until 9 A.M. each day. There was no delay in the melatonin onset or offset until later in the week. Therefore, there was no removal of a suppressant effect of light at either end of the photoperiod. However, there was a delay at the end of the week, consistent with removing bright light from the advance portion of our hypothesized PRC for humans (25).

Our study was the first to demonstrate phase-shifting effects of bright light, independent of the sleep–wake cycle. [Wettenberg (50) may have had some prelimi-

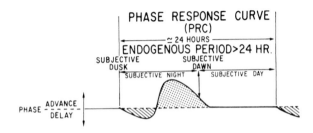

Figure 6-2 Schematic diagram of the hypothesized phase response curve (PRC) for humans. [From Lewy et al. (25), with permission.]

nary, but inconclusive, evidence in this regard.] Our study also indicated that, for determining circadian phase, the melatonin onset should be measured under dim light conditions: the dim light melatonin onset (DLMO) (Fig. 6-3). Subsequent studies in which endogenous circadian rhythms were shifted by shifting the light–dark cycle holding the sleep–wake cycle constant were published by the Boston group (4) and by ourselves (26). Other studies in which circadian rhythms were shifted along with the sleep–wake cycle were done by Wever (52), ourselves (25,30), Eastman (11), Honma (12), and the Boston group (6), although the latter group did not use bright light.

The study by the Boston group (6) provides an excellent review of the field and it is one of many papers (26,52) that discusses the difficulty of attributing phase-shifting to changes in the light–dark cycle (as opposed to changes in social cues); that is, when the light–dark cycle is changed, social cues are also changed. This paper also claims that an absolute light–dark cycle (one in which no light is permitted during the dark phase) is a more effective zeitgeber than the standard (relative) light–dark cycle in which reading lamps are permitted. While this may be true (although their data are not robust), they cannot conclude that the absolute light–dark cycle is a more effective zeitgeber. This is because the absolute light–dark cycle is a powerful social cue: there is a strong temptation to sleep when it is absolutely dark. Furthermore, the Boston group have themselves recently pointed out (4) that their earlier study (6) was inconclusive, given that the sleep–wake cycle was not held constant [a criticism they made about the Wever study (52) as well].

Following our report on the effects of bright light on human melatonin production

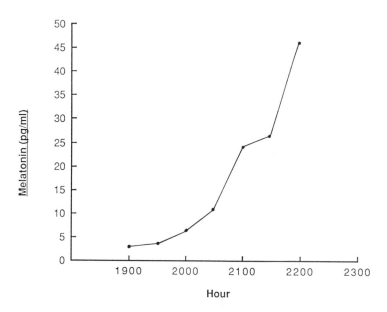

Figure 6-3 Representative dim light melatonin onset (DLMO). Time is given in military time. The subject is kept in dim light after 6 P.M. and blood, drawn through an indwelling venous catheter every 30 min between 7 and 11 P.M., is assayed for melatonin. The time at which the levels rise above 10 pg/ml is considered the DLMO. The DLMO is a useful marker for circadian phase.

(26) and subsequent reports in 1983 (25,52) and 1984 (27) of the effects of bright light on the human circadian system, several other studies (4,11,12,26) have been done that varied the duration, intensity, and timing of the light under a variety of experimental conditions. These studies have produced further evidence for the human PRC we hypothesized in 1983 (25): bright light exposure scheduled in the evening delays circadian rhythms and bright light in the morning advances circadian rhythms. Recently, the Boston group has presented preliminary evidence that bright light can also affect the amplitude of circadian rhythms (5). It is not certain, however, if the strong phase-shifting they report is the result of going through a singularity point. Indeed, Wever and co-workers (52) were able to induce equally rapid phase shifts by using extremely bright light and by shifting the sleep–wake cycle, just as was done in the amplitude reduction paradigm (5).

In summary, the finding that bright light suppresses nighttime melatonin production in humans has ushered in a new way of conceptualizing the human circadian system and has stimulated important contributions from a number of research groups. The capacity of bright light to shift circadian phase has created new ways to experimentally and therapeutically manipulate biological rhythms in humans. Our work with humans has also influenced animal research, such as the comparison of light sensitivity in animals raised in the laboratory to animals raised in the wild (38). (It is perhaps ironic that some chronobiologic studies relevant for animals are best done in humans, such as those that involve holding the sleep–wake cycle constant while shifting the light–dark cycle.)

These findings have also stimulated a reevaluation of the two-pacemaker model. They have certainly influenced us to assume that there need only be one master pacemaker principally entrained by the light–dark cycle. This does not mean that we think that the activity–rest (sleep–wake) cycle is unimportant. Indeed, as will be discussed later, we think that unique characteristics of the sleep–wake cycle may be responsible for certain chronobiologic sleep and mood disorders.

We began our research concerning light treatment of mood disorders in the winter of 1979–1980. As mentioned above, the implications of our just-completed suppression of melatonin by bright light finding suggested that humans may have circadian and seasonal rhythms cued by the natural (bright) light–dark cycle and that these rhythms could be manipulated experimentally, and perhaps therapeutically, using bright light. Our first patient was a 63-year-old man who had a 13-year history of depressions that generally recurred when the days shortened and remitted when the days lengthened. Based on animal studies of seasonal rhythms, we treated him by exposing him to bright (2500 lux) light between 6 and 9 A.M. and between 4 and 7 P.M. Within 4 days of exposure to these two light pulses scheduled to lengthen his day similar to that which normally was associated with a remission, he began to switch out of his depression (21).

Since then, several hundred patients have been similarly treated. Exposure to dim light scheduled at the same times is not effective (39,40). There is general agreement that the light must be of sufficient intensity and of a sufficient duration. An action spectra has also been preliminarily demonstrated: most white sources contain ample representation of the blue-green light (509 nm) optimal for suppression of melatonin production (3). However, two schools of thought have arisen as to the importance of the timing of the light. The Bethesda group has maintained that timing is unimportant (13,14,39,47). Our group, on the other hand, has maintained that timing is critical (25–27).

We based our thinking on our hypothesized phase response curve for bright light's effects in humans (25). Grounded in animal studies (9,36), we thought that humans should have responses to light similar to other animals, except that humans would require brighter light. The common features of PRCs described for several species of animals have indicated that bright light exposure during the subjective day causes relatively small phase shifts. During the first half of subjective night, light causes phase delays that increase in magnitude as the light pulse occurs later and later into the night. During the second half of subjective night, light causes phase advances that increase in magnitude as the light pulse occurs earlier into the night. In the middle of the night, there is an inflection point that separates the greatest phase delays from the greatest phase advances (Fig. 6-2).

Along these lines, we hypothesized that humans should phase delay (shift to a later time) in response to bright light scheduled in the evening and phase advance (shift to an earlier time) in response to bright light scheduled in the morning. As mentioned above, we were the first to demonstrate evidence for such a PRC, holding the sleep–wake cycle constant (27,28). We have further applied our hypothesized PRC to the treatment of chronobiologic sleep and mood disorders by proposing "phase typing" (27,30). By phase typing, we mean that before scheduling a therapeutic trial of bright light, it is best to know if the patient has a phase-advance or a phase-delay type of disorder. Phase-advance disorders should be treated with bright light scheduled in the evening; phase-delay disorders should be treated with bright light in the morning. The phase-advance hypothesis, proposed earlier by Papousek (35), Kripke and co-workers (18), and Wehr and co-workers (48), stated that patients with affective disorders had phase-advanced circadian rhythms. Consequently, our idea that there might be depressed patients with phase-delayed rhythms ran counter to prevailing thought. [It should be mentioned that Kripke and co-workers (18) noted that a small number of manic-depressive patients had phase-delayed circadian rhythms, although Kripke (17) appeared to later minimize this finding.] We thought that our winter depressive patients were generally of the phase-delay type (27).

In the winter of 1984–1985, we studied eight patients and seven normal controls (26). Compared to controls, patients' DLMOs were significantly delayed on the first day of the study and after a week of baseline (adaptation) conditions in which all subjects slept between 10 P.M. and 6 A.M. and avoided bright light between 5 P.M. and 8 A.M. (Fig. 6-4). Subjects' DLMOs advanced in response to a week of morning light, although patients advanced more than normals, and delayed in response to evening light, although controls delayed more than patients. These results are consistent with phase-delayed circadian rhythms in the patients compared to controls. Morning light was significantly more antidepressant than evening light (Fig. 6-5), suggesting that the antidepressant mechanism of action was related, at least in part, to phase-advancing circadian rhythms.

In the winter of 1985–1986, we studied 14 patients and 5 controls: the effects of 0.5 hr and 2 hr of morning light (beginning at 6 A.M.) were compared (32). There were two baseline (adaptation) weeks and a fifth week in which subjects were exposed to the light schedule first administered in the study. The 2-hr morning light exposure was slightly, but statistically insignificantly, more antidepressant than the 0.5 hr of exposure. (A few patients actually did better on the shorter exposure duration.) There was a statistically significant correlation between the antidepressant effect and the degree of

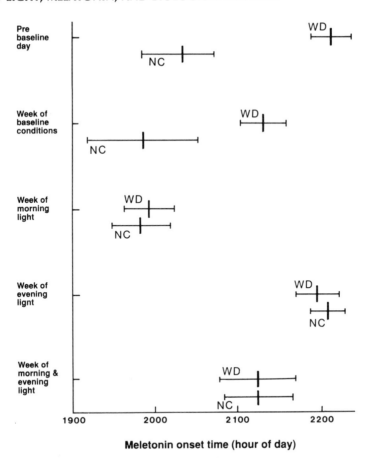

Figure 6-4 Average melatonin onset times in military time ($\pm$SEM) for normal controls (NC) and patients with winter depression (WD) ($n = 6$–8, except $n = 4$ for the prebaseline melatonin values). Subjects slept between 10 P.M. and 6 A.M. for 4 weeks. The first week was a baseline (adaptation) week where bright light was avoided between 5 P.M. and 8 A.M. On weeks 2 and 3, subjects were randomly assigned and crossed over between 2500 lux light scheduled at 6–8 A.M. or at 8–10 P.M. The fourth week subjects were exposed to 2500 lux light at both times. An analysis of variance for repeated measures indicated a significant difference between treatments for both patients ($p = .001$) and normal controls ($p = .009$). Significant paired t tests for the patients were baseline versus A.M. ($p = .001$), baseline versus P.M. ($p = .012$), and A.M. versus P.M. ($p = .001$). Significant paired t tests for the normal controls were baseline versus A.M. + P.M. ($p = .039$), A.M. versus P.M. ($p = .004$), and A.M. versus A.M. + P.M. ($p = .003$). Melatonin onset times of the patients were delayed compared to those of the normal controls at both prebaseline ($p = .02$) and baseline ($p = .05$) (Student's t test). [From Lewy et al. 26), with permission.]

phase advance in the 12 patients for whom complete data sets were available. These results are consistent with our hypothesis that the antidepressant mechanism of action in these patients is related to phase-advancing circadian rhythms. There also was an order effect in this study, in that light was more antidepressant at the end than at the beginning of the study for those patients who began the study without a baseline

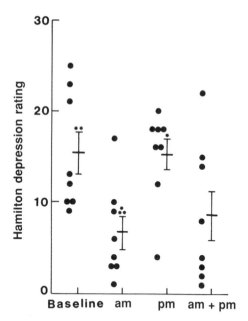

Figure 6-5 Individual and average 21-item Hamilton depression ratings ($\pm$SEM) for the eight patients with winter depression for each of the 4 weeks of the study described in Figure 6-4. An analysis of variance for repeated measures indicated a significant ($p = .026$) difference between treatments. Only the paired t tests comparing the week of morning (A.M.) light and the baseline week (**$p = .004$) and comparing the week of A.M. light and the week of evening (P.M.) light (*$p = .045$) were significant. Average depression ratings ($\pm$SEM) for the seven normal control subjects were 3.0 ± 0.9 at baseline, 2.4 ± 0.3 (A.M. light), 6.1 ± 1.6 (P.M. light), and 4.3 ± 0.9 (A.M. + P.M. light). [From Lewy et al. (26), with permission.]

adaptation week. Although there are several possible explanations for such an order effect, we thought that the most likely explanation was that (before beginning light treatment) patients need several days to adapt their sleep to an advanced schedule or they will not have an antidepressant response by the fourth to seventh day of morning light exposure.

To test this possibility, two inpatient pilot studies were done under extremely well-controlled conditions. In one study, three patients had their sleep delayed 1 hr/day until they were sleeping between 3 and 11 A.M. and then had their sleep advanced 1 hr/day until they were again sleeping between 11 P.M. and 7 A.M. Bright light was scheduled between 11 A.M. and 1 P.M. during the first part of the study and then was advanced when sleep was advanced, so that for the second half of the study patients were always awakening into the light. Patients began to come out of their depressions after a few days of bright light exposure scheduled immediately on awakening.

In another pilot study, two groups of four patients had their sleep delayed and advanced as in the other pilot study. One group awoke into dim light and did not receive their daily 2-hr bright light exposure until 4–8 hr after awakening. The other group received their 2 hr of bright light exposure each day 4 hr after awakening during the first week and immediately after awakening during the second week. By the end of the study, only the latter group remitted.

These findings are consistent with our explanation for the order effect described above. Because circadian rhythms of winter depressives are phase delayed with respect to sleep, these patients can be treated by holding sleep constant and advancing the other rhythms with morning light, or they can be treated by holding the circadian rhythms constant with mid-morning bright light and delaying sleep. If patients have to advance their sleep (to accommodate the morning light exposure), the antidepressant effect may be retarded by a few days to a week.

These findings are also consistent with our hypothesis that in chronobiologic mood disorders, there is an internal phase angle disturbance of the phase-advance or the phase-delay type (30). That is, in these disorders endogenous circadian rhythms are either phase advanced or delayed with respect to real time *and with respect to sleep*. Wehr and co-workers had previously proposed such a theory for the phase-advance hypothesis and presented preliminary evidence that advancing sleep was therapeutic (48). We have extended this theory to include patients whose endogenous circadian rhythms are phase delayed with respect to sleep, and the above data constitute preliminary evidence for the therapeutic effects of delaying sleep in winter depression.

When we first proposed phase typing, we thought that, although most winter depressives were probably phase delayed, a few might be phase advanced. We had one clear-cut (exclusive) evening light responder in the first study (26,32) and thought perhaps we would find more such patients in a follow-up study done during the winter of 1986–1987 (42). In this study, we also scheduled evening light 1 hr earlier than in the 1984–1985 study (7–9 P.M. instead of 8–10 P.M.), to have less of an effect on sleep. Morning light was again significantly more antidepressant than evening light. However, in this study depression ratings were significantly lower compared to the baseline week. We think that 1 week may not be sufficient time for placebo effects to abate. With the earlier evening light, there was less of a phase-delay effect in this study compared to the first study. In that study, we think that the greater phase-delay effect of evening light sufficiently counteracted the placebo effect so that depression ratings after the week of evening light were not lower than those of the baseline week.

When the data from this study were pooled with the data from the previous morning versus evening study (26), patients were statistically significantly delayed compared to controls, on the first day of the study and after a week of baseline conditions. It should be mentioned, however, that these comparisons are not always statistically significant in every study, although most show at least a trend for patients to be phase delayed compared to controls.

In both studies, patients advanced more in response to morning light and delayed less in response to evening light, compared to controls. These differential responses to morning and evening light have perhaps provided another way to phase type individuals. Individuals who are phase delayed should also have PRCs that are phase delayed. Consequently, they should advance more in response to morning light and delay less in response to evening light, compared to individuals who are relatively less phase delayed. Comparing either just the phase-delay response or just the phase-advance response should be sufficient to determine the phase position of the PRC between two individuals. However, should there be a difference in overall light sensitivity between individuals, only one such comparison might be misleading. For example, an individual who is relatively subsensitive to light may have less of a phase advance response to morning light compared to another individual and not necessarily be less phase delayed.

Calculating an advance–delay (A–D) differential (31) obviates this problem. By subtracting the delay response to evening light from the advance response to morning light, an A–D differential can be calculated. The A–D differential takes into account any differences in overall light sensitivity between individuals. Individuals with greater (more positive) A–D differentials should be relatively more phase delayed. A very large shift in a circadian light sensitivity (if such a curve exists to any significant extent in humans) might make this interpretation problematic, providing it is shifted several hours; however, shifts of such magnitude have not been observed.

Consequently, the A–D differential appears to be a highly useful way to phase type individuals and may prove to be more useful than the baseline DLMO, because it takes into account interindividual differences in melatonin physiology (biochemical lag time, amplitude) that might affect comparison of the DLMO among individuals. Nonetheless, the baseline DLMO correlates very well with the A–D differential, as well as the advance response to morning light and the delay response to evening light (32). The later the baseline DLMO, the greater the A–D differential and the advance response to morning light and the less the delay response to evening light; the earlier the baseline DLMO, the less the A–D differential and the phase advance response to morning and the greater the phase delay response to evening light. This suggests that the baseline DLMO may be marking the phase position of the PRC for its endogenous circadian pacemaker and further validates the use of the baseline DLMO as a marker for circadian phase position.

Another way to assess the validity of using melatonin as marker for circadian phase position is to study totally blind individuals (22,43). Most, if not all of these individuals have free-running circadian melatonin rhythms, even though they are sleeping at normal times. Although we have not sampled these individuals every day, a study of one such blind individual over 6 months revealed no effect of the activity–rest cycle on the melatonin onset (41). On the other hand, sleep times seem to be affected by the melatonin onset, depending on the phase angle between the two rhythms. These findings are consistent with a one-pacemaker model and also further validate the use of melatonin as a marker for the phase of its (the) endogenous circadian pacemaker, unaffected by the activity–rest cycle. Cortisol rhythms in these individuals appear to be phase locked with the melatonin rhythm; this further suggests that the melatonin onset is a useful marker for the endogenous circadian pacemaker.

As mentioned earlier, the Bethesda group has maintained that timing is not critical for the antidepressant effect of bright light. We have reviewed this topic elsewhere (23,24). Many studies in this area are not well controlled: in several studies, patients did not have an adapted sleep schedule that remained unchanged during the study and patients did not avoid bright light exposure around twilight. In some controlled studies, patients did not obtain morning light exposure immediately on awakening (13) or were given late evening light that counteracted the antidepressant (phase-advancing) effect of morning light (47).

A recent analysis (44) of pooled data from all studies done to date worldwide agrees with our original hypothesis. Morning plus evening light is no more effective than morning light alone, which are both more effective than evening light. Therefore, the addition of evening light adds nothing to the antidepressant effect of morning light. This study directly disputes the Bethesda group's claim that evening light is as effective as morning plus evening light (14,39) (a treatment that they thought was maximally effective). We are particularly impressed with the findings of the pooled data analysis, given that there were so many methodological differences among studies. What remains a question is whether or not the (modest) antidepressant effect of evening light is real or is just a placebo effect. In the pooled data analysis, bright evening light was slightly more effective than dim evening light. However, dim evening light may not have been an effective placebo control; unlike double-blind pharmacotherapy studies, patients are aware of the intensity of light they are seeing.

As long as the preferential response to morning light remains a consistent finding in well-controlled studies, it is not critical if these patients are shown to be phase delayed compared to a normal control population (although this may be the case as well). This is because the phase-delay disturbance may be ipsative rather than normative (31). An ipsative phase delay means that depressed patients are phase delayed compared to when they are well and not necessarily compared to a normative population. In either case, the phase delay could be a state-dependent marker (for a phase delay disorder). We have preliminary evidence that patients are phase delayed in the winter (when they are depressed) compared to the summer (when they are well).

Winter depression appears to be a biological type of depression. If the biological differences between patients and controls are confirmed over time, this would suggest that patients are biologically different from controls, despite the fact that there appears to be a spectrum of severities of this disorder. It would be interesting to see if subsyndromal patients are phase delayed, perhaps to a lesser extent than the patients who have the more severe disorder. It is hoped that the use of melatonin as a biological marker for circadian phase position and light sensitivity will help to elucidate the biological basis for winter depression and other putative chronobiologic disorders, such as sleep disorders (25,29) and jet lag (8), as well as to help in the understanding and planning of light therapy.

ACKNOWLEDGMENTS

The authors wish to thank Greg Clarke, Mary MacReynolds, Mary Blood, and Joanna Peterson for their technical assistance and Carol Simonton for help with manuscript preparation. This work was supported by NIH Grants MH40161 (AJL) and MH00703 (AJL).

REFERENCES

1. Akerstedt T, Froberg JE, Friberg Y, Wetterberg L. Melatonin secretion, body temperature and subjective arousal during 64 hours of sleep deprivation. *Psychoneuroendocrinology* 1979; 4:219–225.
2. Arendt J. Melatonin assays in body fluids. *J Neural Transm* 1978; 13(Suppl):265–278.
3. Brainard GC, Lewy AJ, Menaker M, Fredrickson RH, Miller LS, Weleber RG, Cassone V, Hudson D. Effect of light wavelength on the suppression of nocturnal plasma melatonin in normal volunteers. *Ann NY Acad Sci* 1985; 453:376–378.

4. Czeisler CA, Allan JS, Strogatz SH, Ronda JM, Sanchez R, Rios CD, Freitag WO, Richardson GS, Kronauer RE. Bright light resets the human circadian pacemaker independent of the timing of the sleep-wake cycle. *Science* 1986; 233:667–671.

5. Czeisler CA, Allan JS, Kronauer RE, Duffy JF. Stong circadian phase resetting in man is effected by bright light suppression of circadian amplitude. *Sleep Res* 1988; 17:367.

6. Czeisler CA, Richardson GS, Zimmerman JC, Moore-Ede MC, Weitzman ED. Entrainment of human circadian rhythms by light-dark cycles: A reassessment. *Photochem Photobiol* 1981; 34:239–247.

7. Daan S, Beersma DGM, Borberly A. Timing of human sleep: Recovery process gated by a circadian pacemaker. *Am J Physiol* 1984; 246:R161–R178.

8. Daan S, Lewy AJ. Scheduled exposure to daylight: A potential strategy to reduce "jet lag" following transmeridian flight. *Psychopharmacol Bull* 1986; 20:566–568.

9. DeCoursey PJ. Daily light sensitivity rhythm in a rodent. *Science* 1960; 131:33–35.

10. Eastman C. Are separate temperature and activity oscillators necessary to explain the phenomena of human circadian rhythms? In MC Moore-Ede and CA Czeisler (eds.), *Mathematical Models of the Circadian Sleep-Wake Cycle*. Raven, New York, 1984: 81–103.

11. Eastman CI. Bright light improves the entrainment of the circadian rhythms of body temperature to a 26-hr. sleep-wake schedule in humans. *Sleep Res.* 1986; 15:271.

12. Honma K, Honma S, Wada T. Phase-dependent shift of free-running human circadian rhythms in response to a single bright light pulse. *Experientia* 1987; 43:1205–1207.

13. Jacobsen FM, Wehr TA, Skwerer RA, Sack DA, Rosenthal NE. Morning versus midday phototherapy of seasonal affective disorder. *Am J Psychiat* 1987; 144:1301–1305.

14. James SP, Wehr TA, Sack DA, Parry BL, Rosenthal NE. Treatment of seasonal affective disorder with evening light. *Br J Psychiat* 1985; 147:424–428.

15. Jimerson DC, Lynch HJ, Post RM, Wurtman RJ, Bunny WE. Urinary melatonin rhythms during sleep deprivation in depressed patients and normals. *Life Sci* 1977; 20:1501–1508.

16. Klein DC. Circadian rhythms in the pineal gland. In DT Krieger (ed.), *Comprehensive Endocrinology Series, Endocrine Rhythms*. Raven, New York, 1979: 203–223.

17. Kripke DF. Critical interval hypotheses for depression. *Chronobiol Int* 1984; 1:73–80.

18. Kripke DF, Mullaney DJ, Atkinson ML, Wolf S. Circadian rhythm disorders in manic-depressives. *Biol Psychiat* 1978; 13:335–351.

19. Kronauer RE, Czeisler CA, Pilato SF, Moore-Ede MC, Weitzman ED. Mathematical model of the human circadian system with two interacting oscillators. *Am J Physiol* 1982; 242:R3–R17.

20. Lewy AJ. Biochemistry and regulation of mammalian melatonin production. In RM Relkin (ed.), *The Pineal Gland*. Elsevier North-Holland, New York, 1983: 77–128.

21. Lewy AJ, Kern HE, Rosenthal NE, Wehr TA. Bright artificial light treatment of a manic-depressive patient with a seasonal mood cycle. *Am J Psychiat* 1982; 139:1496–1498.

22. Lewy AJ, Newsome DA. Different types of melatonin circadian secretory rhythms in some blind subjects. *J Clin Endocrinol Metab* 1983; 56:1103–1107.

23. Lewy AJ, Sack RL. Minireview: Light therapy and psychiatry. *Proc Soc Exp Biol Med*, 1986; 183:11–18.

24. Lewy AJ, Sack RL. Letter to the Editor. *Am J Psychiat* 1988; 145:1041–1042.

25. Lewy AJ, Sack RL, Fredrickson RH, Reaves M, Denney DD, Zielske DR. The use of bright light in the treatment of chronobiologic sleep and mood disorders: The phase-response curve. *Psychopharmacol Bull* 1983; 19:523–525.

26. Lewy AJ, Sack RL, Miller LS, Hoban TM. Antidepressant and circadian phase-shifting effects of light. *Science* 1987; 235:352–354.

27. Lewy AJ, Sack RL, Singer CM. Assessment and treatment of chronobiologic disorders using plasma melatonin levels and bright light exposure: The clock-gate model and the phase response curve. *Psychopharmacol Bull* 1984; 20:561–565.

28. Lewy AJ, Sack RL, Singer CM. Immediate and delayed effects of bright light on human melatonin production: Shifting "dawn" and "dusk" shifts the dim light melatonin onset (DLMO). *Ann NY Acad Sci* 1985; 453:253–259.
29. Lewy AJ, Sack RL, Singer CM. Melatonin, light and chronobiological disorders. In D Evered and S Clark (eds.), *Photoperiodism, Melatonin and the Pineal*. Pitman, London, 1985: 231–252.
30. Lewy AJ, Sack RL, Singer CM. Treating phase typed chronobiologic sleep and mood disorders using appropriately timed bright artificial light. *Psychopharmacol Bull* 1985; 21:368–372.
31. Lewy AJ, Sack RL, Singer CM, White DM. The phase shift hypothesis for bright light's therapeutic mechanism of action: Theoretical considerations and experimental evidence. *Psychopharmacol Bull* 1987; 23:349–353.
32. Lewy AJ, Sack RL, Singer CM, White DM, Hoban TM. Winter depression and the phase shift hypothesis for bright light's therapeutic effects: History, theory and experimental evidence. *J Biol Rhythms* 1988; 3:121–134.
33. Lewy AJ, Wehr TA, Goodwin FK, Newsome DA, Markey SP. Light suppresses melatonin secretion in humans. *Science* 1980; 210:1267–1269.
34. Lynch HJ, Jimerson DC, Ozaki Y, Post RM, Bunney WE, Wurtman RJ. Entrainment of rhythmic melatonin secretion in man to a 12-hour phase shift in the light dark cycle. *Life Sci* 1977; 23:1557–1564.
35. Papousek M. Chronobiological aspects of cyclothymia. *Fortschr Neurol Psychiatr* 1975; 43:381–440.
36. Pittendrigh CS, Daan S. A functional analysis of circadian pacemakers in nocturnal rodents. IV. Entrainment: Pacemaker as clock. *J Comp Physiol* 1976; 106:291–331.
37. Quay WB. Circadian and estrous rhythms in pineal melatonin and 5-OH indole-3-acetic acid. *Proc Soc Exp Biol Med* 1964; 115:710–713.
38. Reiter RJ, Steinlechner S, Richardson BA, King TS. Differential response of pineal melatonin levels to light at night in laboratory-raised and wild-captured 13-lined ground squirrels (Spermophilus tridecemlineatus). *Life Sci* 1983; 32:2625–2629.
39. Rosenthal NE, Sack DA, Carpenter CJ, Parry BL, Mendelson WB, Wehr TA. Antidepressant effects of light in seasonal affective disorder. *Am J Psychiat* 1985; 142:163–170.
40. Rosenthal NE, Sack DA, Gillin JC, Lewy AJ, Goodwin FK, Davenport Y, Mueller PS, Newsome DA, Wehr TA. Seasonal affective disorder. *Arch Gen Psychiat* 1984; 41:72–80.
41. Sack RL, Lewy AJ. Melatonin and affective disorders. In A Miles, D Philbrick and C Thompson (eds.), *Melatonin. Clinical Perspectives*. Oxford, New York, 1988: 205–227.
42. Sack RL, Lewy AJ, White DM, Singer CM, Fireman MJ, Vandiver R. Morning vs evening light treatment for winter depression: Evidence that the therapeutic effects of light are mediated by circadian phase shifts. *Arch Gen Psychiat* 1990; 47:343–351.
43. Sack RL, Lewy AJ, Hoban TM. Free-running melatonin rhythms in blind people: Phase shifts with melatonin and triazolam administration. In L Rensing, U an der Heiden and MC Mackey (eds.), *Temporal Disorder in Human Oscillatory Systems*. Springer-Verlag, Heidelberg, 1987: 219–224.
44. Terman M, Terman JS, Quitkin FM, McGrath PJ, Stewart JW, Rafferty B. Light therapy for seasonal affective disorder: A review of efficacy. *Neuropsychopharmacology* 1989; 2:1–22.
45. Vaughan GM, Bell R, De La Pena A. Nocturnal plasma melatonin in humans: Episodic pattern and influence of light. *Neurosci Lett* 1979; 14:81–84.
46. Vaughan GM, Pelham RW, Pang SF, Loughlin LL, Wilson KM, Sandock KL, Vaughan MK, Koslow SH, Reiter FJ. Nocturnal elevation of plasma melatonin and urinary 5-hydroxyindoleacetic acid: Attempts and modification by brief changes in environmental lighting and sleep and by autonomic drugs. *J Clin Endocrinol Metab* 1976; 42:752–754.

47. Wehr TA, Jacobsen FM, Sack DA, Arendt J, Tamarkin L, Rosenthal NE. Phototherapy of seasonal affective disorder. *Arch Gen Psychiat* 1986; 43:870–875.

48. Wehr TA, Wirz-Justice A, Goodwin FK, Duncan W, Gillin JC. Phase advance of the circadian sleep-wake cycle as an antidepressant. *Science* 1979; 206:710–713.

49. Weitzman ED, Weinberg U, D'Eletto R, Lynch JH, Wurtman RJ, Czeisler CA, Erlich S. Studies of the 24-hour rhythm of melatonin in man. *J Neural Transm* 1978; 13(Suppl):325–337.

50. Wetterberg L. Melatonin in humans: Physiological and clinical studies. *J Neural Transm* 1978; 13(Suppl):289–310.

51. Wever RA. *The Circadian System of Man.* Springer-Verlag, New York, 1979.

52. Wever RA, Polasek J, Wildgruber CM. Bright light affects human circadian rhythms. *Pflugers Arch* 1983; 396:85–87.

7

Twilight Therapeutics, Winter Depression, Melatonin, and Sleep

MICHAEL TERMAN AND DAVID S. SCHLAGER

Daily light stimulation of physiologic systems is determined both by natural light–dark (LD) cycles and by factors that affect exposure to those cycles. Such factors include timing of rest and activity (e.g., nocturnal vs diurnal), natural habitat (e.g., open-plain, underground, or indoor living), and anatomic features (e.g., eyelids, extraretinal photoreceptors). Patterns of illumination in the laboratory often contrast arbitrarily with those outdoors. Such deviations, along with alterations in habitat or behavior often produce unintended differences between experimental and naturally occurring LD stimulation.

LD signals produced for experimental protocols have typically consisted of a set intensity of light of specific duration, with abrupt transitions to and from darkness as produced by conventional electrical switching. In contrast, light signals in nature are embedded in graded light–dark profiles spanning an approximate 8 log unit range of illuminance, from starlight to midday maxima (cf. Fig. 7-1).

The earth's year-long orbit around the sun gives rise to an annual cycle of variation in the timing and shape of the natural illuminance profile. Daily and monthly differences can be measured in both absolute levels of illumination and momentary rates of change throughout the day. Seasonal variation in these parameters increases as a function of distance from the equator and, in the temperate zones, gives rise to easily observable changes in photoperiod—the duration of daylight between sunrise and sunset.

The relation between LD cycles and seasonal rhythms in biology (e.g., hibernation, migration, annual reproductive cycles) has been studied with a focus on variation in photoperiod. This perspective overlooks any significance of the complex, graded light signals before sunrise and after sunset (Fig. 7-1). Biological sensitivity to twilight stimulation—dawn and dusk—has been suggested in animal experiments using natural outdoor lighting (18,27) and indoor simulations (24,25,56). In rats, self-selected exposure to naturalistic lighting shows distinct patterns of twilight stimulation, with specific circadian phase-shifting effects (56). Such reduced exposure contrasts markedly with both the protracted light exposures under LD cycles and the bright-light skel-

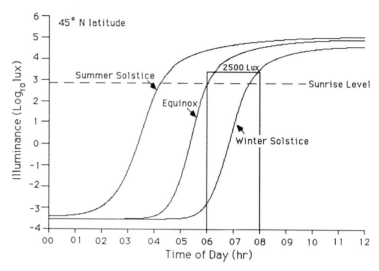

Figure 7-1 Algorithmic representation, at 45° N latitude, of dawn twilight illuminance patterns at summer solstice, autumnal equinox, and winter solstice. The standard bright-light therapy signal of 2500 lux administered for 2 hr on awakening at 6 A.M. is superimposed. Also denoted is the illuminance at the point of sunrise. Note differences in shape as well as position among the different curves.

eton photoperiods applied in laboratory studies, and suggests that the latter provide supernormal stimulation of the circadian system.

In humans, indoor living reduces light availability and stimulation compared with outdoor living conditions (42). Nonetheless, studies of clinical and physiologic effects of light have concentrated on exposure to bright light that exceeds normal indoor levels. Furthermore, such bright-light exposure has been delivered through open eyes in awake subjects. The significance of early-morning dim-light exposure, such as occurs through bedroom windows during sleep–wake transitions, has not previously been investigated.

A clinical syndrome of seasonal affective disorder (SAD) has recently been described in the temperate zones, in which depression is recurrent in the late fall or winter with spontaneous remission in the spring. The depression is associated with increases in sleep duration and daytime drowsiness, along with prominent changes in energy, activity, appetite, and weight (45). Rapid clinical remissions are induced within a few days of exposure to artificial light whose intensity matches outdoor daylight levels [>2000 lux; for reviews see (32,54)]. Depending on the time of day, exposure to such light intensities can also produce suppression and phase shifts of pineal melatonin secretion (28,31,51). Of various lighting regimens, early-morning exposures have generally yielded the strongest therapeutic response, which may reflect corrective circadian phase advances given an abnormally delayed baseline in winter.

It is generally thought that the light intensity needed to produce such effects substantially exceeds the intensity of normal indoor illumination (<500 lux); in contrast, most animals are sensitive to lower intensities (44). One can ask whether the relative insensitivity to early-morning, indoor-level light observed in humans is an artifact of abrupt switching on of the lights after awakening in relative darkness. Specifically, might indoor levels of illumination produce antidepressant effects and alterations of melatonin secretion equivalent to that using bright light, if the signal shape more closely approximated naturally occurring early-morning light during spring and summer periods of spontaneous remission?

This chapter explores effects of simulated dawn twilight exposures on a group of winter depressives. We ask whether high daylight intensities are necessary to achieve the antidepressant effect if a more naturalistic exposure pattern is provided in the bedroom. We also consider the role of the gradual dawn signal in the regulation of melatonin secretion and the sleep–wake pattern.

METHODS

Subjects

Eight subjects in the New York City area were selected with a diagnosis of major affective disorder, depressed, seasonal type, winter pattern by DSM-III-R criteria (4). Three of them (subjects 1, 2, and 3) had an established history of responsiveness to conventional bright-light therapy. Clinical status throughout the trial was assessed using the SIGH–SAD structured interview (60), which consists of the 21-item Hamilton Depression Rating Scale (HAM-D) and eight additional items that assess atypical vegetative changes common in SAD. On entry into the study, baseline HAM-D score was greater than 8, and total SIGH-SAD score was greater than 18 (Table 7-1). Clinician-rated measures of severity and change were based on the Clinical Global Impressions Scale [CGI; (38)].

Apparatus

The lighting system included an encased bright fluorescent light source, light-attenuation mechanism, microprocessor controller, and photosensor feedback loop. A compre-

Table 7-1 Timing of Dawn Twilight Treatment and SIGH–SAD Ratings for Baseline, Treatment, and Withdrawal Phases

Subject	Profile	Light onset[a] (A.M.)	Sunrise (A.M.)	Baseline	Treatment	Withdrawal
1 (RT)	May 5[a]	3:05	4:53	14/18[b]	5/3	10/5
2 (RR)	May 5[a]	3:05	4:53	10/20	13/18	—[c]
3 (LS)	May 5[a]	3:05	4:53	13/10	7/3	13/12
4 (JM)	Equinox[d]	4:45	5:30	12/16	5/1	12/13
5 (IS)	Equinox[d]	4:45	5:30	15/16	1/1	17/12
6 (AH)	Equinox[d]	4:45	5:30	9/13	0/3	10/15
7 (ND)	Equinox[d]	4:45	5:30	16/17	6/2	18/10
8 (EH)	Equinox[d]	4:45	5:30	16/12	2/2	13/8

[a]At 45° N latitude.

[b]Component scales: HAM-D/atypical symptoms.

[c]Subject was not withdrawn, given lack of treatment response.

[d]At the equator (0° latitude).

hensive reference-generating algorithm was used to specify the expected momentary level of horizontal illumination on the earth's surface—from skylight, sunlight, and starlight sources (and, optionally, from moonlight)—across the 24-hr day at any specified day of year and geographic latitude. By means of a precision motor-control interface, the algorithm drove the attenuator (a set of finely crafted rotating vanes), producing the naturalistic illumination patterns. The photosensor measured the light received, and sent the empirical result to the computer, to adjust illumination level dynamically for optimum fit to the algorithm specifications. The structure of the algorithm—which has been validated against outdoor measurements under clear-sky conditions—is described elsewhere (53). For the present experiments, the system was positioned on a rack at the patient's bedside. The photosensor was mounted close to a diffusing screen in front of the attenuator vanes.

Procedure

While in their depressed state during December through March the subjects were exposed, in 7- to 14-day home trials, to simulated twilight profiles delivered at the bedside. Graded illuminance, as measured by the photosensor, spanned astronomical twilight (approximately 0.001 lux) through sunrise to a maximum intensity of approximately 2000 lux, with some contamination from variable ambient room light through the night. Maximum illuminance at the subject's pillow, 3 feet farther from the light source than the photosensor, was in the range of 100–500 lux. Illuminance at the eye was not measured directly and depended on the subject's head position and whether the eyes were open or closed.

The morning light signals consisted of dawn profiles whose latitude, calendar date, and timing varied among the subjects (Table 7-1). In all cases, the timing of the twilight signal corresponded to a calendar date well past the onset of natural remission for the subject. The light profiles, determined by the algorithm, progressed to a maximum illuminance approximately 1 min after sunrise, a level maintained until the subject left bed. All subjects were instructed to awaken spontaneously and to arise at will as early as they felt ready. However, awakening was at times forced by an alarm clock as dictated by the subjects' workday schedules or other responsibilities.

Overnight plasma melatonin patterns were measured in subjects 1 and 2 in our sleep laboratory before, during, and after twilight exposure phases, using a radioimmunoassay technique (51). Lighting conditions during laboratory overnights consisted of incandescent light of <200 lux from 8:00 to 11:00 P.M., and <1 lux from 11:00 P.M. to 3:00 A.M. After 3:00 A.M., the subjects were exposed to either continuing darkness (<1 lux) or a dawn twilight probe whose timing and profile sometimes differed from that used during home treatment.

Subjects were asked to maintain daily sleep–wake logs with 15-min resolution. One noncompliant subject, #2, failed to submit logs.

RESULTS AND DISCUSSION

Clinical Response

After 2 weeks of daily dawn twilight exposure, six of the eight subjects showed full remissions of SAD symptoms (Table 7-1). Subject 3 showed a large reduction in SIGH–SAD score although the CGI rating indicated only partial improvement. Subject

2 showed no antidepressant response, although she had previously responded to 30 min of postawakening light therapy at 10,000 lux intensity. All six responders relapsed within 2 weeks of discontinuation of the twilight regimen and return to normal bedroom conditions.

Subjects reported awakening spontaneously and briefly during the early reaches of dawn, returning to sleep easily despite gradually increasing illuminance, and awakening finally some point after the moment of sunrise. The interval of exposure to the maximum postsunrise illuminance therefore varied. Most of the twilight exposure occurred during sleep, with subjects usually reporting only brief periods (<15 min) in bed after final awakening. Other factors influencing total light received—head orientation, eyelid closure—must also be considered in future research to specify the effective signal.

Naturalistic dawn exposures, timed to correspond to calendar dates during natural remission, appeared to be effective in alleviating symptoms of winter depression. Such antidepressant responses suggest that conventional bright light treatment (>2000 lux, administered for up to several hours after awakening) may not be required, and that some component of the complex dawn signal other than its maximum illuminance—its timing, gradual progression, specific seasonal and latitudinal profile—is effective even with exposure during sleep, with the eyelids closed.

Both antidepressant and circadian effects of light involve retinal phototransduction. Retinal mediation of postawakening bright light—for which the antidepressant "dose" can be adjusted throughout the range of 2000–10,000 lux (50)—must involve photopic (cone) mechanisms, given a full and rapid bleach of rhodopsin in the highly sensitive rods, which are specialized for nighttime and twilight scotopic and mesopic vision (56). On the other hand, circadian rhythm phase adjustment, which may underlie the light-therapeutic response in SAD (32), would be expected to involve scotopic activity during the dawn interval critical for obtaining phase advances (43). Our findings imply that dim light—which is therapeutically ineffective when administered to the light-adapted eye after awakening—can produce antidepressant and circadian responses if delivered in a way that promotes scotopic mediation by the dark-adapted eye. An implication is that conventional early-morning bright-light treatment provides a supernormal stimulus for the transition to photopic vision, with a sudden bleach of rhodopsin contrasting with the gradual desensitization of rods and concurrent onset of cone activity within the mesopic twilight range. However, to the extent that duration of bright-light exposure up to several hours constitutes a dosing dimension for clinical response (55), photopic mechanisms are likely also to be involved.

Circadian Phase Responses to Dawn

The timing of nocturnal melatonin secretion was used as a marker for the circadian phase. Measured under identical dim light conditions (<200 lux), both subjects 1 and 2 showed phase advances in the rising limb of melatonin secretion after 8–14 days of home exposure to sunrise signals, relative to the pretreatment baseline conditions (Fig. 7-2a and c). In subject 2, under conditions of early-morning darkness (<1 lux), the spontaneous decline of morning melatonin was also phase-advanced (Fig. 7-2c).

Contraction of photoperiod during winter in the temperate zones is marked by delays of up to several hours in the early-morning dark-to-light transition. SAD patients tend to show wintertime phase delays in melatonin secretion relative to normals (33), perhaps reflecting the effects of early-morning light deprivation. An exaggerated internal phase angle difference, or misalignment, between sleep and other circadian processes may thus be primary to the pathogenesis of the syndrome. Individuals vulnerable to SAD may rely on early-morning, phase-advancing light signals to forestall the appearance of depressive changes (33).

One might then seek to attribute the therapeutic response to this circadian adjustment, as has been done for bright-light treatment (32,51). Of the two subjects showing phase advances, however, only one showed a significant clinical improvement (Table 7-1, subject 1) while the other showed no discernible response other than improved morning energy and arousal (subject 2).

The discordance between phase response and clinical response in the refractory patient might indicate that the two effects, though coincident in SAD patients treated with morning light, are not functionally connected. Alternately, the phase advance of the nonresponder may have been "too large" or "too small" relative to the sleep cycle to promote remission [cf. (34)], or both sleep and melatonin may have phase shifted together with no net change in internal phase angle. Nonetheless, it seems heuristically valuable to question how phase advances might be dissociable from the clinical response. One could speculate that the phase shift is necessary, but not by itself sufficient, to induce remission of symptoms.

Demonstration of circadian sensitivity to dawn twilights forces attention to the specific features of naturally occurring light exposure responsible for spontaneous remissions of SAD in the spring. Does the high intensity of artificial bright-light therapy mimic therapeutic springtime light exposure during periods of natural remission?

Differences, across the seasons, in momentary outdoor illuminance during twilight can reach 10^7 lux. For example, at 6:00 A.M. at 45° N latitude (e.g., Boston, Massachusetts), outdoor illuminance is approximately 0.001 lux on December 21, and 10,000 lux on June 21. However, by the time most people actually go outdoors in the morning (e.g., after 7:30 A.M.), illuminance has surpassed 2000 lux—even in winter. Early-morning indoor illumination varies within a much smaller range across the seasons. Such lighting is composed of degraded outdoor light signals through windows and artificial room light, rarely exceeding a net illuminance of 750 lux in any season. Thus, as a result of indoor living habits, natural expansion of the photoperiod in the spring produces increased early-morning light exposure to a maximum of only approximately 750 lux.

The phase-shift hypothesis seems paradoxical in observing that only bright artificial morning light (>2000 lux) has shown antidepressant effects, while at the same time implying that springtime morning light exposure, as received indoors to a maximum of 750 lux, is responsible for natural remission. The paradox becomes more apparent than real when considering the responsiveness to twilight illumination. Full suppression and subsequent entrainment of melatonin secretion were obtained with simulated twilight exposure well below the thresholds for clinical and circadian-phase responses previously demonstrated in SAD patients using postawakening bright light. Furthermore, our data suggest that the human circadian system is sensitive to seasonally varying, naturally occurring indoor levels of light, given the gradual twilight profile. Equivalent exposure to constant light levels might be ineffective, as in the "dim light control" of many light therapy studies [cf. (54)].

The general role of the light–dark (LD) cycle as a zeitgeber in human circadian rhythms has been questioned in the past two decades. Early studies suggested that dim, indoor LD cycles alone could not provide stable entrainment in temporal isolation (59). More recent studies in depressed patients and normals have suggested that light can directly phase shift and entrain the circadian pacemaker, but only at intensities exceeding 2000 lux (17,31,59). The phase-shifting effect of dawn twilight exposure seen in this study would appear to be at odds with the notion that ordinary room-intensity illumination (200–500 lux) is insufficient to produce entrainment. However, Czeisler et al. (16), in a temporal isolation study using strictly imposed LD cycles of ordinary room light with gradual dark-to-light transitions, did show entrainment. This was attributed to prevention of self-selected light exposure, but a specific twilight sensitivity may have contributed.

Immediate Effects of Dawn on Melatonin Secretion

Pineal secretion of melatonin is under circadian control, its rhythm preserved even in a constant environment (58). At the same time, nocturnal secretion can be immediately suppressed by light exposure to the eyes (e.g., 28). We wondered whether dawn exposure would suppress melatonin and, if it did, whether such early-morning twilight suppression represents a daily event with effects on mood and sleep.

Subject 1 showed an exponential decline of early-morning plasma melatonin during the first night of simulated dawn exposure (equinox profile, sunrise at 6 A.M.; Fig. 7-2a), while depressed. After 12 days of treatment consisting of daily exposure to equinox dawn, sunrise at 4:53 A.M., the same subject again showed suppression of melatonin secretion, albeit now phase-advanced. Given continued suppression of early-morning melatonin, even while in a stable remission state, a role for active suppression in maintenance of the clinical response (51) must be considered.

Subject 2, the clinical nonresponder, also showed immediate suppression during dawn exposure, in this case compared to a morning-darkness control on the following night, both measured in the baseline depressed state (Fig. 7-2b).

In both subjects, the decline of plasma melatonin followed a time course indicative of complete termination of pineal secretory activity [$t_{1/2}$ approx. 45 min; (51)]. Previous studies of nocturnal exposure to abruptly-switched artificial light have suggested that illuminance >2000 lux is needed to trigger complete melatonin suppression in humans. Yet, under the artificial dawn, such suppression was observed for cases in which illuminance never exceeded 250 lux at the pillow. Although recent studies indicate a wide range of light sensitivity among individuals, and a dose-dependent relationship between illuminance and degree of melatonin suppression (9,14,30,39), complete suppression has not been previously demonstrated with the relatively low levels of light that normally occur in the bedroom during early-morning hours.

The dawn-suppression effect was observed whether the twilight signal continued past the moment of sunrise (Fig. 7-2a) or was artificially truncated to darkness just prior to sunrise (Fig. 7-2b), suggesting that the induced elimination of melatonin from the circulation need not, in itself, occur in the presence of light. Pineal activity thus appeared to terminate for the day in response to the pre-sunrise dawn signal. In contrast, previous studies of humans receiving suddenly-switched bright light have noted a rebound of melatonin secretion upon return to darkness, as late as 5 A.M. [e.g., (39)]. It is possible

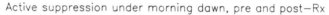

(a) Subject 1

Active suppression under morning dawn, pre and post—Rx

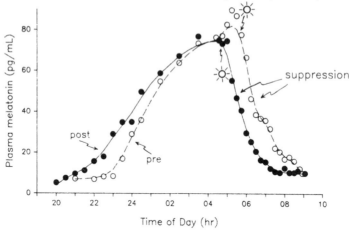

(b) Subject 2

Pre—treatment, consecutive nights:
Morning dawn (truncated at sunrise) vs morning darkness

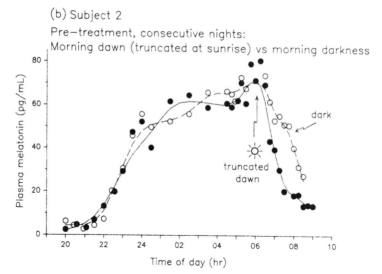

Figure 7-2 (a) Subject 1. Phase advance in melatonin secretion after 8 days of home exposure to the May 5 dawn signal. Secretion profiles were measured in the presence of evening dim light (<200 lux) before sleep and <1 lux during sleep until onset of the dawn signal. Pretreatment dawn signal for this overnight melatonin assessment was of equinox profile, 45° N latitude, with light onset 4:21 A.M. and sunrise (sun symbol) at 6:00 A.M. Posttreatment dawn for the overnight test was an identical profile but with light onset at 3:15 A.M. and sunrise at 4:53 A.M. Both dawns progressed beyond sunrise to a maximum, steady signal of approximately 250 lux at the pillow, reached within 1 min of sunrise and maintained until the end of plasma sampling. (b) Subject 2. Early morning suppression of nocturnal melatonin secretion in the depressed state in the presence of simulated equinox dawn signal, truncated suddenly to darkness, compared to baseline, morning-darkness conditions on two consecutive nights. Truncated equinox dawn had light onset at 4:21 A.M. and sunrise at 6:00 A.M. (c) Subject 2. Phase advance measured under evening dim light conditions and morning darkness, before and after 2 weeks of home exposure to May 5 dawn. Curve fits are based on an iterated running median.

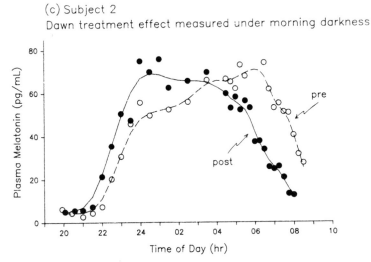

(c) Subject 2
Dawn treatment effect measured under morning darkness

Figure 7-2 (*Continued*)

that pineal suppression sensitivity is influenced by specific components of the dawn signal that are absent in abruptly-switched bright light, such as gradual onset, seasonally-defined time anchor, or presentation while asleep. Thus, naturally-occurring early-morning bedroom light exposure may play a role in the regulation of mood and vegetative state, as seen in SAD.

The active component of the dawn twilight suppression effect remains to be determined and distinguished from individual sensitivity to low intensities of abruptly switched light. We are currently comparing responses to dawn and abruptly switched light at corresponding intervals. With total photon exposure controlled, failure of a discrete pulse of fixed-intensity light to suppress melatonin secretion would support a specific sensitivity to dynamic twilight parameters. We have also tested three SAD patients with a standard bright light automatically switched on at the bedside 1 hr before morning rise time: this procedure is clearly inadequate for a clinical response in comparison to postawakening exposure.

Light, Melatonin, and Sleep

Under dawn twilights most subjects showed phase advances of awakening as well as smaller advances of sleep onset, decreased total sleep duration, and consolidation of disturbed sleep compared with baseline depressed conditions (e.g., Fig. 7-3a and c). Earlier wake-up times were uniformly accompanied by reports of increased subjective energy and ease of arising, suggesting an effect other than simple sleep disruption by the procedure (as, for example, with an alarm clock). Subject 3 (Fig. 7-3b), who was schedule-bound to arise early for work during baseline period, did not show an advance of sleep termination under the dawn signal, yet still reported increased energy and arousal on awakening. This subject also chose to sleep later on weekends, despite the presence of the light.

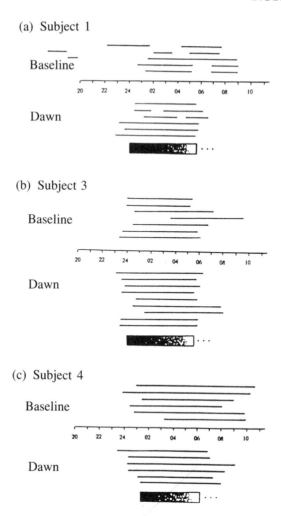

Figure 7-3 (a–c) Self-rating daily sleep records illustrating phase adjustments and changes in total sleep duration under dawn twilight exposure.

Such changes in sleep–wake timing and duration are similar to those seen in studies of bright-light therapy of SAD (56,51). It is impossible in this situation to determine if there is a direct effect of light exposure on sleep timing or if improved sleep is secondary to the antidepressant effect. However, one subject reported earlier awakening and increased morning energy in the absence of any antidepressant response, suggesting that modification of sleep by light is independent of overall mood state. Early-morning bright light exposure in awake subjects has been observed to influence subsequent spontaneous morning awakening in normals (20,21) and to advance sleep onset and termination in individuals with delayed sleep-phase disorder [(29), N.E. Rosenthal, personal communication, M. Terman, unpublished observations].

The effect of light on sleep may involve melatonin responses to the dawn signal.

Early-morning suppression and subsequent phase advance of melatonin secretion was observed to occur under dim, indoor-level lighting conditions. The signal mimicked naturally occurring spring and summertime light patterns transmitted through the window into the bedroom. To our knowledge, this is the first demonstration of early-morning suppression and phase shifts of melatonin secretion in response to light exposure during sleep. A role for light transduction during sleep has been suggested for cats, in whom rapid eye movements (REM) were thought to potentiate photic transmission to the central nervous system (48). In rats, surgical disruption of extraocular movements underlying the REM response abolished entrainment to LD cycles (36).

The timing of nocturnal melatonin secretion in our study shows a general correlation with the timing of sleep as measured by sleep–wake logs during comparable home-treatment phases. Under the dawn signal, phase advances of sleep onset paralleled phase advances of melatonin onset when compared to pretreatment conditions. Similarly, phase advances in awakening paralleled those of the spontaneous melatonin decline under darkened test conditions as well as during active suppression under the dawn signal. Group-average correlations between the timing of sleep and various measures of melatonin secretion also have been observed under bright-light exposure in SAD subjects (51) and normals (21). However, statistically significant correlations of these variables have not yet been observed within individual subjects or for individual sleep episodes. Such analyses of correlations between sleep timing and melatonin secretion have considered nocturnal melatonin as a marker of circadian phase, similar to rhythms of body temperature in other circadian sleep studies [e.g., (49,59)]. Circadian influence on sleep–wake timing has been supported by numerous findings (discussed below). Thus, parallel changes in timing of sleep and melatonin secretion seen in the present study, and in other studies of SAD subjects and normals, could be coincidental—both processes independently controlled by the circadian pacemaker. If so, the entraining effect of LD exposure in humans (17) could explain any correlation between melatonin and sleep changes produced by manipulation of light exposure. It is also possible, however, that melatonin is involved in neurochemical mediation between circadian entrainment by light and sleep–wake timing.

Circadian Control of Sleep

A circadian basis for sleep–wake timing is evident from studies in both animals and humans. Clear disruptions in sleep–wake rhythms have been observed, for example, in rats with lesions of the suprachiasmatic nucleus [e.g., (23)]. In humans, evidence for circadian regulation of sleep comes mainly from studies in temporal isolation and after sleep deprivation. In temporal isolation, during internal synchronization, sleep–wake cycles free-run with a period equal to that of other circadian functions [e.g., (59)]. During internal desynchronization, the sleep–wake rhythm appears to break away from other rhythms, and assumes an unstable phase relationship to body temperature (8). However, further analyses have shown that even during internal desynchronization, sleep onset is clearly confined to specific intervals within the circadian temperature cycle (19,49). Sleep-deprivation studies, measuring unrestricted recovery sleep following systematically delayed bedtimes, have shown sleep duration to be determined largely by the degree to which a sleep period coincides with the nighttime phase of the circadian cycle (2).

The two-process model of sleep regulation (11,13,19) indicates that sleep onset and duration in humans are determined jointly by circadian phase and accumulated sleep debt. The circadian contribution to total sleep propensity is represented by separate oscillating thresholds for sleep onset and awakening.

A neurochemical mediator for the circadian regulation of sleep has not been definitively identified, though many have been considered [e.g., (22)]. In this context, melatonin has been a candidate (12,61), given its nocturnal pattern and control by both direct light exposure (28) and circadian phase (37). In humans, pharmacologically induced increases in plasma melatonin have increased sleepiness and fatigue (5,35) and induced sleep (15,57). Stimulation of endogenous release of melatonin with a psoralen compound causes drowsiness associated with physiologic increases in plasma melatonin (47). Self-ratings of fatigue/sleepiness during sleep deprivation or after recovery sleep show increases in the late evening, peaks in the early morning (3:00 A.M.), and decreases in the late morning (1,2), covarying with urinary melatonin excretion (3). Finally, in a case study of a retinally blind person given oral melatonin at 11 P.M., correlations were observed between spontaneous sleep and melatonin availability (6).

Other findings have not been consistent with a generalized role for melatonin as a direct modulator of circadian regulation of sleep. Pinealectomy in mammals does not disrupt the rest–activity rhythm under constant conditions [for review see (7)], although one study (41) showed dampening or elimination of the diurnal rhythm of paradoxical sleep in rats. Furthermore, there is preliminary evidence in humans (6,46) and animals (7) that exogenously administered melatonin can produce circadian phase shifts so that any direct links between melatonin and sleep must be distinguished from those mediated by the circadian pacemaker.

Melatonin is not likely to function as a direct hypnogen since it is secreted during the active phase in nocturnal species. Melatonin might, however, be understood as a modulator of putative endogenous sleep substances, several of which have been identified (26). Alternatively, melatonin may function as an internal zeitgeber through which a secondary sleep–wake oscillator system might be synchronized (7). Light exposure could influence sleep–wake timing, then, through both its suppressive and entraining effects on melatonin secretion. More specifically, the effects of dawn exposure on early-morning melatonin secretion may affect the circadian wake-threshold.

In our study, early morning suppression and phase-advance of melatonin secretion were often observed in association with similar advances in spontaneous awakenings in the presence of the twilight signal. Subjects awakened by alarm, who showed no clear advance in posttreatment wake-up times, reported increased subjective energy on awakening with the artificial dawn. Such increased postawakening arousal might mirror the earlier decline of plasma melatonin than occurs under pretreatment conditions. Furthermore, naturally occurring annual cycles of sleep–wake timing, seen in the course of SAD and its subsyndromal variant (52), might be explained on the basis of melatonin secretion patterns controlled by seasonally varying early-morning light exposure (10).

Conclusion

Exposure to certain patterns of naturalistic, early-morning light appears able to promote an antidepressant response in SAD as well as changes in sleep timing and duration.

Early-morning suppression and phase-advance of nocturnal melatonin secretion are affected by such light exposure, suggesting a specific sensitivity of the circadian pacemaker to graded twilight signals. There may be functional links between the shape and timing of the melatonin profile and the 24-hr rhythm of sleep propensity. It will be important to determine the specificity of natural, graded twilight signals in eliciting such effects in SAD patients, those suffering nonseasonal sleep disorders, and normal controls.

ACKNOWLEDGMENTS

Research supported by NIMH Grants K02 MH00461, R01 MH42931, R43 MH40584, T32 MH18264, and MHCRC MH30906, and New York State Science and Technology Foundation. We thank Stephen Fairhurst, Joel Levitt, Bill Perlman, and Brian Rafferty for their work in developing and maintaining the twilight apparatus; Thomas Cooper and Ee Sing Lo for developing and conducting the melatonin assays; Jack Gorman and the staff of our Biological Studies Unit for assistance in conducting overnight sessions; and Martha Link, Jiuan Su Terman, and Anna Wirz-Justice for comments on the manuscript.

REFERENCES

1. Åkerstedt T, Froberg JE. Psychophysiological circadian rhythms in women during 72 h of sleep deprivation. *Waking Sleeping* 1977; 1:387–394.
2. Åkerstedt T, Gilberg M. The circadian variation of experimentally displaced sleep. *Sleep* 1981; 4:159–169.
3. Åkerstedt T, Gilberg M, Wetterberg L. The circadian covariation of fatigue and urinary melatonin. *Biol Psychiat* 1982; 17:547–554.
4. American Psychiatric Association. *Diagnostic and Statistical Manual of Mental Disorders*, 3rd ed.-rev., DSM–III–R. American Psychiatric Association, Washington, DC, 1987.
5. Arendt J, Borbély AA, Franey C, Wright J. Effects of chronic, small doses of melatonin given in the late afternoon on fatigue in man: A preliminary study. *Neurosci Lett* 1984; 45:317–321.
6. Arendt J, Aldhous M, Wright J. Synchronization of a disturbed sleep-wake cycle in a blind man by melatonin treatment. *Lancet* 1988; 2:772–773.
7. Armstrong SM. Melatonin: The internal zeitgeber of mammals? *Pineal Res Rev* 1989; 7:157–202.
8. Aschoff J. Circadian rhythms in man. *Science* 1965; 148:1427–1432.
9. Bojkowski C, Aldhous M, English J, Franey C, Poulton AL, Skene DJ, Arendt J. Suppression of nocturnal plasma melatonin and 6-sulphatoxymelatonin by bright and dim light in man. *Horm Metab Res* 1987; 19:437–440.
10. Bojkowski CJ, Arendt J. Annual changes in 6-sulphatoxymelatonin excretion in man. *Acta Endocrinol* 1988; 117:470–476.
11. Borbély AA. A two process model for sleep regulation. *Human Neurobiol* 1982; 1:195–204.
12. Borbély AA. Endogenous sleep-substances and sleep regulation. *J Neural Transm* 1986 [Suppl]; 21:243–254.
13. Borbély AA. The two-process model of sleep regulation: Implications for sleep in depression. In DJ Kupfer, TH Monk, and JD Barchas (eds.), *Biological Rhythms and Mental Disorders*. Guilford Press, New York, 1988: 55–81.

14. Brainard GC, Lewy AJ, Menaker M, Frederickson RH, Miller LS, Weleber RG, Cassone V, Hudson D. Dose-relationship between light irradiance and the suppression of plasma melatonin in human volunteers. *Brain Res* 1988; 454:212–218.

15. Cramer H, Rudolph J, Consbruch U, Kendel K. On the effects of melatonin on sleep and behavior in man. *Adv Biochem Psychopharmacol* 1974; 11:187–191.

16. Czeisler CA, Richardson GS, Zimmerman JC, Moore-Ede MC, Weitzman ED. Entrainment of human circadian rhythms by light-dark cycles: A reassessment. *Photochem Photobiol* 1981; 34:239–247.

17. Czeisler CA, Allan JS, Strogatz SH, Ronda JM, Sánchez R, Ríos D, Freitag WO, Richardson GS, Kronauer R. Bright light resets the human circadian pacemaker independent of the timing of the sleep-wake cycle. *Science* 1986; 233:667–671.

18. Daan S, Aschoff J. Circadian rhythms of locomotor activity in captive birds and mammals: Their variations with season and latitude. *Oecologia* 1975; 18:269–316.

19. Daan S, Beersma GM, Borbély AA. Timing of human sleep: Recovery process gated by a circadian pacemaker. *Am J Physiol* 1984; 15:R161–178.

20. Dijk DJ, Visscher CA, Bloem GM, Beersma DGM, Daan S. Reduction in human sleep duration after bright light exposure in the morning. *Neurosci Lett* 1987; 73:181–186.

21. Dijk DJ, Beersma DGM, Daan S, Lewy AJ. Bright morning light advances the human circadian system without affecting NREM sleep homeostasis. *Am J Physiol* 1989; 256: R106–111.

22. Ehlers CL, Kupfer DJ. Hypothalamic peptide modulation of EEG sleep in depression: A further application of the S-process hypothesis. *Biol Psychiatry* 1987; 22:513–517.

23. Ibuka N, Inouye S, Kawamura H. Analysis of sleep-wakefulness rhythms in male rats after suprachiasmatic lesions and ocular enucleation. *Brain Res* 1977; 122:33–47.

24. Kavaliers M, Ross DM. Twilight and day length affect the seasonality of entrainment and endogenous circadian rhythms of a fish, Couesius plumbieus. *Can J Psychol* 1980; 59:1326–1334.

25. Kavanau JL. Activity and orientational responses of white-footed mice to light. *Nature (London)* 1968; 218:245–252.

26. Krueger JM, Obal F Jr, Opp M, Cady AB, Johannsen L, Toth L, Majde J. this volume.

27. Laakso ML, Porkka-Heiskanen T, Alila A, Peder M, Johansson G. Twenty-four hour pattern of pineal melatonin and pituitary and plasma prolactin in male rats under "natural" and artificial lighting conditions. *Neuroendocrinology* 1988; 48:308–313.

28. Lewy AJ, Wehr TA, Goodwin FK, Newsome DA, Markey SP. Light suppresses melatonin secretion in humans. *Science* 1980; 210:1267–1269.

29. Lewy AJ, Sack RL, Fredrickson RH, Reaves M, Denney DD, Zielske DR. The use of bright light in the treatment of chronobiologic sleep and mood disorders: The phase response curve. *Psychopharm Bull* 1983; 19:523–525.

30. Lewy AJ, Nurnberger JI, Wehr TA, Pack D, Becker LE, Powell R-L, Newsome DA. Supersensitivity to light: Possible trait marker for manic-depressive illness. *Am J Psychiat* 1985; 142:725–727.

31. Lewy AJ, Sack RL, Singer CM. Immediate and delayed effects of bright light on human melatonin production: Shifting "dawn" and "dusk" shifts the dim light melatonin onset (DLMO). *Ann NY Acad Sci* 1985; 453:253–259.

32. Lewy AJ, Sack RL. Minireview: Light therapy and psychiatry. *Proc Soc Exp Biol Med* 1986; 183:11–18.

33. Lewy AJ, Sack RL, Miller S, Hoban TM. Antidepressant and circadian phase-shifting effects of light. *Science* 1987; 235:352–354.

34. Lewy AJ, Sack RL, Singer CM, White DM, Hoban TM. Winter depression and the phase-shift hypothesis for bright-light's therapeutic effects: History, theory, and experimental evidence. *J Biol Rhythms* 1988; 3:121–134.

35. Lieberman HR, Waldhauser F, Garfield G, Lynch HJ, Wurtman RJ. Effects of melatonin on human mood and performance. *Brain Res* 1984; 323:201–207.

36. Livermore AH Jr, Stevens JR. Light transducer for the biological clock: A function for rapid eye movements. *J Neural Transm* 1988; 72:37–42.

37. Lynch HJ, Wurtman RJ, Moskowitz MA, Archer MC, Ho MH. Daily rhythm in human urinary melatonin. *Science* 1975; 187:169–171.

38. McGlashan T (ed.). *The Documentation of Clinical Psychotropic Drug Trials.* National Institutes of Health, Rockville MD, 1973.

39. McIntyre IM, Norman TR, Burrows GD, Armstrong SM. Human melatonin suppressed by light is intensity dependent. *J Pineal Res* 1989; 6:149–156.

40. McIntyre IM, Norman TR, Burrows GD, Armstrong SM. Human melatonin response to light at different times of the night. *Psychoneuroendocrinology* 1989; 14:187–193.

41. Mouret J, Coindet J, Chouvet G. Effet de la pinealectomie sur les états et rhythmes de sommeil du rat male. *Brain Res* 1974; 81:97–105.

42. Okudaira N, Kripke DF, Webster JB. Naturalistic studies of human light exposure. *Am J Physiol* 1983; 14:R613–615.

43. Pittendrigh CS, Daan S. A functional analysis of circadian pacemakers in nocturnal rodents. IV. Entrainment: Pacemaker as clock. *J Comp Physiol* 1976; 106:291–331.

44. Reiter RJ. Action spectra, dose-response relationships and temporal aspects of light's effects on the pineal gland. *Ann NY Acad Sci* 1985; 453:215–230.

45. Rosenthal NE, Sack DA, Gillin JC, Lewy AJ, Goodwin FK, Davenport Y, Mueller PS, Newsome DA, Wehr TA. Seasonal affective disorder: A description of the syndrome and preliminary findings with light therapy. *Arch Gen Psychiat* 1984; 41:72–80.

46. Sack RL, Lewy AJ. Melatonin advances circadian rhythms in humans. Paper presented at American Psychiatric Association meeting, Montreal, Quebec, 1988.

47. Souêtre E, Salvati E, Belugou JL, Krebs B, Darcourt G. 5-Methoxypsoralen increases sleepiness in humans: Possible involvement of melatonin secretion. *Europ J Pharm* 1989; 36:91–92.

48. Stevens JR, Livermore A Jr. Eye blinking and rapid eye movement: Pulsed photic stimulation of the brain. *Exp Neurol* 1978; 60:541–556.

49. Strogatz SH, Kronauer RE, Czeisler CA. Circadian regulation dominates homeostatic control of sleep length and prior awake length in humans. *Sleep* 1986; 9:353–364.

50. Terman JS, Terman M, Schlager D, Rafferty B, Rosofsky M, Link MJ, Quitkin FM. Efficacy of brief, intense light exposure for treatment of winter depression. *Psychopharmacology Bulletin* 1990, 26:3–8.

51. Terman M, Terman JS, Quitkin FM, Cooper TB, Lo ES, Gorman JM, Stewart JW, McGrath PJ. Response of the melatonin cycle to phototherapy for seasonal affective disorder. *J Neural Transm* 1988; 72:147–165.

52. Terman M, Botticelli SR, Link BG, Link MJ, Quitkin FM, Hardin TE, Rosenthal NE. Seasonal symptoms patterns in New York: Patients and population. In C Thompson and T Silverstone (eds.), *Seasonal Affective Disorders.* CRC Clinical Neuroscience, London, 1989, pp. 77–95.

53. Terman M, Fairhurst S, Perlman B, McCluney RM. Daylight deprivation and replenishment: A psychobiological problem with a naturalistic solution. In *Proceedings II. Second International Daylighting Conference: Architecture and Natural Light.* American Society of Heating, Refrigerating, and Air Conditioning Engineers, Atlanta, 1989, pp. 438–445.

54. Terman M, Terman JS, Quitkin FM, McGrath PJ, Stewart JW, Rafferty B. Light therapy for seasonal affective disorder: A review of efficacy. *Neuropsychopharmacology* 1989; 2:1–22.

55. Terman M, Terman JS, Quitkin FM, Stewart JW, McGrath PJ, Nunes EV, Wager SG, Tricamo E. Dosing dimensions of light therapy: Duration and time of day. In C Thompson

and T Silverstone (eds.), *Seasonal Affective Disorders*. CRC Clinical Neuroscience, London, 1989, pp.187–204.

56. Terman M, Remé CE, Wirz–Justice A. The visual input stage of the mammalian circadian pacemaking system. II. The effect of light and drugs on retinal function. *J Biol Rhythms* (submitted).

57. Vollrath L, Semm P, Gammel G. Sleep induction by intranasal application of melatonin. *Biosciences* 1981; 29:327–329.

58. Weitzman ED, Weinberg U, D'Eletto R, Lynch HJ, Wurtman RJ, Czeisler CA, Erlich S. Studies of 24 hour rhythms of melatonin in man. *J Neural Transmission* 1978; 13 (suppl): 325–337.

59. Wever R. Use of light to treat jet lag: Differential effects of normal and bright artificial light on human circadian rhythms. *Ann NY Acad Sci* 1985; 453:282–304.

60. Williams JBW, Link MJ, Rosenthal NE, Terman M. *Structured Interview Guide for the Hamilton Depression Scale—Seasonal Affective Disorder version (SIGH-SAD)*. New York State Psychiatric Institute, 1988.

61. Wurtman RJ, Lieberman HR. Melatonin secretion as a mediator of circadian variations in sleep and sleepiness. *J Pineal Res* 1985; 2:301–303.

II
SLEEP

8

Brainstem Cholinergic Systems
and Models of REM Sleep Production

ROBERT W. MCCARLEY

This chapter first briefly reviews earlier work on cholinergic induction of REM sleep, and then presents recent data from our laboratory on brainstem projections of cholinergic systems and *in vitro* actions of cholinergic compounds on medial pontine reticular formation neurons. It concludes with a discussion of the implications of these findings for models of REM sleep control.

PHARMACOLOGICAL INDUCTION OF REM SIGNS
BY MICROINJECTIONS OF CHOLINERGIC AGONISTS

Cholinergic agonists, when locally injected into the pontine reticular formation (PRF), are the single class of agents capable of reliable induction of a phenomenologically complete REM sleep-like state (see reviews in 44 & 46). In contrast, numerous trials of other putative neurotransmitters/neuromodulators have not been able to produce an adequate pharmacological model of REM sleep. Cholinergic induction of an REM sleep-like state was originally reported in the 1960s (see 8 and 9), was documented with respect to completeness of mimicry of REM sleep (i.e., presence of muscle atonia, EEG desynchronization, pontogeniculooccipital (PGO) waves, rapid eye movements, hippocampal theta, etc.) and has been subsequently confirmed by workers in a number of laboratories (1, reviewed in 4 & 46). This REM sleep-like state is produced in a dose-dependent manner by neostigmine microinjections in PRF, and this neostigmine effect is blocked by atropine (3) suggesting the effect may occur via endogenous acetylcholine (ACh) acting on muscarinic receptors. With respect to localization, carbachol-induced signs of REM sleep are produced by microinjections in PRF, particularly in the giant cell field, but not by microinjections in bulbar reticular formation (BRF) or mesencephalic reticular formation (MRF). (It should be mentioned that not all regions of the BRF have been explored and that both in this region and in MRF elicitation of competing behaviors may have interfered with production of REM sleep effects.) Within PRF, there is always a delay (more than 1 min) before the microinjection produces REM sleep effects, suggesting recruitment of neural populations is a necessary feature of pharmacological induction of REM sleep. Latency to effects depends on the locus of the particular aspect of REM sleep machinery being analyzed: for example, muscle atonia is most quickly elicited by injections in dorsolateral reticular formation, lateral geniculate PGO waves by injections near the brachium conjunctivum (the zone that includes the cholinergic pedunculopontine tegmental nucleus, to be discussed below), and eye movements by injections near more medial reticular structures that include the horizontal saccade generation system. Thus, a simple, and probably accurate conceptualization of the effect of these injections is that they are able to activate various aspects of the neuronal machinery normally involved in REM sleep production, and that, with activation of the total set of REM sleep components, one has the full-blown REM sleep syndrome. Localization of effects is further discussed in Baghdoyan et al. (5).

These *in vivo* microinjection data thus suggest that the full set of REM sleep phenomena can be triggered by pontine cholinoceptive mechanisms, but they cannot specify if PRF is the natural trigger zone and ACh the natural neurotransmitter, nor indeed if the pharamacological effects occur at physiological concentrations of agonists or are direct effects on PRF neurons, as opposed to effects that are synaptically mediated. The presence of increased amounts of ACh in cortex during REM sleep does suggest however that natural REM sleep has at least some cholinergic component (18).

In view of the responsiveness to ACH agonists, it is not surprising that all studies evaluating the presence of acetylcholinesterase (AChE) have found heavy concentrations in PRF and BRF neurons (e.g., 7,21,39). However, recent studies using monoclonal antibodies to choline acetyltransferase (ChAT), a presumptive indicator of cholinergic neurons, have found only a few ChAT-positive neurons in pontobulbar RF, and these principally in BRF. The principal pontine concentration of ChAT-positive neurons is in two zones in rat (2,30) and in cat (19). The Ch5 group defined by Mesulam and co-workers (30) is composed of neurons "in and around" the superior cerebral peduncle in the pedunculopontine tegmental nucleus (PPT) and the Ch6 group lies in the lateral part of central gray, primarily in the laterodorsal tegmental nucleus (LDT). [There is an interesting question as to whether, on structural grounds, PPT should be labeled a "reticular nucleus" and Newman (35) so designates it; we use PRF to designate core RF and so do not include PPT.]

Given this information on PRF and cholinergic responsiveness, it appeared to us to be a plausible hypothesis that Ch5–6 neurons might project to pontine RF and might be a "natural" source of ACh triggering or reinforcing REM sleep—in addition to being the source of the ACh responsible for neostigmine REM sleep induction. For support of this hypothesis one needs to demonstrate (a) cholinergic connectivity, (b) appropriate *direct* synaptic action of *physiological concentrations* of ACh on pontine RF, and (c) a Ch5–6 discharge so timed as to induce or facilitate the induction of REM sleep. The next section addresses the question of cholinergic projections to pontine reticular formation, and in particular to the giant cell field portion of PRF, termed the gigantocellular tegmental field (FTG) by Berman (6), constituting the medial portion of PRF and corresponding to the nucleus reticularis pontis caudalis in alternative terminology.

CHOLINERGIC PROJECTIONS TO PONTINE RETICULAR FORMATION

Double Labeling Study

The basic plan of the immunohistochemical study in cats was straightforward; a detailed description of this study is in Mitani et al. (32). Small volume (10–30 nl) pressure injections of wheat germ agglutinin–horseradish peroxidase (WGA–HRP) from a micropipette syringe (so as to reduce leakage along the needle track) were placed in the pontine portion of FTG (PFTG, Fig. 8-1D). Choline acetyltransferase (ChAT) immunoreactivity was identified using monoclonal antibody AB8 localized by the unlabeled secondary antiserum/peroxidase–antiperoxidase (PAP) method, with diaminobenzidine (DAB) as the chromogen. The neurons that were double-labeled with ChAT immunoreactivity and retrogradely transported WGA–HRP were identified by the presence of a black granular deposit scattered in the cytoplasm (tetramethylbenzidine, TMB, was the chromogen for retrogradely transported WGA–HRP) and a diffuse brown DAB deposit indicated ChAT immunoreactivity.

Double-labeled neurons were observed bilaterally in the LDT and PPT (Fig. 8-1A–D). Of all ChAT immunoreactive neurons in the LDT (black dots in Fig. 8-1), 6.9% were double-labeled (as indicated by open triangles in Fig. 8-1), with 10.2% of ChAT-positive neurons being double-labeled ipsilateral to the WGA–HRP injection site and 3.7% contralateral. Double-labeled neurons were observed throughout the rostrocaudal extent of the LDT, and no apparent preferential localization was observed in the nucleus. Of all ChAT immunoreactive neurons in the PPT (black dots in Fig. 8-1), 3.1% were double-labeled (open triangles), with 5.2% ipsilateral and 1.3% contralateral to the WGA–HRP injection site. Double-labeled neurons were observed throughout the rostrocaudal extent of the PPT, with no apparent preferential localization. In addition to the retrograde labeling in LDT and PPT, WGA–HRP labeling was observed (not illustrated in Fig. 8-1) in contralateral PFTG, bilateral bulbar FTG, and the other sites previously shown to project to PFTG (41).

Anterograde Transport Study

To confirm the double-labeling results and to provide information on the pathway of the fibers from LDT and PPT to PRF we performed an anterograde labeling study in cats utilizing *Phaseolus vulgaris* leukoagglutinin (PHA-L) injected via a micropipette into LDT and PPT; this study is described in detail in Mitani et al. (31). PHA-L was visualized by the PAP method with a primary antibody to PHA-L.

After PHA-L injections in the LDT, PHA-L-positive fibers projecting into the PFTG spread ventrally from the injection site and entered the ipsilateral PFTG (Fig. 8-2). Some of them crossed the midline and entered the contralateral PFTG (Fig. 8-2A–C). On both sides of the PFTG, the PHA-L-positive fibers gave rise to bouton-like varicosities. PHA-L-positive fibers and varicosities were also observed in the raphe nucleus and contralateral LDT. In all cases of PHA-L injections in the PPT, PHA-L-positive fibers projecting into the PFTG coursed ventromedially from the injection site (Fig. 8-3A), and entered the ipsilateral PFTG. Some of them crossed the midline and entered the contralateral PFTG (Fig. 8-3A–C). In both sides of the PFTG, the

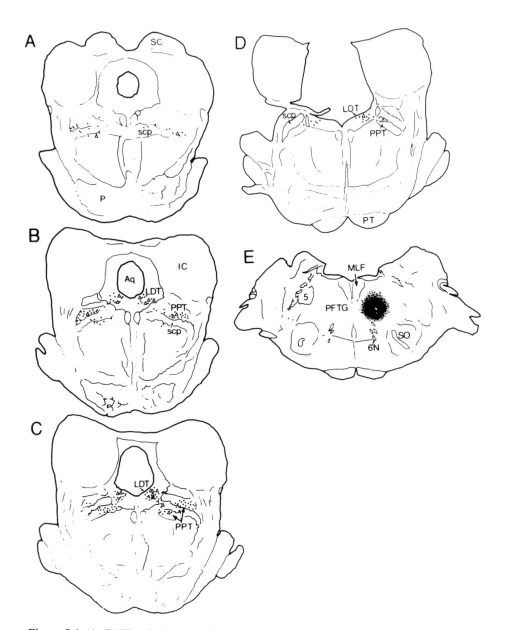

Figure 8-1 (A–D) The distribution of LDT and PPT neurons double-labeled with both retrogradely transported WGA-HRP and ChAT immunocytochemistry (open triangles), and single-labeled with ChAT immunocytochemistry (black dots). Note: non-ChAT positive neurons with retrogradely transported WGA-HRP are *not* represented. (E) Representation of the PFTG injection site of WGA-HRP. IC, inferior colliculus; LDT, laterodorsal tegmental nucleus; MLF, medial longitudinal fasciculus; P, pontine nuclei; PFTG, pontine gigantocellular tegmental field; PPT, pedunculopontine tegmental nucleus; PT, pyramidal tract; SC, superior colliculus; scp, superior cerebellar peduncle; SO, superior olive; 5, trigeminal nucleus; 6N, abducens nerve.

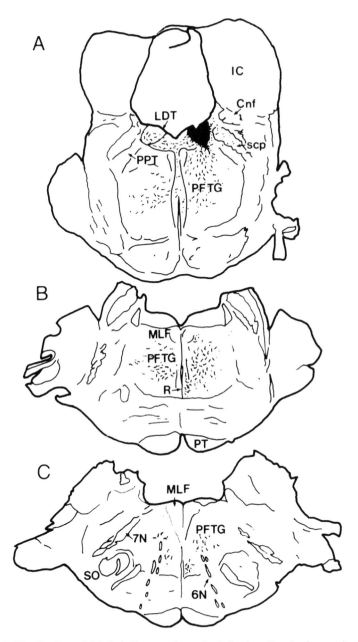

Figure 8-2 Distribution of labeled fibers and terminal (broken lines) after an iontophoretic injection of PHA-L into the laterodorsal tegmental nucleus. Injection site is represented in A. Cnf, cuneiform nucleus; R, raphe nucleus; 7N, facial nerve. Other abbreviations as in Figure 8-1.

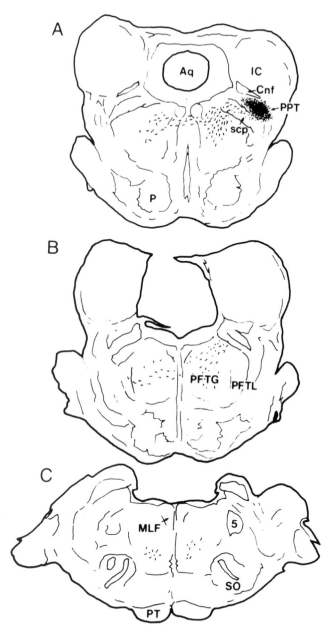

Figure 8-3 Distribution of labeled fibers and terminals (broken lines) after an iontophoretic injection of PHA-L into the pars compacta of the pedunculopontine tegmental nucleus. Injection site is represented in A. PFTL, pontine lateral tegmental field. Other abbreviations as in Figure 8-1.

fibers gave rise to bouton-like varicosities. Fewer PHA-L-positive fibers and varicosities were labeled after PHA-L injections in PPT than in LDT.

In summary, our group (31) has identified the LDT and PPT as sources of cholinergic inputs to the PFTG in the cat; this complements previous reports of ascending
projections of these nuclei (15,40). As most previous studies have emphasized the
rostral projections of LDT/PPT, it may be useful to underline the density of the caudal
projections to PRF. As measured by the percentage of double-labeled cholinergic
neurons, the density of cholinergic LDT to PFTG projections observed in the present
study appeared to approximate that of cholinergic LDT to thalamus projections in rat
(15), where, ipsilaterally, a mean of 10% of ChAT-positive LDT neurons was double-
labeled after WGA–HRP injections of comparably small size in thalamus ($N = 28$
injections, range = 1–26%; percentages computed by Dr. A. Hallanger from data of
her previously published study), as compared with the ipsilateral percentage of about
10% in the present LDT–PFTG study. Cholinergic PPT to PFTG projections in the
present study appeared to be somewhat less dense than described for PPT to thalamus
in rat, where ipsilateral double-labeling averaged 22% of PPT neurons (range 3–47%;
percentages computed by Dr. Hallinger from data of her previously published study),
and also for PPT to bulbar FTG projections in the rat (36) where the percentage of
ipsilateral PPT double-labeling following one bulbar FTG injection was 18%. These
percentages should, of course, be taken only as approximate comparisons of projection
strengths, since the species were different and the size of WGA–HRP injections in the
zones of interest varied; however the basic techniques of injection, processing, and
counting were similar. It is important to note that the findings of cholinergic LDT and
PPT to PRF projections described here have recently been confirmed by Shiromani and
co-workers (42).

In summary, there seems rather clear anatomical evidence for fairly dense cholinergic projections to pontine reticular formation. The next section addresses the
important question for cholinergic theories of REM induction of whether cholinergic
agonists act directly on reticular neurons and do so in physiological concentrations.

ACTIONS OF CHOLINERGIC AGONISTS ON MEDIAL PRF NEURONS *IN VITRO*

With respect to the physiology of excitatory cholinergic effects, the presence of a slow
depolarizing, excitatory response to ACh with a decreased potassium conductance in
cortex (22) and in guinea pig and cat medial and lateral geniculate nuclei (29) has been
described, but effects on PRF were unknown. Microwire extracellular recordings during cannula applications of carbachol in quantities sufficient to produce REM sleep
signs (4 μg) suggested that PRF neurons have heterogeneous responses to cholinergic
compounds, some neurons increasing and some decreasing discharge (43).

However, serious interpretive problems arise when the concentration of the agent
applied to the recorded neuron is not controlled and when the direct effects of the agent
cannot be distinguished from effects of the agent on neurons presynaptic to the recorded neuron. For example the usual concentration of microinjected carbachol is
about 1 μg/μl or in the millimolar range, a *thousand-fold* greater than the usual
micromolar concentrations used in assessing pharmacological effects. Unfortunately,

with high concentrations of agents, there is the possibility that nonphysiological concentrations may act on different receptors and/or they may cause nonphysiological effects. For example, agents causing depolarization may, in sufficiently high concentrations, lead to depolarization blockade. That is, the neuron may not generate an action potential because sufficient repolarization does not take place following a spike to deinactivate the sodium current responsible for the action potential. In fact, tests using intracellular depolarizing test currents demonstrate that depolarization blockade is readily elicited in PRF neurons (Greene, Gerber, and McCarley, unpublished data). Even *in vivo* extracellular iontophoretic studies have problems in terms of being unable to specify site of action, the mechanisms of effects, and the precise concentrations of agents. Thus, the findings of Greene and Carpenter (11), who used these techniques in cat, needed to be confirmed *in vitro;* these workers found both suppressive and long-duration excitatory responses, as well as biphasic responses of some PRF neurons to carbachol.

The ability to control the medium bathing PRF neurons while doing intracellular recordings was a strong motivation for development of the pontine reticular formation slice preparation (12) and its use for the evaluation of cholinergic effects (13). In this study, brainstem slices from young Sprague–Dawley rats were perfused with a modified Ringer's solution. Anatomical localization of recording and stimulating electrodes was confirmed by marker lesions followed by Nissl staining of the slice. Drugs were bath applied except for five experiments in which carbachol was applied by puffer, employing glass pipettes with tip diameters of 10–50 μm placed submerged in media but above the surface of the slice. Pressurized nitrogen was used to eject the drug. The only difference in response between these techniques was in a shorter time to onset of carbachol action with the puffer, a difference consonant with closer proximity to the neuron. Voltage clamp recordings were obtained with a sample and hold circuit (electrode resistance 50–70 MΩ). Only neurons that maintained robust and stable electrophysiological properties throughout the wash-in (2–5 min) and wash-out (10 min) periods were used in this study.

Of the 21 neurons in the medial pontine reticular formation exposed to carbachol at concentrations of 0.5–1.0 μM in the bath or 1–10 mM in puffer electrodes, over three-fifths (N = 13, 62%) responded with a depolarization of 16 $\pm$ 7 mV SD associated with an increase of input resistance of 21 $\pm$ 18% SD (Fig. 8-4A). A biphasic

---

Figure 8-4 Carbachol depolarization response is mediated by a decrease in a voltage-insensitive conductance and is blocked by atropine. (A) Chart record of a typical depolarizing response of an medial PRF neuron to bath application of carbachol (0.5 μM during time indicated). Downward deflections were due to intracellular current pulses (400 msec, 200 pA) applied to assess input resistance. At arrows, membrane potential was returned to the baseline potential of -74 mV by dc hyperpolarizing current to avoid voltage-sensitive changes of the membrane resistance not specific to carbachol. (B) Atropine (0.5 μM) blocks the depolarizing response to carbachol. (C) Decreased membrane conductance during pressure application of carbachol from a micropipette (arrow) is indicated by the decreased amplitude of downward deflections in the upper current record in response to 10-mV, 400-msec membrane potential shift commands (lower record) in a neuron under voltage clamp control. (D) I/V plot generated by a constant depolarization of the membrane potential (1 mV/200 msec) from -100 to -50 mV during control conditions and during exposure to 0.5 μM carbachol in the perfusate. Note the voltage insensitivity of the carbachol current.

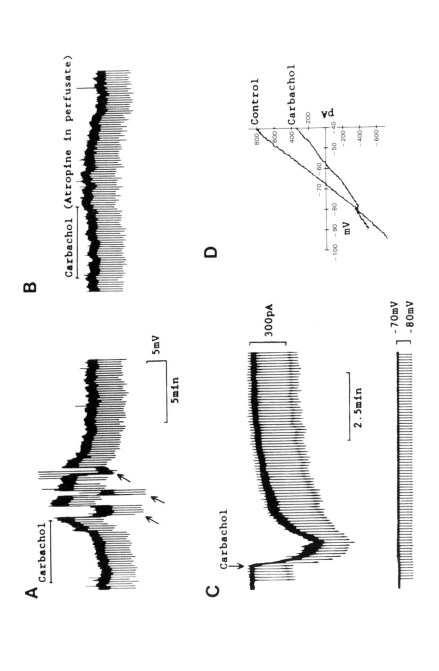

B

Carbachol (Atropine in perfusate)

D

Control

Carbachol

pA

800
600
400
200

-100 -90 -80 -70 -60 -50 -40

mV

-200

-400

-600

A

Carbachol

5mV

5min

C

300pA

2.5min

Carbachol

-70mV
-80mV

response consisting of a shorter duration hyperpolarization followed by longer duration depolarization was found in three neurons. Thus, overall, a depolarizing response was present in over three-fourths of the neurons (16/21, 76%). In four neurons (19%) there was a hyperpolarization associated with a decrease in input resistance. Only one neuron did not respond to carbachol.

These were direct, nonsynaptically mediated effects, as indicated by their presence with bath application of tetrodotoxin (1 μM), which prevents sodium action potential-dependent synaptic activity ($N = 12$). Both depolarized and hyperpolarizing carbachol effects, without any preferential localization, were observed on members of each of the main classes of mPRF neuron, the low threshold burst neurons and the nonburst neurons (10).

The depolarizing response was further analyzed as to its pharmacological and voltage sensitivities. The addition of atropine (0.5 μM) to the perfusate ($N = 4$) resulted in complete blockade of the carbachol-evoked depolarization, indicating the effect was muscarinic (Fig. 8-4B). Under voltage clamp control of the membrane potential, carbachol evoked a net inward current associated with a decrease in chord conductance, as indicated by a decrease in the amount of current required to hyperpolarize the membrane potential 10 mV (Fig. 8-4C). The voltage sensitivity of the current evoked by carbachol was measured by subtraction of the current recorded during carbachol from that during control over a membrane potential range of -100 to -50 mV and the slope of the I/V plot of this current was found to be constant over the measured range, and thus indicative of a voltage insensitive conductance change (Fig. 8-4D). The reversal potential was -98 ± 17 mV SD ($[K+]_o = 3.25$ mM).

We next examined effects of carbachol on neuronal excitability and reticulo-reticular postsynaptic potential (PSP) amplitude to determine if these paralleled those seen in normal REM sleep (15). The depolarization response evoked by carbachol was accompanied by an increase in neuronal excitability, since identical amplitude and duration depolarizing current pulses elicited from 1.3- to 4-fold as many action potentials during carbachol application as compared with control. The effect was due to the steady-state inward current elicited by carbachol, since combined carbachol application with intracellular injection of a hyperpolarizing dc current sufficient to return the membrane potential to control level did not increase excitability.

It is known that enhanced depolarizing PSPs are obtained by reticular stimulation during natural REM sleep as contrasted with slow-wave sleep (16). In the slice preparation, we found that the depolarizing PSPs evoked by electrical stimulation of the contralateral mPRF (10–100 μA amplitude) were enhanced in carbachol-depolarized neurons and that this PSP enhancement was blocked in the presence of atropine.

An initial analysis of the hyperpolarizing response showed a nonlinear current–voltage relationship of the carbachol-evoked current (in the presence of tetrodotoxin 1 μM). It was characterized by the presence of inward rectification (characteristic of the anomalous rectifier current (14,20), that is, slope conductance was greater at membrane potential levels negative to the reversal potential.

In summary, over two-thirds of mPRF neurons responded to carbachol with a strong depolarizing response that was associated with an increase in input resistance. There was an increase in excitability as measured by an increased number of spikes to the same depolarizing current and enhancement of PSPs elicited by electrical stimulation of the contralateral pontine reticular formation. Atropine blockade of carbachol effects suggests mediation by a muscarinic receptor. The remaining third responded with either a biphasic hyperpolarization–depolarization or hyperpolarization alone.

IMPLICATIONS FOR MODELS OF REM SLEEP CONTROL

In 1975 McCarley & Hobson (23) proposed a structural and mathematical model of REM sleep control that depended on neuronal populations that became active preceding and during REM sleep ("REM-on neurons") and reciprocally interacted with neuronal populations whose discharge activity diminished or ceased preceding and during REM sleep ("REM-off") neurons. The REM-on neurons were postulated to be excitatory and to play an active role in production of REM sleep phenomena, whereas the REM-off neurons were suggested to be inhibitory to REM-on neurons in waking and, when the REM-off neurons ceased firing, to disinhibit the REM-on neurons as the time of REM sleep onset approached. This idea of interaction of REM-off and REM-on neurons to control the sleep cycle has been found to be useful by other groups (see, for example, discussions by Sakai (38)), and the mathematical model based on this structure has similarly been found useful (see discussion in McCarley and Massaquoi (28) and Steriade & McCarley (44)).

Results from subsequent work on identifying the neurotransmitters, the locations, and the connectivity of REM-off and REM-on neurons have indicated the appropri-

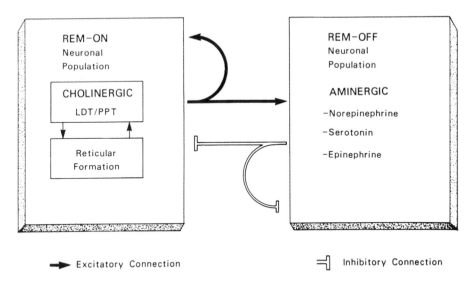

Figure 8-5 Reciprocal interaction model for REM sleep control. Solid-head arrows represent excitatory connections and open bars represent inhibitory connections. The dynamics of the REM-on and REM-off population interactions are described in the text. Note each population has, in addition to connections with the other population, a feedback- or self-connection of the same sign. The neurochemical identity of the REM-off aminergic populations is listed in the box. For the REM-on populations, the possible mode of interaction of the cholinergic neurons in the laterodorsal tegmental nucleus (LDT) and the pedunculopontine tegmental nucleus (PPT) with the pontobulbar reticular neurons is described in the text.

ateness of extensions and modifications of the 1975 model, although the basic postulates of REM-off and REM-on interaction and their mathematical description are conserved [for a recent description and elaboration of the mathematics and the dynamics of the model, see McCarley and Massaquoi (28)]. Figure 8-5 represents our current working version of this model. It illustrates the fact that the set of REM-off neurons likely includes a wide variety of aminergic neurons with the discharge activity profile of decreasing discharge activity preceding REM sleep and a very low level of activity or even of silence during the REM sleep episode. Brainstem neurons with this discharge activity profile include those utilizing norepinephrine, epinephrine, and serotonin as neurotransmitters and located in the locus coeruleus, dorsal raphe, and peribrachial region, and those scattered elsewhere in the brainstem. [It is possible that histaminergic neurons in the hypothalamus may play an analogous role, since discharge rates are maximal in waking and are greatly reduced in REM sleep (45); they are not included in the Figure 8-3 model, however, since brainstem transection experiments indicate they are not necessary for REM sleep.]

Since advances in immunohistochemistry have made it clear that the principal sources of cholinergic neurons in brainstem are LDT and PPT, and that, although pontine reticular neurons are likely cholinoceptive, few are cholinergic, the major locus of cholinergic REM-on neurons postulated by the 1975 model has been shifted to the LDT/PPT (Fig. 8-5). Note that this figure includes both LDT/PPT and PRF neurons in the category of "REM-on" neurons. As will be made clear below, the exact relationship of these two groups of neurons and their respective roles in REM sleep are matters of current intense investigation.

Postulated Steps in Production of a REM Sleep Episode

Before discussing details of the interaction of LDT/PPT and reticular neurons, it may be useful to outline the model's postulate of steps in production of an REM sleep episode and the repetition of this REM sleep cycle.

1. The slowing and near cessation of firing of REM-off neurons disinhibit the population of REM-on neurons.
2. As a result of this disinhibition, the population of REM-on neurons becomes increasingly active and this activity is augmented because of the excitatory interconnections in this REM-on population until the REM sleep episode is produced.
3. The REM-off population becomes active as a result of excitatory input from the REM-on population. When the REM-off population becomes sufficiently active, the REM sleep episode is terminated because of the REM-off neurons' inhibition of the REM-on population.
4. The population of REM-off neurons is postulated to become less active because of inhibitory feedback, and this leads to step 1 and a resumption of the cycle.

We hasten to emphasize that this sequence is only a model and much additional work will be needed before it can be said to be grounded in solid data. Our reading is, however, that the currently available behavioral, pharmacological, and cellular neurophysiological data indicate the model is plausible, although a full discussion of the evidence for and against various postulates of the model is considerably beyond the scope of this chapter. [We are however, discussing these data elsewhere (44).] The astute reader will also have noticed that the oscillatory system as described continues to oscillate indefinitely; a more detailed account of the model (28) describes the turning on and off of the oscillator through interaction with circadian systems. In this chapter we want to discuss several points relevant to the LDT/PPT and their input to reticular formation.

The first point is that from the perspective of *in vivo* intracellular recording the principal phenomenon related to the REM episode is the membrane potential depolarization of virtually all members of the "medial pontine reticular pool" (16). The membrane potential depolarization begins in many PRF neurons even before the onset of PGO waves (which occurs prior to REM onset) and progresses to the 7–10 mV membrane potential depolarization seen in REM relative to slow-wave sleep. This membrane potential depolarization is present throughout the REM episode and, in the neurons thus far recorded, is followed by a repolarization on transition to the state of waking (W). During W there may be membrane potential depolarization of specific sets of neurons in association with specific waking events—for example, eye or somatic movements, but the reticular population as a whole does not have a depolarized MP throughout W, in contrast to the situation during REM sleep. We have suggested that this reticular neuronal population membrane potential depolarization during REM sleep (and consequent action potential production) is responsible for activation of the neuronal machinery contained within the PRF, and causes the events of REM sleep, including rapid eye movements, pontine component of PGO waves, muscle twitches, and, for the dorsolateral PRF, muscle atonia (24). Viewed in this manner the question then becomes what processes act to produce this membrane potential depolarization, and the data presented in this chapter suggest that cholinergic influences on PRF may be important. The presence of reticuloreticular excitatory synapses that may be important in the spread of this REM sleep-associated activation has been documented elsewhere (17,27,32,33).

Interaction between LDT/PPT Neurons and Reticular Neurons

Figure 8-5 shows that the "REM-on" set of neurons has an internal structure: there are excitatory connections between LDT/PPT and reticular formation neurons. These LDT/PPT projections to PRF and the excitatory effects of cholinergic agonists have of course been described in the preceding two sections of this chapter. Figure 8-5 also indicates the possibility of excitatory reticular projections to LDT/PPT; there is anatomical evidence for these projections, although it is not known if they are excitatory.

At this point it is useful to mention that, from an *a priori* point of view, there appear to be two principal possible modes of action of LDT/PPT neurons on reticular neurons involving the production of a REM sleep episode.

1. *Trigger.* If the pre-REM time of onset of LDT/PPT neuronal discharge is early enough then they might act to "trigger" the population membrane depolarization and increased action potential discharge observable in PRF neurons prior to REM sleep. This possibility is indicated in Figure 8-5 by the excitatory projection to PRF.

2. *Latch.* Even if LDT/PPT neuronal discharge begins at the same time or later than PRF neuronal discharge, the cholinergic excitatory input to PRF may act to enhance the membrane depolarization of PRF neurons. Further, as indicated in Figure 8-5, it is possible that members of the LDT/PPT and reticular populations may form a mutually augmenting network during REM, as indicated by the mutually excitatory projections between the two groups of neurons. We have termed this mode of interaction as a "latch," since the activation of reticular neurons would be augmented and then "latched" at a high level by the interaction with LDT/PPT neurons. Note that the trigger and latch modes are not mutually exclusive.

Data on Discharge Activity of LDT/PPT Neurons

We emphasize at the outset that we think it likely that the discharge activity of LDT/PPT neurons may *not* be homogeneous, and that there may be several different types of cholinergic neuronal discharge patterns. Much empirical work clearly remains to be done in this area.

Cholinergic Neurons and PGO Wave Production

The present evidence is most clear for a role in PGO wave production. Studies in several laboratories have now clearly found the presence of "PGO burst neurons" in and around the brachium conjunctivum (24,37,34), which discharge in a stereotyped way just prior to a large PGO wave in the ipsilateral LGN. These PGO burst neurons have been demonstrated to project to the thalamus and are localized to "in and around the brachium conjunctivum," that is, the zone of the PPT cholinergic neurons. Sakai has also briefly noted finding PGO burst neurons in LDT, although this finding has not been fully documented (38). Thus, there is circumstantial evidence that the "PGO burst neurons" may be cholinergic neurons. [We must caution, unfortunately, there have been no physiological recordings of identified Ch5–6 cholinergic neurons; for certainty of identification there must be a marker stain of the recorded neuron combined with a ChAT stain for double labeling. Although the reader may think the demanded technical virtuosity may render this a moot point, the author believes that rapid advancement of techniques will make such double labeling commonplace within the next 5 years.] These PGO burst neurons might, through projections to PRF as well as to thalamus, act to increase the excitability of PRF neurons. However, several factors suggest that PRF excitation from PGO burst neurons alone would not explain most of the observed PRF excitation in REM. First, PRF neurons discharging in association with PGO waves do so with 30–300 msec lead times, much longer than the 12–15 msec of the PGO burst neurons, and thus the burst neurons could not cause the preceding activation (26,34); second, the membrane potential depolarization of PRF neurons is present throughout the REM sleep period and not just during the periods where PGO waves occur.

From recordings of unidentified neurons in PPT we know that non-PGO burst neurons are also found in the area and these increase discharge rate in anticipation of and during REM sleep (McCarley, unpublished data), although the precise timing of the onset of REM-anticipatory discharge and waking discharge properties of this group are incompletely characterized. Obviously systematic characterization of the discharge activity of LDT and PPT neurons with reticular projections (identified by antidromic activation) is an important current task. (Recent work by Steriade & coworkers is described in Steriade and McCarley [44]).

Evidence supporting a role of the Ch5–6 neuronal zone in production of REM sleep phenomena has recently been obtained by bilateral kainic acid lesions of this zone (47). These lesions markedly diminished PGO waves, REM sleep muscle atonia, the rapid eye movements, and the overall percentage of REM sleep (from a control value of 13 to 8.5% 28 days postlesion). Furthermore, some cholinergic specificity was suggested by the fact that postlesion REM sleep percentage and PGO spike rate correlations were highest with the number of ChAT positive neurons destroyed (Pearson's $r = -.69$ and $-.66$, respectively) than the correlations with the total volume of the lesion (r's $= -.53$ and $-.32$) or with the number of tyrosine hydroxylase-positive neurons destroyed (r's $= -.18$ and $-.27$). This study is thus encouraging in suggesting a role for this region in REM sleep; however, such histochemically nonspecific lesions cannot offer final proof as to whether these effects are mediated through ChAT-positive or nearby non-ChAT-positive neurons. Cellular physiological studies utilizing double labeling techniques, as described above, will likely be required for definitive conclusions. Despite the need for much additional work, we conclude that the current excitement about and ferment of work on cholinergic systems in REM sleep are indicative of a scientifically very promising line of investigation.

ACKNOWLEDGMENTS

Supported by a Veterans Administration Medical Investigator award & grant to RWM and by NIMH R37 39,683. Collaborators in the more recent work described here are Drs. K. Ito, A. Mitani, A. Hallanger, B. H. Wainer (immunohistochemical study and *in vivo* work), R. W. Greene, U. Gerber, H. L. Haas (*in vitro* study), and S. Massaquoi (modeling). We thank Marie Fairbanks for administrative assistance.

REFERENCES

1. Amatruda TT, Black DA, McCarley RW, Hobson JA. Sleep cycle control and cholinergic mechanisms: Differential effects of carbachol injections at pontine brain stem sites. *Brain Res* 1975; 98:501–515.
2. Armstrong DM, Saper CB, Levey AI, Wainer BH, Terry RD. Distribution of cholinergic neurons in rat brain: Demonstrated by the immunocytochemical localization of choline acetyltransferase. *J Comp Neurol* 1983; 216:53–68.
3. Baghdoyan HA, Monaco AP, Rodrigo-Angulo ML, Assens F, McCarley RW, Hobson JA. Microinjection of neostigmine into the pontine reticular formation enhances desynchronized sleep signs. *J Pharm Exp Therap* 1984; 231:173–180.
4. Baghdoyan HA, McCarley RW, Hobson JA. Cholinergic manipulation of brainstem reticular systems: Effects on desynchronized sleep generation. In A Waquier, J Monti, JP Gaillard, and M Radulovacki (eds.), *Sleep: Neurotransmitters and Neuromodulators*. Raven, New York, 1985: 15–27.
5. Baghdoyan HA, Rodrigo-Angulo ML, McCarley RW, Hobson JA. A neuroanatomical gradient in the pontine tegmentum for the cholinoceptive induction of desynchronized sleep signs. *Brain Res* 1987; 414:245–261.

6. Berman AI. *The Brain Stem of the Cat. A Cytoarchitectonic Atlas with Stereotaxic Coordinates.* University of Wisconsin Press, Madison, 1968.

7. Butcher LL, Marchand R, Parent A, Poirier LJ. Morphological characteristics of acetyl-cholinesterase-containing neurons in the CNS of DFP-treated monkeys. Part 3. Brain stem and spinal cord. *J Neurol Sci* 1977; 32:169–185.

8. Cordeau JP, Moreau A, Beaulnes A, Laurin C. EEG and behavioral changes following microinjections of acetylcholine and adrenaline in the brain stem of cats. *Arch Ital Biol* 1983; 101:30–47.

9. George R, Haslett WL, Jenden DJ. A cholinergic mechanism in the brainstem reticular formation: Induction of paradoxical sleep. *Int J Neuropharmacol* 1964; 3:541–552.

10. Gerber U, Greene RW, McCarley, RW. Repetitive firing properties of medial pontine reticular formation neurones of the rate recorded in vitro. *J Physiol (London)* 1989; 410:533–560.

11. Greene, RW, Carpenter DO. Actions of neurotransmitters on pontine medial reticular formation neurons of the cat. *J Neurophysiol* 1985; 54:520–531.

12. Greene RW, Haas HL, McCarley RW. A low threshold calcium spike mediates firing pattern alterations in pontine reticular neurons. *Science* 1986; 234:738–740.

13. Greene RW, Gerber U, McCarley RW. Cholinergic activation of medial pontine reticular formation neurons in vitro. *Brain Res* 1989; 476:154–159.

14. Hagiwara S, Takahashi S. The anomalous rectification and cation selectivity of the membrane of a starfish egg cell. *J Membr Biol* 1974; 18:61–80.

15. Hallanger AE, Levey AI, Lee HJ, Rye DB, Wainer BH. The origins of cholinergic and other subcortical afferents to the thalamus in the rat. *J Comp Neurol* 1987; 262:105–124.

16. Ito K, McCarley RW. Alterations in membrane potential and excitability of cat medial pontine reticular formation neurons during naturally occurring sleep-wake states. *Brain Res* 1984; 292:169–175.

17. Ito K, McCarley RW. Physiological studies of brainstem reticular connectivity; I. Responses of mPRF neurons to stimulation of bulbar reticular formation. *Brain Res* 1987; 409:97–110.

18. Jasper HH, Tessier J. Acetylcholine liberation from cerebral cortex during paradoxical (REM) sleep. *Science* 1971; 172:601–602.

19. Jones BE, Beaudet A. Distribution of acetylcholine and catecholamine neurons in the cat brain stem studied by choline acetyltransferase and tyrosine hydroxylase immunohisto-chemistry. *J Comp Neurol* 1987; 261:15–32.

20. Katz B. Les constantes électriques de la membrane du muscle. *Arch Sci Physiol* 1949; 3:285.

21. Kimura H, McGeer PL, Peng JH, McGeer EG. The central cholinergic system studied by choline acetyltransferase immunohistochemistry in the cat. *J Comp Neurol* 1981; 200:151–201.

22. Krnjevic K, Pumain R, Renaud L. The mechanism of excitation by acetylcholine in the cerebral cortex. *J Physiol (London)* 1971; 215:247–268.

23. McCarley RW, Hobson JA. Neuronal excitability modulation over the sleep cycle: A structural and mathematical model. *Science* 1975; 189:58–60.

24. McCarley RW, Nelwon JP, Hobson JA. PGO burst neurons: Correlative evidence for neuronal generators of PGO waves. *Science* 1978; 201:209–262.

25. McCarley RW, Ito K. Desynchronized sleep-specific changes in membrane potential and excitability in medial pontine reticular formation neurons: Implications for concepts and mechanisms of behavioral state control. In D McGinty, R Drucker-Colin, A Morrison, and PL Parmeggiani (eds.), *Brain Mechanisms of Sleep.* Raven, New York, 1985: 63–80.

26. McCarley RW, Ito K. Intracellular evidence linking medial pontine reticular formation neurons to PGO wave generation. *Brain Res* 1983; 280:343–348.

27. McCarley RW, Ito K, Rodrigo-Angulo ML. Physiological studies of brainstem reticular

connectivity: II. Responses of mPRF neurons to stimulation of mesencephalic and contralateral pontine reticular formation. *Brain Res* 1987; 409:111–127.

28. McCarley RW, Massaquoi SG. A limit cycle mathematical model of the REM sleep oscillator system. *Am J Physiol* 1986; 251:R1011–R1029.

29. McCormick DA, Prince DA. Actions of acetylcholine in the guinea-pig and cat medial and lateral geniculate nuclei, *in vitro. J Physiol (London)* 1987; 392:147–165.

30. Mesulam M-M, Mufson EJ, Wainer BH, Levey AI. Central cholinergic pathways in the rat: An overview based on an alternative nomenclature (Ch1-Ch6). *Neuroscience* 1983; 10:1185–1201.

31. Mitani A, Ito K, Hallanger AE, Wainer BH, Kataoka K, McCarley RW. Cholinergic projections from the laterodorsal and pedunculopontine tegmental nuclei to the pontine gigantocellular tegmental field in the cat. *Brain Res* 1988; 451:397–402.

32. Mitani A, Ito K, Mitani Y, McCarley RW. Morphological and electrophysiological identification of gigantocellular tegmental field neurons with descending projections in the cat. I. Pons. *J Comp Neurol* 1988; 268:529–545.

33. Mitani A, Ito K, Mitani Y, McCarley RW. Morphological and electrophysiological identification of gigantocellular tegmental field neurons with descending projections in the cat. II. Bulb. *J Comp Neurol* 1988; 274:371–386.

34. Nelson JP, McCarley RW, Hobson JA. REM sleep burst neurons, PGO waves and eye movement information. *J Neurophysiol* 1983; 50:784–797.

35. Newman DB. Distinguishing rat brainstem nuclei by their neuronal morphology. II. Pontine and mesencephalic nuclei. *J Hirnforsch* 1985; 26:385–418.

36. Rye DB, Saper CB, Lee HJ, Wainer BH. Medullary and spinal efferents of the pedunculopontine tegmental nucleus and adjacent mesopontine tegmentum in the rat. *J Comp Neurol* 1988; 269:315–341.

37. Sakai K, Jouvet M. Brain stem PGO-on cells projecting directly to the cat dorsal lateral geniculate nucleus. *Brain Res* 1980; 194:500–505.

38. Sakai K. Neurons responsible for paradoxical sleep. In A Wauquier, JM Gaillard, JM Monti, and M Radulovacki (eds.), *Sleep: Neurotransmitters and Neuromodulators.* Raven, New York, 1985; 29–42.

39. Satoh K, Armstrong DM, Fibiger HC. A comparison of the distribution of central cholinergic neurons as demonstrated by acetylcholinesterase pharmacohistochemistry and choline acetyltransferase immunohistochemistry. *Brain Res Bull* 1983; 11:693–720.

40. Satoh K, Fibiger HC. Cholinergic neurons of the laterodorsal tegmental nucleus: Efferent and afferent connections. *J Comp Neurol* 1986; 253:277–302.

41. Shammah-Lagnado SJ, Negrao N, Silva BA, Richardo JA. Afferent connections of the nuclei reticularis pontis oralis and caudalis: A horseradish peroxidase study in the rat. *Neuroscience* 1987; 20:961–989.

42. Shiromani PJ, Armstrong DM, Gillin JC. Cholinergic neurons from the dorsolateral pons project to the medial pons: a WGA-HRP and choline acetyltransferase immunohistochemical study. *Neurosci Lett* 1988; 95:19–23.

43. Shiromani PJ, McGinty DJ. Pontine neuronal response to local cholinergic infusion: Relation to REM sleep. *Brain Res* 1986; 386:20–31.

44. Steriade M, McCarley RW. *Brainstem Control of Wakefulness and Sleep.* Plenum, New York, 1990.

45. Vanni-Mercier G, Sakai K, Jouvet M. Neurones specifiques de l'éveil dans l'hypothalamus postérieur du Chat. *CR Acad Sci Paris* 1984; 298:195–200.

46. Waquier A, Monti J, Gaillard JP, Radulovacki, eds. *Sleep: Neurotransmitters and Neuromodulators.* Raven, New York, 1985.

47. Webster, HH, Jones BE. Neurotoxic lesions of the dorsolateral pontomesencephalic tegmentum-cholinergic area in the cat. II. Effects upon sleep-waking states. *Brain Res* 1988; 458:285–302.

9

Brainstem Genesis and Thalamic Transfer of Internal Signals during Dreaming Sleep: Cellular Data and Hypotheses

MIRCEA STERIADE AND DENIS PARÉ

Pontogeniculooccipital (PGO) waves are stigmatic events of the stage of sleep with rapid eye movements (REMs). They consist of spiky, initially negative field potentials in the brainstem, thalamus, and depth of the cerebral cortex. Interest in PGO waves stemmed from the discovery that eye movement direction is related to gaze direction in dream imagery of humans (5) coupled with data from animal experiments showing that saccadic REMs are coincident with PGO waves (24). Although PGO waves have not yet been detected in humans, parietooccipital potentials recorded from the human scalp during REM sleep share some similarities with PGO waves of animals, including lateralization according to eye movements (35). These observations led to the consensus that PGO waves are physiological correlates of brain activation during dreaming sleep (14), the stuff that dreams are made off.

PGO waves herald REM sleep by about 30–90 sec and continue throughout the state of REM sleep in cat (Fig. 9-1). This and other aspects of PGO phenomenology have been repeatedly confirmed since their description in the early 1960s (cf. 23). In contrast, very little knowledge has been gained concerning the brainstem generation of PGO events and their thalamic transfer. It is the purpose of this chapter to examine the present status of this problem, to reveal some inconsistencies within current hypotheses, to report what we have done recently, and to indicate the paths for future research on brainstem and thalamic mechanisms underlying PGO activity.

BRAINSTEM GENESIS

The brainstem neurons that transfer PGO waves to thalamocortical systems are located in the pedunculopontine nucleus of the upper reticular core, in and around the brachium conjunctivum (hereafter termed peribrachial, PB, area). Although the PGO waves

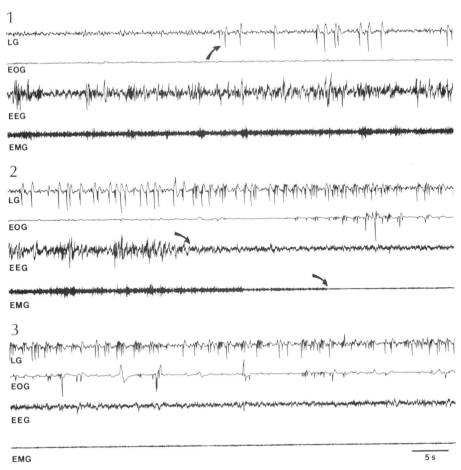

Figure 9-1 Electrographic criteria of sleep states in the cat. 1–3: contiguous epochs. The four ink-written traces represent electrical activity of the LG nucleus recorded by a coaxial electrode, ocular movements (EOG), EEG waves recorded from the anterior suprasylvian gyrus, and electromyographic activity (EMG). The arrow in 1 indicates the start of the pre-REM epoch, beginning with the first PGO wave. The first arrow in 2 points to EEG desynchronization, while the second arrow indicates complete muscular atonia during REM sleep. [From Steriade et al. (53).]

were initially regarded as confined to the visual system, there is now evidence that these phasic events transcend the lateral geniculate (LG) thalamic nucleus and the occipital cortex, since they can be recorded in a variety of nonvisual thalamocortical systems.

Two series of data obtained from experiments conducted in cat have indicated that at least some of the PB cells give rise to the final common path of the brainstem-generated PGO waves: (a) the induction versus reduction or suppression of PGO waves following stimulation versus lesions of the PB area (45,59); and (b) the fact that PB neurons discharge brief bursts of high-frequency spikes 10–20 msec before the wave onset in the LG thalamic nucleus (34,37,44). Although there is no direct evidence for the cholinergic nature of the recorded brainstem neurons that transfer PGO waves to the thalamus, this is likely to be so since (a) the PB area is a major group of cholinergic neurons (22,57) that projects to the visual thalamus (3,49) as well as to all major relay, associational (54), and intralaminar (39) thalamic nuclei of cat; (b) 80% of the PB cells projecting to the LG nucleus are cholinergic (3,49); and (c) thalamic PGO waves induced by PB stimulation are abolished by iontophoretic injections of nicotinic antagonists into the cat LG nucleus (17).

Concerning the brainstem mechanism of PGO genesis, the current hypothesis favored by most authors involves the reciprocal discharge of two pontine (cholinergic and monoaminergic) neuronal groups. Assuming that monoaminergic neurons of the locus coeruleus (LC) and dorsal raphe (DR) nuclei exert inhibitory actions on REM-on cholinergic neurons, it was proposed that during REM sleep the enhanced excitability of brainstem cholinergic neurons occurs through a disinhibitory process consequent to the suppressed activity of LC and DR neurons (15,31,41,42, and chapter 8, this volume).

This hypothesis still awaits direct testing. Although disinhibition could eventually account for tonic excitatory phenomena observed in numerous mesopontine neurons throughout REM sleep, it is not adequate to explain the genesis of PGO-related spike bursts. Indeed, as a rule, the mechanism of such stereotyped events, characterized by short duration (20–30 msec) and high intraburst frequency, is a slow, calcium-mediated, low-threshold spike (LTS), deinactivated by membrane hyperpolarization, and crowned by high-frequency, fast, sodium-mediated, conventional action potentials (see 52, for a review). The LTS was discovered in the inferior olive (30) and was thereafter found in various thalamic neurons (6,20,21,40,51,56) as well as pontine (9), lateral parabrachial (29), and laterodorsal tegmental (60) brainstem neurons. Since LTSs appear at hyperpolarized levels, PGO-related bursts should be generated by any impulse impinging on a hyperpolarized, rather than a disinhibited, PB neuron.

We then hypothesize that PGO-related bursts of PB neurons are generated by any excitatory volley reaching the cells during a steady hyperpolarized state and/or are induced by phasic hyperpolarizations of sufficient amplitudes to trigger a rebound excitation. The former mechanism (steady hyperpolarization) would operate in PGO-on bursting neurons that are otherwise silent during REM sleep, such as already described (37,44), whereas the latter mechanism (phasic hyperpolarizations) would sculpture PGOs from a background of tonic discharge during REM sleep, as we have detected in current experiments.

Where should we search for the progenitors of the hyperpolarization of PB and other possible PGO-command cells during REM-sleep?

1. The GABAergic neurons of the substantia nigra pars reticulata (SNr) may represent one of the inhibitory sources acting on PGO generators. The connections between SNr and PB have been established by means of tracing techniques (2) and electrophysiological analyses (37a,46). SNr neurons contact pedunculopontine neurons with terminals containing pleomorphic vesicles at symmetrical synaptic junctions, that is compatible with the idea of inhibitory SNr-PB actions. To test this hypothesis, simultaneous recordings of thalamically projecting PB neurons and SNr cells antidromically identified from the PB area should be performed. The prediction is that the period of silence preceding the PGO-related bursts in PB neurons would be associated

with phasically increased activity of GABAergic SNr neurons. The source of the hypothesized spike barrages of SNr cells during REM sleep remains to be determined.

This idea extends the demonstrated role played by SNr cells in waking orienting reactions to a similar role during the other brain-activated state, REM sleep. It is now established that GABAergic SNr neurons decrease their firing rates on novel sensory stimuli during the waking state. One consequence of this reduced firing of SNr cells is disinhibition of their superior collicular targets, thus eventually leading to excitation of premotor ocular neurons through colicullopontine projections and to eye movements directed toward the stimulus (11,12). PGO waves may be regarded as a sign of brain responses to internally generated signals during REM sleep, an "inside" orienting reaction whose external reflection is aborted because of motoneuronal hyperpolarization. This view is supported by the oneiric behavior of animals with adequate dorsolateral pontine lesions to suppress muscular atonia during REM sleep (10,25). In addition, the entire repertoire of hallucinatory behaviors similar to those occurring during REM sleep (watching imaginary enemies, fear, groping movements, and attack) can be elicited by microinjections of glutamate analogues into and near the PB area of awake animals (27). Thus, similar behaviors can be released in REM sleep and wakefulness. As to the underlying mechanisms, however, the activity of collicular-projecting SNr neurons related to orienting reactions during wakefulness should be different from that of PB-projecting SNr cells possibly involved in PGO-burst genesis during REM sleep, since the former are silenced on sensory orienting stimuli whereas the latter are hypothesized to discharge upon internally generated signals.

2. The other, nonexclusive possibility is that hyperpolarization of some PGO-burst PB neurons results from the tonic firing of the majority of cholinergic PB cells during REM sleep (50a). The latter would hyperpolarize adjacent PGO-on burst cells through local axonal collaterals, taking into consideration data from *in vitro* experiments indicating that acetylcholine hyperpolarizes brainstem neurons in some areas surrounding the brachium conjunctivum, an action that is due to activation of a potassium conductance via an M2 muscarinic receptor (29a).

Although the PGO-on burst cells in and near the PB area are commonly regarded as representing the unique class of neurons for the transfer of PGO signals to the thalamus, little can be found in the literature about their activity in relation to other behavioral states and about their incidence among brainstem neurons. The only indications are that some of the PGO-burst neurons also display short bursts (44) or single spikes (37) in association with eye-movement potentials (EMPs) during wakefulness. Puzzlingly, the study (37) in which the number of PGO-on cells out of the total sample of brainstem elements is provided forces us to conclude that neurons that selectively discharge in close temporal relation with thalamic PGO waves represent the exception, rather than the rule, in the upper brainstem core. In our experiments (53a), microelectrode tracks are identified on NADPH-diaphorase-stained sections, where cholinergic cells of the PB and laterodorsal tegmental (LDT) nuclei can be readily identified (see 58). This method allows us to emphasize the very low proportion (less than 5%) of PGO-on burst cells among PB and LDT as well as noncholinergic neurons of adjacent brainstem reticular fields.

What is, then, the PGO-related behavior of the overwhelming majority of mesopontine neurons? We have recently detected at least three other neuronal types that increase or cease their discharges in close temporal relation with PGO waves recorded from the LG thalamic nucleus (53a).

1. Some brainstem PB neurons discharge high-frequency spike bursts related to every PGO wave but, unlike the otherwise silent PGO-burst cells discussed before, they also exhibit a tonic increase in spontaneous firing during REM sleep. Moreover, these PGO-related bursts are preceded by an acceleration of background firing and their incidence is higher with increasing frequencies of spontaneous discharges, thus raising the intriguing possibility that these bursts are generated at relatively depolarized levels (Fig. 9-2A). This is clearly different from the mechanism of the already described PGO-related burst that, as we have postulated above, probably represents an LTS deinactivated by membrane hyperpolarization. The type of burst depicted in Figure 9-2A has been characterized in medial mammillary neurons studied in vitro as a calcium-dependent plateau potential (1) that may be generated in dendrites, by contrast with the somatic genesis of the LTS.

2. The activity of other neurons is exclusively related to PGO events. They display a progressive increase in firing rate, reaching quite high discharge frequencies (over 100 Hz), reliably preceding by hundreds of msec clusters of PGO waves and related ocular saccades. Such precursor signs occur much earlier than those reported for the short-lead PGO-on burst cells (about 10–20 msec before the thalamic PGO waves) or for the somewhat longer lead (50–300 msec) neurons recorded from the medial pontine reticular formation (32). Various chronological steps in the development of PGO-related discharges do probably reflect, at least partially, the cascade of excitatory connections within reticuloreticular networks (19,33,43).

3. Still another type of mesopontine neurons discharges tonically, at high rates, during epochs of REM sleep without PGO events and decreases their discharges about 300 msec before and during the PGO wave (Fig. 9-2B). Such PGO-off neurons are obviously not aminergic because all available data indicate that LC and DR neurons are virtually silent during REM sleep (cf. 16). The discovery of GABAergic neurons in the LDT nucleus (28) raises the possibility that those PGO-off neurons are GABAergic and that their silenced firing during PGO waves could disinhibit the adjacent cholinergic cells displaying tonically increased firing during PGO waves, as we have encountered in current experiments. The PGO-off (not REM-off) neurons may belong to the same family of inhibitory neurons known as the eye-movement-related omnipause neurons located near the midline in the caudal pons (38,55). According to the current view, omnipause neurons would disinhibit premotor ocular neurons by ceasing their tonic discharge (6a,26,36). Whether the cell depicted in Figure 9-2B is an omnipause cell whose silence leads to a saccade and consequently to a corrolary discharge generating a PGO wave, and whether the decreased firing of PGO-off cells can disinhibit PGO-on neurons independently of any eye movement, remains to be elucidated. As known, PGO waves do not exclusively occur in relation with REMs, since they appear during the pre-REM epoch, without concomitant ocular saccades (see Fig. 9-1).

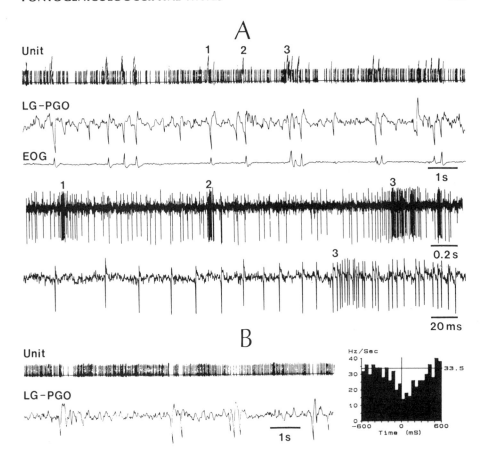

Figure 9-2 PGO-related discharges of two (A and B) cat brainstem reticular neurons during REM sleep. (A) Neuron in the dorsal part of the pedunculopontine nucleus discharging high-frequency spike bursts (over a tonically increased background firing) in close time relation with PGO waves recorded from the LG thalamic nucleus and eye movements. Three of such bursts (1, 2, 3 on the top ink-written record) are depicted with original spikes at two speeds. See text. (B) Neuron in the medial part of the pedunculopontine nucleus, diminishing its rate of spontaneous firing or ceasing its discharges during PGO waves recorded from the LG thalamic nucleus. Peri-PGO histograms (50-msec bins) obtained from 20 singly or clustered PGO events. The rate of spontaneous rate is indicated (33.5 Hz). [Modified from Steriade et al. (53a.).]

All of the above observations and hypotheses point to the great variety of brainstem neurons involved in PGO genesis and the complexity of the underlying mechanisms. The electrophysiological properties of PGO-on neurons should now be investigated intracellularly in simplified, brainstem-transected preparations.

THALAMIC TRANSFER

The cellular mechanisms of thalamic PGO waves have been investigated in our laboratory in two types of experiments conducted in the LG-perigeniculate thalamic complex of cat. The general methodology of these studies is discussed below.

1. The first type of experiments involved the intracellular recording of LG responses to brainstem-generated PGO volleys, to shed light on the neuronal classes involved in the excitatory and inhibitory events related to various components of PGO thalamic field potentials. By necessity, the best experimental condition would be the chronically implanted animal that displays spontaneous fluctuations of waking and sleep states. Although a few such experiments have been carried out in the LG thalamic nucleus (8,13), they did not reveal the electrophysiological bases of thalamic PGO events. In fact, intracellular analyses of thalamic neurons in naturally sleeping and arousing animals meet the extreme difficulty to have stable recordings and to adequately monitor the resting membrane potential of neurons under an intense synaptic bombardment, as is the case in the unanesthetized, brain-intact animal. Hence, precise questions concerning the electrophysiological bases of thalamic PGO waves should be answered in acute, simplified experimental conditions. At least two requirements must be fulfilled in such studies. (a) First, both retinae and ipsilateral visual cortex must be removed to suppress the intense activity in major afferent projections to the LG nucleus and to preclude the possibility that LG responses to brainstem PB stimulation are mediated by circuitous pathways, especially involving the visual cortex. (b) The second point concerns the choice of the anesthetic. Previous intracellular studies were conducted under barbiturate anesthesia and the conclusion was drawn that the brainstem-induced increase in LG-cell excitability is the result of a process of disinhibition, rather than a direct excitation of LG cells (47,48). It is now known that even very small (2 mg/kg) doses of barbiturate abolish the acetylcholine (ACh)-induced excitation of LG neurons (7). Since the brainstem-generated PGO volley is transferred to the thalamus through a cholinergic pathway, we used urethane as anesthetic, while PGO waves were induced by reserpine (a monoamine depletor that precipitates PGO waves) or by electrical stimulation of the brainstem PB area in reserpinized preparations (18).

2. In the second type of experiments, extracellular recordings of LG and perigeniculate neurons (physiologically identified by their typical responses to optic chiasm stimulation) were performed in chronically implanted, naturally sleeping cats (53). Here, the major concern was the comparison of LG-cell responses to the PGO volleys during two distinct stages of the sleep cycle: the pre-REM epoch, with PGO waves occurring over a background of EEG synchronization and the fully developed REM sleep with all its major signs, including EEG desynchronization (see Fig. 9-1). The rationale behind our searching for distinct activity patterns in LG neurons during these two sleep stages was that EEG-synchronized versus EEG-desynchronized behavioral states are characterized by opposed firing mode and excitability of thalamic cells (50,52). It was particularly expected that the thalamic response to the PGO volley during the pre-REM epoch with EEG synchronization when LG neurons are hyperpolarized (13) begins with a spike burst, whereas the burst would be inactivated during REM sleep when the membrane potential of LG relay cells is relatively depolarized (see previous details on LTS). As shown below, this is indeed the case and it can explain the higher amplitudes of PGO field potentials during the pre-REM epoch, as

compared to REM sleep. This and other data related to the signal-to-noise ratio (PGO signal-to-background firing) led us to speculate about the vivid imagery of dream mentation during the epoch immediately preceding REM sleep.

Intracellular Data in Acute Experiments

The reserpine- or brainstem-induced PGO waves are biphasic, initially negative field potentials. A second negative deflection or a negative notch may be superimposed on the rising phase of the late, longer lasting field positivity (Fig. 9-3). Intracellular recordings of LG neurons in the vicinity of the macroelectrode used for field potentials revealed that (a) the initial negativity of the PGO wave was associated with a depolarizing potential (with occasional spikes) lasting about 200–300 msec, increasing on cell

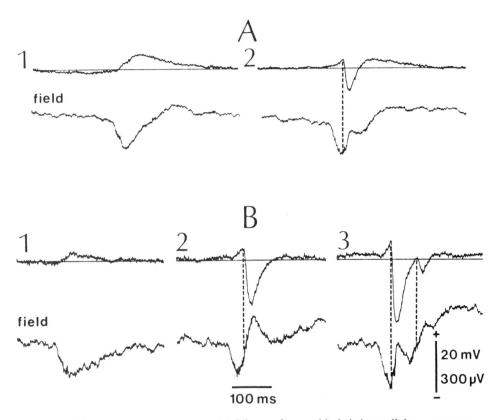

Figure 9-3 Sample of reserpine-induced PGO waveforms with their intracellular counterparts taken from two LG neurons of cat (A and B). Urethane anesthesia. Negative PGO waves showing a smooth return toward the baseline were usually correlated with pure depolarizing events in LG neurons (A1 and B1). When the negativity was interrupted by a positive going deflection, a prominent IPSP was always present in the intracellular traces (A2, B2–3). Double notched PGO waveforms were correlated with the appearance of a second IPSP in the traces (B3). Vertical lines indicate the IPSP onset and emphasize the close time relation between IPSPs and the positive upswing in the field potentials. All cells were slightly hyperpolarized to prevent spike discharges. [From Hu et al. (18).]

hyperpolarization, and eventually triggering an LTS; (b) when the negative phase of the PGO was interrupted by a sharp positive deflection, a prominent inhibitory postsynaptic potential (IPSP) appeared (Fig. 9-3, A2, B2–3); this IPSP became depolarizing on intracellular chloride injection; (c) the late, slow field positivity could not be related to a distinct intracellular event. Intracellular injections of hyperpolarizing current pulses demonstrated a 25–40% drop in input resistance during PGO waves, even when the PGO-related intracellular events lacked their hyperpolarizing component.

These intracellular events indicate that both relay neurons and at least some local-circuit LG neurons are excited by the brainstem-generated PGO volley. The early depolarization of relay cells is probably nicotinic in nature as iontophoretic application of nicotonic antagonists (mecamylamine or hexamethonium) blocks the PGO field potentials in the LG as well as the PGO-related early excitation of LG relay cells (17). On the other hand, the unitary chloride-dependent IPSP that interrupts the early depolarization of relay cells is generated within the LG nucleus and is probably mediated through a parallel activation of GABAergic local-circuit elements. This assumption is supported by the fact that the other class of GABAergic neurons operating on LG thalamocortical neurons in a recurrent inhibitory circuit, namely the perigeniculate cells, was very infrequently activated by the PGO volley in the acute conditions under which these experiments were performed. As shown below, the PGO cholinergic volley consistently excites GABAergic PG neurons in the chronically implanted animal, possibly because such an excitation is voltage dependent and requires the powerful excitatory impingement of the corticothalamic projection.

Extracellular Data in Chronically Implanted, Naturally Sleeping Animals

Whereas perigeniculate neurons discharged bursts of action potentials superimposed on the peak negativity of PGO field potentials during both pre-REM and REM sleep, the activity of LG neurons was quite different in these two sleep stages. (a) During the pre-REM epoch, the activity of LG relay cells started with a short (7–15 msec), high-frequency (300–500 Hz) spike burst coinciding with the negativity of the PGO field potential, and continued with a train of single spikes at 50–80 Hz, lasting for 200–400 msec, superimposed on the declining phase of the negative field potential and the subsequent slow positivity. (b) During REM sleep, the rate of LG-cells' spontaneous discharges was 1.5- to 3-fold higher than in pre-REM, the peak-to-peak amplitudes of PGO waves were 2–3 times lower, and the PGO-related activity of LG neurons lacked the initial high-frequency burst that characterized the pre-REM epoch (Fig. 9-4). The peri-PGO histograms of unit discharges in the two LG cells depicted in Figure 9-5 show that the signal-to-noise ratio reached values of about 6 to 7 during the pre-REM epoch, whereas the values during REM sleep were between about 1.5 and 2.5.

Two main findings emerge from our study. They relate to the presence of initial spike bursts and to the higher PGO-to-spontaneous firing ratio during the pre-REM epoch, as compared to REM sleep.

If the initial high-frequency spike bursts that initiate the PGO-related activity of LG neurons were occurring synchronously in pools of LG cells, it would explain why PGO field potentials of the pre-REM epoch have a significantly higher amplitude than PGO waves of the REM sleep.

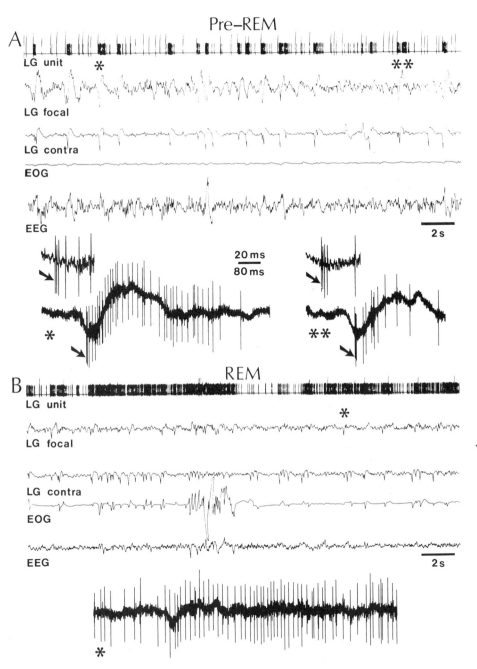

Figure 9-4 PGO-related activity of an LG neuron during the pre-REM epoch (A) and REM sleep (B) in the chronically implanted cat. In both pre-REM and REM sleep, the ink-written records depict unit discharges (deflections exceeding the common level of single spikes represent high-frequency bursts), focal waves recorded by the same microelectrode in the LG nucleus, electrical activity in the contralateral LG nucleus recorded by a coaxial electrode, eye movements (EOG), and EEG rhythms over the neocortical surface. In both pre-REM and REM sleep, PGO-related activity is depicted with original spikes below each ink-written recording. Asterisks mark corresponding PGOs in ink-written and oscilloscopic recordings. Note the tonically increased firing rate in REM sleep, the smaller amplitudes of PGO field potentials in REM sleep (compared to pre-REM epoch), and the absence of PGO-related spike bursts in REM sleep (contrasting with their presence, arrows, in pre-REM). [From Steriade et al. (53).]

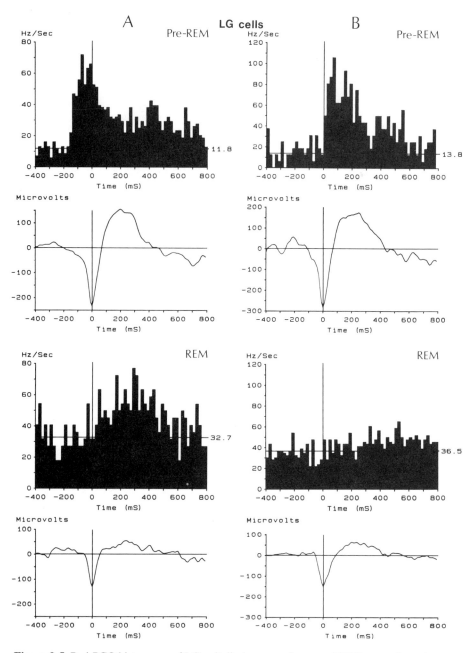

Figure 9-5 Peri-PGO histograms of LG unit discharges and averaged PGO waves from the same epochs during pre-REM and REM sleep. (A and B) Two cells. The average level of spontaneous discharges (11.8 Hz, etc.) is also indicated in each histogram. (A) Nineteen PGO events in pre-REM and 11 PGO events in REM-sleep; (B) 8 PGO events in pre-REM and 23 PGO events in REM-sleep. [From Steriade et al. (53).]

The higher signal-to-noise ratio observed in the pre-REM epoch suggests that vivid imagery may appear well before REM sleep, during a period of apparent EEG-synchronized sleep. For those who may be reluctant to envisage dreaming mentation in relation to experiments conducted in cats, let us mention again that, if adequate pontine lesions are made to prevent muscular atonia, cats display an oneiric behavior during REM sleep (see details under "Brainstem Genesis"). These speculations on the vividness of dreaming mentation during the pre-REM epoch corroborate earlier experiments by Dement and colleagues (1969) on the rebound (or compensation) after REM sleep deprivation. Instead of depriving cats of REM sleep (the standard deprivation), they interrupted sleep immediately after the occurrence of the first PGO wave and eliminated about 20 sec of the EEG-synchronized sleep that precipitates into the fully developed REM sleep. This comparison between classical REM sleep deprivation and "PGO deprivation" led to the conclusion that "the crucial factor in the so-called REM-sleep deprivation–compensation phenomenon is the deprivation of phasic events." And the increase in total REM sleep time after deprivation was regarded "as a response to an accumulated need for phasic events, rather than a response to the loss of REM-sleep per se" (4, pp. 310–311). Researches are now invited to explore the dreaming imagery during the period immediately preceding REM sleep in humans.

ACKNOWLEDGMENTS

This work was supported by the Medical Research Council of Canada (Grant MT-3689). D. Paré is an MRC fellow.

REFERENCES

1. Alonso A, Llinás R. Electrophysiology of guinea pig mammillary bodies *in vitro. Soc Neurosci Abstr* 1987; 13:536.
2. Beckstead RM. Long collateral branches of substantia nigra pars reticulata axons to the thalamus, superior colliculus and reticular formation in monkey and cat. Multiple retrograde neuronal labeling with fluorescent dyes. *Neuroscience* 1983; 10:767–779.
3. DeLima AD, Singer W. The brainstem projection to the lateral geniculate nucleus in the cat: Identification of cholinergic and monoaminergic elements. *J Comp Neurol* 1987; 259:92–121.
4. Dement W, Ferguson J, Cohen H, Barchas J. Nonchemical methods and data using a biochemical model: the REM quanta. In A Mandell and MP Mandell (eds.), *Psychochemical Research in Man—Methods, Strategy and Theory.* Academic Press, New York, 1969:275–325.
5. Dement W, Kleitman N. The relation of eye movements during sleep to dream activity: An objective method for the study of dreaming. *J Exp Psychol* 1957; 53:339–346.
6. Deschênes M. Paradis M, Roy JP, Steriade M. Electrophysiology of neurons of lateral thalamic nuclei in cat: Resting properties and burst discharges. *J Neurophysiol* 1984; 51:1196–1219.
6a. Evinger C, Kaneko CRS, Johanson GW, Fuchs AF. Omnipause cells in the cat. In R Baker and A Berthoz (eds.), *Control of Gaze by Brain Stem Neurons. Developments in Neuroscience,* Vol. 1. Elsevier/North-Holland Biomedical Press, Amsterdam, 1977: 337–340.

7. Eysel UT, Pape HC, van Schayck R. Excitatory and differential disinhibitory actions of acetylcholine in the lateral geniculate nucleus of the cat. *J Physiol London* 1986; 370:233–254.

8. Fourment A, Hirsch JC, Marc ME. Oscillations of the spontaneous slow-wave sleep rhythm in lateral geniculate nucleus relay neurons of behaving cats. *Neuroscience* 1985; 14:1061–1075.

9. Greene RW, Haas HL, McCarley RW. A low-threshold calcium spike mediates firing pattern alterations in pontine reticular neurons. *Science* 1986; 234:738–740.

10. Hendricks JC, Morrison AR, Mann GL. Different behaviors during paradoxical sleep without atonia depend on pontine lesion site. *Brain Res* 1982; 239:81–105.

11. Hikosaka O, Wurtz RH. Visual and oculomotor functions of monkey substantia nigra pars reticulata. Relation of visual and auditory responses to saccades. *J Neurophysiol* 1983; 49:1230–1253.

12. Hikosaka O, Wurtz RH. Visual and oculomotor functions of monkey substantia nigra pars reticulata. IV. Relation of substantia nigra to superior colliculus. *J Neurophysiol* 1983; 49:1285–1301.

13. Hirsch JC, Fourment A, Marc ME. Sleep-related variations of membrane potential in the lateral geniculate body relay neurons of the cat. *Brain Res* 1983; 259:308–312.

14. Hobson JA. *The Dreaming Brain*. Basic Books, New York, 1988: 319.

15. Hobson JA, McCarley RW, Wyzinski PW. Sleep cycle oscillation: Reciprocal discharge by two brainstem neuronal groups. *Science* 1975; 189:55–58.

16. Hobson JA, Steriade M. The neuronal basis of behavioral state control. In VB Mountcastle and FE Bloom (eds.), *Handbook of Physiology, The Nervous System, Sect. 1, Vol. IV, Internal Regulatory Systems*. American Physiological Society, Bethesda, 1986: 701–823.

17. Hu B, Bouhasssira D, Steriade M, Deschênes M. The blockage of ponto-geniculo-occipital waves in the cat lateral geniculate nucleus by nicotinic antagonists. *Brain Res* 1988; 473:394–397.

18. Hu B, Steriade M, Deschênes M. The cellular mechanism of thalamic ponto-geniculo-occipital (PGO) waves. *Neuroscience* 1989; 31:25–35.

19. Ito K, McCarley RW. Physiological studies of brainstem reticular connectivity. I. Responses of mPRF neurons to stimulation of bulbar reticular formation. *Brain Res* 1987; 309:97–110.

20. Jahnsen H, Llinás R. Electrophysiological properties of guinea-pig thalamic neurones: An *in vitro* study. *J Physiol London* 1984; 349:205–226.

21. Jahnsen H, Llinás R. Ionic basis for the electroresponsivenes and oscillatory properties of guinea-pig thalamic neurones *in vitro*. *J Physiol London* 1984; 349:227–247.

22. Jones BE, Beaudet A. Distribution of acetylcholine and catecholamine neurons in the cat brain stem studies by choline acetyltransferase and tyrosine hydroxylase immunohisto-chemistry. *J Comp Neurol* 1987; 261:15–32.

23. Jouvet M. Neurophysiology of the state of sleep. *Physiol Rev* 1967; 47:117–177.

24. Jouvet M. The role of monoamines and acetylcholine-containing neurons in the regulation of the sleep-waking cycle. *Ergebn Physiol* 1972; 64:166–307.

25. Jouvet M, Delorme JF. Locus coeruleus et sommeil paradoxal. *CR Soc Biol Paris* 1965; 159:895–899.

26. Keller EL. Control of saccadic eye movements by midline brain stem neurons. In R Baker and A Berthoz (eds.), *Control of Gaze by Brain Stem Neurons. Developments in Neuroscience*, Vol 1. Elsevier/North-Holland Biomedical, Amsterdam, 1977: 327–336.

27. Kitsikis A, Steriade M. Immediate behavioral effects of kainic acid injections into the midbrain reticular core. *Behav Brain Res* 1981; 3:361–380.

28. Kosaka T, Kosaka K, Hataguchi Y, Nagatsu I, Wu JY, Ottersen OP, Storm-Mathisen J, Hama K. Catecholaminergic neurons containing GABA-like and/or glutamic acid decarbox-

ylase-like immunoreactivities in various brain regions of the rat. *Exp Brain Res* 1987; 66:191–210.

29. Leonard CS, Llinás R. Low threshold calcium conductance in parabrachial reticular neurons studied *in vitro* and its blockade by 1-octanol. *Soc Neurosci Abstr* 1987; 13:1012.

29a. Leonard CS, Llinás R. Electrophysiology of thalamic-projecting cholinergic brainstem neurons and their inhibition by ACh. *Soc Neurosci Abstr* 1988; 14:297.

30. Llinás R, Yarom Y. Electrophysiology of mammalian inferior olivary neurones *in vitro*. *J Physiol London* 1981; 315:549–567.

31. McCarley RW, Hobson JA. Neuronal excitability modulation over the sleep cycle: A structural and mathematical model. *Science* 1975; 189:58–60.

32. McCarley RW, Ito K. Intracellular evidence linking medial pontine reticular formation neurons to PGO wave generation. *Brain Res* 1983; 280:343–348.

33. McCarley RW, Ito K, Rodrigo-Angulo ML. Physiological studies of brainstem reticular connectivity. II. Responses of mPRF neurons to stimulation of mesencephalic and contralateral pontine reticular formation. *Brain Res* 1987; 409:111–127.

34. McCarley RW, Nelson JP, Hobson JA. Ponto-geniculo-occipital (PGO) burst neurons: Correlative evidence for neuronal generators of PGO waves. *Science* 1978; 201:269–272.

35. McCarley RW, Winkelman JW, Duffy FH. Human cerebral potentials associated with REM sleep rapid eye movements: Links to PGO waves and waking potentials. *Brain Res* 1983; 274:359–364.

36. Nakao S, Curthoys IS, Markham CH. Direct inhibitory projection of pause neurons to nystagmus-related pontomedullary reticular burst neurons in the cat. *Exp Brain Res* 1980; 40:283–293.

37. Nelson JP, McCarley RW, Hobson JA. REM sleep burst neurons, PGO waves, and eye movement information. *J Neurophysiol* 1983; 50:784–797.

37a. Noda T, Oka H. Nigral inputs to the pedunculopontine region: intracellular analysis. *Brain Res* 1984; 322:223–227.

38. Ohgaki T, Curthoys IS, Markham CH. Anatomy of physiologically identified eye-movement-related pause neurons in the cat: Pontomedullary region. *J Comp Neurol* 1987; 266:56–72.

39. Paré D, Smith Y, Parent A, Steriade M. Projections of brainstem core cholinergic and non-cholinergic neurons of cat to intralaminar and reticular thalamic nuclei. *Neuroscience* 1988; 25:69–86.

40. Paré D, Steriade M, Deschênes M, Oakson G. Physiological properties of anterior thalamic nuclei, a group devoid of inputs from the reticular thalamic nucleus. *J Neurophysiol* 1987; 57:1669–1685.

41. Pompeiano O, Hoshino K. Central control of posture: Reciprocal discharge by two pontine neuronal groups leading to suppression of decerebrate rigidity. *Brain Res* 1976; 116:131–138.

42. Pompeiano O, Valentinuzzi M. A mathematical model for the mechanism of rapid eye movements induced by an anticholinersterase in the decerebrate cat. *Arch Ital Biol* 1976; 114:103–154.

43. Ropert N, Steriade M. Input-output organization of the midbrain reticular core. *J Neurophysiol* 1981; 46:17–31.

44. Sakai K, Jouvet M. Brain stem PGO-on cells projecting directly to the cat dorsal lateral geniculate nucleus. *Brain Res* 1980; 194:500–505.

45. Sakai K, Petitjean F, Jouvet M. Effects of ponto-mesencephalic lesions and electrical stimulation upon PGO waves and EMPs in unanesthetized cats. *Electroenceph Clin Neurophysiol* 1976; 41:49–63.

46. Scarnati E, Proia A, DiLoreto S, Pacitti C. The reciprocal electrophysiological influence between the nucleus tegmenti pedunculopontinus and the substantia nigra in normal and decorticated rat. *Brain Res* 1987; 423:116–124.

47. Singer W. The effect of mesencephalic reticular stimulation on intracellular potentials of cat lateral geniculate neurons. *Brain Res* 1973; 61:35–54.

48. Singer W. Control of thalamic transmission by corticofugal and ascending reticular pathways in the visual system. *Physiol Rev* 1977; 57:386–420.

49. Smith Y, Paré D, Deschênes M, Parent A, Steriade M. Cholinergic and non-cholinergic projections from the upper brainstem core to the visual thalamus in the cat. *Exp Brain Res* 1988; 70:166–180.

50. Steriade M. The excitatory-inhibitory response sequence in thalamic and neocortical cells: State-related changes and regulatory systems. In GM Edelman, WE Gall, and WM Cowan (eds.), *Dynamic Aspects of Neocortical Function*. Wiley-Interscience, New York, 1984: 107–157.

50a. Steriade M, Datta S, Paré D, Oakson G, Curró Dossi R. Neuronal activities in brain-stem cholinergic nuclei related to tonic activation processes in thalamocortical systems. *J Neurosci* 1990 (in press).

51. Steriade M, Deschênes M, Domich L, Mulle C. Abolition of spindle oscillations in thalamic neurons disconnected from nucleus reticularis thalami. *J Neurophysiol* 1985; 54:1473–1497.

52. Steriade M, Llinás RR. The functional states of the thalamus and the associated neuronal interplay. *Physiol Rev* 1988; 68:649–742.

53. Steriade M, Paré D, Bouhassira D, Deschênes M, Oakson G. Phasic activation of lateral geniculate and perigeniculate thalamic neurons during sleep with ponto-geniculo-occipital waves. *J Neurosci* 1989; 9:2215–2229.

53a. Steriade M, Paré D, Datta S, Oakson G, Curró Dossi R. Different cellular types in mesopontine cholinergic nuclei related to ponto-geniculo-occipital waves. *J Neurosci* 1990 (in press).

54. Steriade M, Paré D, Parent A, Smith Y. Projections of cholinergic and non-cholinergic neurons of the brainstem core to relay and associational thalamic nuclei in the cat and macaque monkey. *Neuroscience* 1988; 25:47–67.

55. Strassman A, Evinger C, McCrea RA, Baker RG, Highstein SM. Anatomy and physiology of intracellularly labelled omnipause neurons in the cat and squirrel monkey. *Exp Brain Res* 1987; 67:436–440.

56. Thompson AM. Inhibitory postsynaptic potentials evoked in thalamic neurons by stimulation of the reticularis nucleus evoke slow spikes in isolated rat brain slices. *Neuroscience* 1988; 25:491–502.

57. Vincent SR, Reiner PB. The immunohistochemical localization of choline acetyltransferase in the cat brain. *Brain Res Bull* 1987; 18:371–415.

58. Vincent SR, Sato K, Armstrong DM, Fibiger HC. NADPH-diaphorase: A selective histochemical marker for the cholinergic neurons of the pontine reticular formation. *Neurosci Lett* 1983; 43:31–36.

59. Webster HH, Jones BE. Neurotoxic lesions of the dorsolateral pontomesencephalic tegmentum-cholinergic cell area in the cat. II. Effects upon sleep-waking states. *Brain Res* 1988; 458:285–302.

60. Wilcox KS, Grant SJ, Cristoph GR. Electrophysiological properties of lateral dorsal tegmental neurons *in vitro*. *Soc Neurosci Abstr* 1987; 13:537.

10

Putative Sleep Neuromodulators

JAMES M. KRUEGER, FERENC OBÁL, JR., MARK OPP,
ALAN B. CADY, LARS JOHANNSEN, LINDA TOTH, AND
JEANNINE MAJDE

The postulate that a sleep-promoting substance(s) (sleep factor: SF) accumulates in the brain during wakefulness had its origin in the ancient observation that prolonged wakefulness results in a strong propensity for sleep. The intense efforts to characterize SFs over the past 20 years have been stimulated by the expectation that such investigations would help to elucidate the function and brain mechanisms of sleep. Early in the twentieth century, the groups of Ishimori (66) and Pieron (98) demonstrated the presence of sleep-promoting substances in cerebrospinal fluid. Over the next 50 years, some attempts to repeat these experiments were successful (51,123,134). Within the past few years, a variety of substances have been proposed as putative SFs (reviewed, 87; also see Fig. 10-2), and other SFs have been described but are not yet characterized. Therefore, the field of SFs is in a very active phase, and some of the proposed SFs have already yielded new hypotheses for the functions of sleep (94).

The existence of multiple endogenous substances with the capacity to promote sleep has undermined the original hypothesis postulating a single specific factor with actions confined to sleep. One solution to this dilemma is to assume that only one of the reported sleep-promoting substances (or yet another unidentified substance) is the true SF, and that the effects of the others can be attributed to special experimental conditions. In the discussion that follows, we will argue that such an assumption is unwarranted on both theoretical and experimental grounds.

There are many variables that have a great impact on sleep–wake activity in addition to the influences of prior wakefulness and time of day. For example, sleep is promoted by food intake, mildly warm ambient temperature, infectious diseases, and immobility; all these conditions provide separate inputs for sleep regulation. Electrical or chemical stimulations of many structures in the brain elicit sleep or sleep-like encephalographic (EEG) activity. Lesions in various brain regions induce insomnia followed by partial or complete recovery of sleep. McGinty concluded that sleep is regulated via numerous independent neuronal networks at all levels of the neuraxis (105). Sleep involves changes in the function of most behavioral, psychological, and physiological variables. The various brain areas implicated in sleep regulation may be modulated by such variables. Signals from all these functions may also serve as inputs for sleep regulation. This regulation, with its complex organization and many inputs, is not likely to occur exclusively via one substance. Instead, sleep, like all other physiological systems, is probably regulated by multiple endogenous substances that also have multiple physiological actions.

We will discuss sleep regulation by SFs within the context of two models. The first model (Fig. 10-1) presents a view of how several SFs may interact to induce sleep. The discussion of this model brings SFs into focus in terms of their specificity to sleep, organization of neuronal networks in reference to sleep, and what bearing this organization has on SFs. The second model (Fig. 10-2) attempts to tie together the actions of several putative SFs on the basis of their known interactions in the brain and other physiological systems. For the involvement of monoaminergic and other transmitter systems in sleep regulation, we refer to the model proposed by Koella (78).

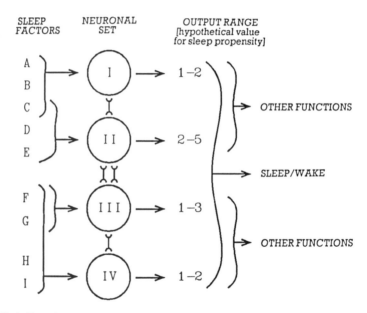

Figure 10-1 Sleep factor interaction with neuronal sets. A sleep factor is defined as a substance that can enhance or inhibit sleep under appropriate conditions and whose concentration–metabolism–receptors are dependent, in part, on past sleep–wake activity. A neuronal set is defined as a collection of neurons that responds to a set of SFs. Although unlikely, any given neuronal set may be associated with a specific neurotransmitter. Because certain SFs (e.g., IL-1, GRF) induce the synthesis–release of certain mitogens (e.g., IL-2) and/or growth factors (e.g., GH), it is likely that neuronal sets are similar to Edelman's concept of neuronal groups (45) that are selected on the basis of common differentiation signals and reciprocal interconnections. These actions of SFs have further implications in terms of sleep function if one considers CNS plasticity (e.g., synaptic turnover, astrocyte activation). Output range values shown are purely hypothetical; they are meant to illustrate that (a) the output from any set is variable, (b) not all sets are equally important for sleep, and (c) no single set is necessary for sleep, although all are necessary for normal sleep. For the sake of discussion, in the text we assume that once a total value of 7 is reached, sleep ensues.

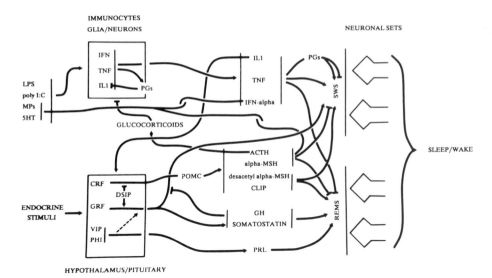

Figure 10-2 Simplified scheme of interaction between putative sleep factors. LPS, lipopolysac-charide; poly I:C, polyriboinosinic:polyribocytidylic acid; MPs, muramyl peptides; 5HT, sero-tonin; IFN, interferon; TNF, tumor necrosis factor; IL1, interleukin-1; PGs, prostaglandins; CRF, corticotropin-releasing factor; GRF, growth hormone-releasing factor; VIP, vasoactive intestinal peptide; PHI, histidine-isoleucine containing peptide; DSIP, delta sleep-inducing pep-tide; POMC, proopiomelanocorticotropin; α-MSH, α-melanocyte-stimulating hormone; CLIP, corticotropin-like intermediate lobe peptide; GH, growth hormone; PRL, prolactin; SWS, slow-wave sleep; REMS, rapid eye movement sleep. Arrows indicate enhancement, perpendicular lines indicate inhibition, and wavy lines indicate binding.

Neuronal Sets: One View of Brain Organization

Four different neuronal sets are illustrated as circles in Figure 1. Each set is involved in at least one aspect of sleep and is defined as a sleep set. Any substance that acts on these sets to modulate sleep–wake cycles should be considered a SF. Each sleep set can also be defined anatomically as a neuronal group with common differentiation signals and reciprocal interconnections (45).

A single neuronal set interacts with more than one SF (labeled A–I, Fig. 10-1), and the degree of stimulation impinging on a specific set depends on the concentration of the SFs interacting with it. Some SFs interact with more than one neuronal set. The interaction of an SF with one neuronal set may be different from its interaction with another neuronal set; in one it may be excitatory and in another inhibitory. Further-more, the affinity of one neuronal set for a SF may be substantially different from that of another neuronal set for the same SF. Such interactions are well known and are used as a pharmacological basis for receptor classification. These latter two points allow one to easily envision a mechanism to explain why certain putative SFs (e.g., adenosine) have sleep-promoting activity only in a narrow dose range. Perhaps at an optimal dose, an SF binds to and maximally stimulates a specific neuronal set; as the dose is in-creased, it approaches the optimal dose of a second neuronal set and has an effect opposite to that in the neuronal set, thus reducing the propensity to sleep. One can further refine such an approach by assuming some interaction between neuronal sets, as illustrated in Fig. 1, although the degree of interconnection between neuronal sets would be less than within a neuronal set.

For the purpose of illustration, we have assigned hypothetical numerical values to the outputs from each neuronal set. These values are meant to represent the relative contribution of individual neuronal sets to sleep propensity. It is assumed that a total value of 7 from all neuronal sets must be reached before sleep can ensue and that the output from any individual neuronal set is variable and dependent on the relative degree of SF stimulation. Thus, the interaction of several SFs on sleep can be envisioned as follows:

1. Some neuronal sets are more important (have larger output values) in regard to sleep than others; hence, some SFs are more important (have larger effects) than others.
2. If all sets are operating at a minimal level, the total neuronal output is less than 7, and the animal will not sleep.
3. It is possible to hold the output of three neuronal sets constant, maximally stimulate the fourth neuronal set, and reach sleep threshold, for example, the exogenous administration of an SF may cause excess sleep.
4. In contrast, no matter how much set I is stimulated by SFs A and B, if sets II, III, and IV are at minimal output levels, SFs A and B will not initiate sleep (although they could if sets II, III, and IV were operating at a higher level).
5. Lesioning one set would reduce the total propensity for sleep; thus, over time, there would be less sleep. However, sleep may still be possible if the remaining sets are driven to a greater degree, for example, sleep or sleep-like EEG can be induced in animals with insomnia produced by CNS lesions (137) or by pharmacological treatment (147) if exogenous SF is administered or if an SF is allowed to accumulate endogenously during sleep deprivation.
6. An inherent feature of the model is that no single neuronal set is necessary for sleep, although each is necessary to reach "normal" sleep propensity. Similarly, one could envision sleep recovery after a lesion due to a gradual increase in SFs that drive the nonlesioned sets or altered receptor affinities for remaining SF receptors (also see 105).

Another major concept illustrated in Figure 10-1 is that any particular neuronal set is involved in physiological functions other than sleep. Experimental support for this concept can be found in many physiological regulatory systems. Boulant, for example, showed that anterior hypothalamic neurons can alter their firing rates if stimulated by one or more regulatory stimuli, that is, glucose, osmotic pressure, changes in temperature, and sex steroids (140,141). Further, almost all putative SFs (more than 30 have been proposed; reviewed, 87) have biological activities in addition to their ability to enhance sleep. Also, because effectors for various physiological systems are different, it is theoretically possible to separate these activities from the sleep-inducing activity of an SF (e.g., see 92).

Another degree of complexity can be added to this model if one assumes there are multiple sites in the brain that are hierarchically arranged to regulate sleep. At each level, one could draw a scheme similar to that of Figure 10-1. However, the complexity is likely to be far greater at the top of any such hierarchical order than at the bottom. Thus, at the highest levels, one would anticipate multiple neuronal sets, each integrating information from a variety of physiological systems. Many of the inputs (e.g., SF concentration) into these neuronal sets would be dependent on past sleep–wake activity. No set would be specific for any function, and all would be involved in regulation of two or more physiological variables.

From a theoretical point of view, it is important to consider the outputs of the neuronal sets illustrated in Figure 10-1, as it has bearing on whether it is reasonable to postulate the existence of an SF specific for sleep. If the outputs from these neuronal sets either diverge or operate in parallel to produce sleep, there would be very little chance of finding an SF with biological activity confined to sleep, because the same model would apply to the subsequent parallel–divergent pathways. On the other hand, if the outputs from the model converge to affect a single final common pathway leading to sleep, then it would be possible that the summated output of sets I–IV affects the levels of some substance contained within that pathway, which in turn regulates its own output, sleep. Such a substance might conceivably have actions specifically in that pathway and, thus, if made available to the appropriate intracellular sites, could enhance sleep. However, such a brain construction (single final common pathway for a vigilant state) is unlikely for any complex behavior such as sleep in view of the effects of sleep on many functions of the body. The underlying paradigm for such a construction is one gene:one peptide/enzyme/neurotransmitter:one receptor:one animal behavior. The absurdity of such linear thinking is reviewed elsewhere (101).

Finally, from a biochemical point of view, each SF will have its own anabolic and catabolic pathways. The regulations of these biochemical pathways are likely to be interwoven with one another, as well as influenced by neuronal traffic within and among neuronal sets.

Sleep Factors and Their Interactions

On the basis of numerous experimental results, we have developed a simplified scheme relating the interactions of several putative SFs to their effects on sleep–wake cycles (Fig. 10-2). It is important to emphasize a few major points concerning Figure 10-2.

1. This is a greatly simplified scheme [see reference (58,76,104) for a more expanded discussion of neuroendocrine regulation and its multilevel feedback loops or references (37,39) for a more in-depth review of interleukin-1 (IL-1) regulation].
2. We emphasize that some of the possible interactions shown are postulated based on information obtained *in vitro* using cells that were not of central nervous system (CNS) origin.
3. The role of classical neurotransmitters is not illustrated, with the exception of serotonin (5HT). This neurotransmitter is discussed because of its structural similarity to muramyl peptides (MPs) (128), and there is experimental evidence suggesting it is involved in interactions with other putative SFs illustrated in Figure 10-2.
4. We emphasize that almost every substance shown in Figure 10-2 has been described as a normal constituent of the brain.

5. Many substances and regulatory events that are known to be involved in sleep–wake regulation are not shown in Figure 10-2 because they have been reviewed elsewhere. For example, the effects of IL-1 on calcium metabolism are described by Dinarello (37), and circadian influences on sleep–wake cycles are reviewed elsewhere in this book.

6. The cells involved in the events illustrated on the left side of Figure 10-2 include neurons, glia, pituitary, and immunocytes. One major hypothesis we wish to emphasize is that glia may be involved in sleep regulation. This is postulated because many of the SFs shown in Figure 10-2 either bind to or are produced by glia (reviewed 83,91).

IMMUNE RESPONSE MODIFIERS AND SLEEP

Infectious Disease

Despite the common observation that people often experience increased lassitude or sleepiness during infectious disease, there has been relatively little research applied to this phenomenon. In fact, to our knowledge, there are no published reports in which quantitative measurements of sleep were made over the course of an infectious disease. Consequently, we carried out a study in which we inoculated rabbits with viable *Staphylococcus aureus* (*S. aureus*) and monitored their sleep for 2 days (149). We found that slow-wave sleep (SWS) was enhanced beginning 4–6 hr after *S. aureus* inoculation, and this enhancement continued for up to about 18 hr postinoculation. After this time, SWS decreased compared to that during the control period. SWS returned to normal levels about 30–40 hr after inoculation. Accompanying this biphasic effect, we also observed increases and decreases in EEG slow-wave amplitudes coincident with increased or decreased SWS. Rapid eye movement (REM) sleep was inhibited throughout much of the 48-hr recording period after an initial delay of 4–6 hr.

S. aureus is a gram-positive bacterium containing MPs in its cell wall peptidoglycan. In other studies, we have examined the effects of *Escherichia coli,* a gram-negative bacterium containing MPs and endotoxin (lipopolysaccharide, LPS) in its cell walls. *E. coli* inoculation also altered sleep patterns, though the effects were rapid in onset and of short duration compared to the effects observed after *S. aureus*. Likely candidates for the mediation of these bacterial effects on sleep include the MPs and LPS, as discussed below, as well as a number of endogenous immune response modifiers such as IL-1, tumor necrosis factor (TNF), and interferon (IFN).

Bacterial Products: Muramyl Peptides and Lipopolysaccharides

MPs were first recognized as somnogenic agents when they were described as sleep-promoting substances in brain and urine extracts (84). These studies had their origin in the observation that sleep-promoting activity accumulated in cerebrospinal fluid (CSF) during wakefulness (123). The materials isolated from brain and urine possess chromatographic and sleep-promoting activities indistinguishable from those described for the CSF material (122,88). The most active component isolated from urine is NAG-1,6-anhydro-NAM-ala-glu-dap-ala; 1 pmol given intracerebroventricularly (ICV) to rabbits enhanced SWS for several hours (84). Subsequently, several analogs of this substance, for example, muramyl dipeptide (NAM-L-ala-D-isogln) (MDP), were also found to be somnogenic in several species (89,93,65,133,159,72,103). Although MDP is less active somnogenically (minimum effective dose, about 100 pmol ICV in rabbits) than the materials isolated from brain and urine, its profile of activities resembles that of the MPs isolated from mammalian tissues (84), and it is readily available from commercial sources.

MDP was first isolated as the minimal structure capable of replacing the mycobacterial component of Freund's complete adjuvant (48). MPs are the monomeric building blocks of bacterial cell wall peptidoglycan; within peptidoglycan, MPs are extensively cross-linked to each other via peptide and glycosidic bonds. Mammalian macrophages have the capacity to phagocytoze bacteria and partially digest their cell walls (153). During this process, the macrophages release biologically active monomeric MPs (69). This is particularly important because some of the components of MPs, for example, diaminopimelic (dap) and muramic acid, do not have known mammalian synthetic pathways. Such an identifiable source of MPs is necessary if they are to be considered as putative endogenous SFs. This processing of peptidoglycans by macrophages is probably also important in the initiation and amplification of the immune response to bacteria. It has also been proposed that MPs are vitamin-like, in that they are required by, but cannot be synthesized by, the host (2,70) since (a) muramic acid (161) and dap (68) in hydrolyzable linkage and MPs themselves (88) are present in normal mammalian tissue, (b) mammals are constantly exposed to bacteria, and (c) MPs have numerous biological activities.

In addition to their capacity to alter sleep–wake activity, MPs have a wide variety of other biological actions (reviewed 8,30,31). Indeed, the most extensively studied activities of MPs are their effects on the immune system and temperature regulation. An important point is that these activities can be separated, in part, from their somnogenic activities. Thus, certain MPs, for example, NAM-L-ala-D-gln OMe (murametide) are active as immune adjuvants but have little somnogenic activity (93). More important for sleep regulation is that the pyrogenic actions of MPs (89,103) can be separated from their somnogenic activities. Thus, certain MPs are pyrogenic but somnogenic (90,93). In rabbits, MDP is less pyrogenic if given at nighttime than if given during daylight hours, but is somnogenic at both times (139). In rabbit neonates, MDP enhances quiet sleep, the precursor to SWS, without inducing simultaneous increases in body temperature (36). In rats, low doses of MDP are somnogenic but not pyrogenic (72). Further, acetaminophen attenuated MDP-induced febrile response without altering its somnogenic action (89). Finally, although certain MPs are pyrogenic, they do not affect brain temperature (T_{br}) changes that are tightly coupled to states of vigilance (81).

It is important to ascertain whether MPs can be moved from one physiological compartment to another. It is likely, although currently unknown, that MPs are present in the intestinal lumen, which contains a large number of bacteria (about 1.5 kg in humans). The passage of MPs from the intestinal lumen into the blood has been described (124). Further, the passage of MPs from the blood to the brain via a carrier-mediated system has also been reported (91). Thus, regardless of whether MPs reach the blood after macrophage processing of bacteria or by passage from the gut into the blood, they will have access to immunocytes as well as to the CNS. Whether MPs undergo further modification once they reach the CNS or immunocytes remains unknown. However, from MP structure–activity studies (81,89,93), it is known that hydration of the 1,6-anhydro moiety of muramic acid contained within the urine-derived sleep-promoting substance reduces somnogenic potency about 10-fold (84). Perhaps more important, if terminal carboxyl groups of several somnogenic MPs are converted to unsubstituted amides (e.g., MDP to NAM-L-ala-D-glu[NH$_2$]$_2$), somnogenic activity is completely lost (89,90). This latter finding may be important in view of the fact that the biological activity of several peptides is regulated by amidation–deamidation reactions. Thus, it is possible that once MPs reach the brain, their somnogenic activity may be regulated via enzymes capable of hydration–dehydration or amidation–deamidation of MPs.

Cellular sites responsible for the biological action of MPs have only recently been studied. Binding sites for MPs on macrophages and glia have been described (Fig. 10-2) (142,143). MP binding to these tissues occurs at both high- and low-affinity sites with K_D values lying within a physiological range (50–1000 pM and 3.5 μM). The state of activation of macrophages influences the kinetics of interaction of MPs with these cells. Thus, *Listeria monocytogenes*-activated macrophages exhibited high-affinity binding sites with a higher K_D and higher maximal binding capacity than did resident macrophages (143). In addition, the binding to macrophages of several different MPs of varying somnogenic and immune activities is correlated with their biological activities. Perhaps most important in regard to CNS function, MP binding to glia was shown to be dependent, in part, on where in the brain glia were obtained (142). Thus, glia from the diencephalon possessed a higher binding capacity for MPs than did glia obtained from the neocortex (142). Further, it was shown that 5HT could compete with MPs for these binding sites (144). Interestingly, the kinetics of 5HT binding to brain homogenates are altered after sleep deprivation (158), although whether these sites are also MP binding sites remains unknown. Another interesting binding phenomenon is that both MPs and 5HT can bind to IFN, melanocyte-stimulating hormone α-MSH, and adrenocorticotropic hormone (ACTH) (Fig. 10-2) (discussed below).

MPs may also have direct action on neurons. Thus, in a preliminary study, it was shown that MDP can alter neuronal firing rates in different brain regions (41). In addition, lesions to the raphe system alter MDP-induced sleep and febrile actions (72,73) and enhance MDP-immunoadjuvant activity (103). Further, pyrogenic doses of MDP increase 5HT turnover in the brainstem, midbrain, and hypothalamus (103). This increased 5HT turnover is antagonized by indomethacin, although this treatment does not alter the effects of MPs on sleep (103). In another study, the somnogenic and pyrogenic actions of MDP were studied in animals with lesions to the preoptic area of the hypothalamus. After such lesions, the animals slept less than normal and were hyperthermic. After MDP treatment, the lesioned animals exhibited increased SWS and body temperature (137). It is, of course, possible that all these CNS effects of MPs result from MP–glia interaction since MPs induce glia to produce IL-1; IL-1 is known to have direct action on neurons (135).

In addition to MPs, other bacterial products are also known to be somnogenic. LPS, for example, is a component of gram-negative bacterial cell walls composed of a polysaccharide chain and a glycolipid region (lipid A). Like MPs, LPS possesses a wide variety of biological activities in addition to promoting sleep, including pyrogenicity and immunoactivity (reviewed, 79). The lipid A moiety is necessary for most of these biological activities, and, indeed, lipid A by itself is immunoactive, pyrogenic, and somnogenic (79,85). In general, the actions of LPS/lipid As are categorized as toxic or potentially beneficial (immunostimulatory). It is worthwhile to note that mammalian cells, including macrophages, possess enzymes that can remove acyloxyacyl groups from and dephosphorylate the lipid A moiety of LPS (111). The removal of such groups reduces toxicity, although similarly modified lipid As retain some immunomodulatory (79) and somnogenic (25,85) actions. Such processes are most likely important during gram-negative infections. However, as in the case of MPs, whether such processing of these microbial products and their subsequent biological actions are integral parts of normal sleep regulation remains to be determined.

Viruses and Viral Products: Poly(I:C)

Viral diseases have played a relatively important role in sleep research. Historically, the study of CNS lesions produced during viral infections led von Economo to describe sleep as an active process mediated by specific brain regions (44). Indeed the specific hypothalamic areas identified by von Economo are now widely recognized as being involved in sleep–wake regulation (reviewed, 110). More recently, viral infections have been associated with a wide range of maladies, each associated with sleep disorders. These include fibrositis (fibromyalgia) syndrome (57,109), chronic fatigue syndrome (23,64), excessive daytime sleepiness (62), sudden infant death syndrome (9,63,61), apnea in young children (1,6,160), and human affective disorders (5). Despite this long list of possible sleep disorders associated with viral infection, there are no reports in the literature in which sleep was monitored systematically over the course of an acute viral infection.

Three distinct pathological processes are recognized during an acute viral disease: (a) direct localized cell destruction induced by the replicating virus, (b) nonspecific or specific inflammatory responses to the virus and/or injured cells, and (c) systemic toxicity. The molecular basis for the latter effect has not been completely elucidated, though certain desoxyribonucleic acid (DNA) viral classes have been found to produce characteristic protein toxins. Further, double-stranded RNA ribonucleic acid (dsRNA) produced during replication of RNA viruses may mediate some of the systemic symptoms associated with these viral infections (28). This hypothesis is based, in part, on the observation that many systemic symptoms associated with viral disease are also elicited by the injection of synthetic dsRNA substances such as polyriboinosinic : polyribocytidylic acid [poly(I:C)]. Poly(I:C) injected either intravenously (IV) or ICV into rabbits increased body temperature and duration of SWS and decreased REM sleep, but failed to raise plasma copper levels (86).

Cytokines: Effects on Sleep and Interrelationships with the Neuroendocrine Axis

The bacterial and viral products discussed above have the capacity to alter the production of a variety of cytokines. These cytokines may, in turn, mediate many of the immune-related and CNS activities induced by bacterial and viral products. To date, the somnogenic activities of four cytokines have been determined: interleukin-1α (IL-1α), interleukin-1β (IL-1β), interferon α_2 (IFN-α_2), and tumor necrosis factor β

(TNF-β). Each of these substances has wide-ranging effects on the immune response (reviewed, 37,39,119) and enhances SWS (82,92,138). Each has also been cloned, and recombinant (r) forms of these cytokines are commercially available. For the purpose of this discussion, we will focus on IL-1β since it has been studied more extensively than the other cytokines in regard to sleep and brain localization.

IL-1 refers to a family of polypeptides of 13,000–17,500 Da; distinct forms of IL-1 are produced by individual species, although IL-1 from one species is often active in another species. IL-1 was initially characterized as a macrophage product that was synthesized and released in response to certain pyrogens and stimulants of the immune response (reviewed, 37). More recently, a variety of cell types, including astrocytes (52,53), microglia (56), and keratinocytes (55), have also been shown to produce IL-1. IL-1 is found in a variety of physiological fluid compartments, including CSF (59), milk (112), and plasma (26,27). Farrar et al. (49) used *in situ* hybridization histochemistry techniques, and showed that IL-1β-messenger (m) RNA is produced in the normal brain, although IL-1α-mRNA is not. IL-1β-mRNA was found throughout the rat brain, although the choroid plexus and the granular cell layer of the hippocampus were most darkly stained. The authors emphasized that the mRNA found was not associated with blood cells in vascular areas. The distribution pattern of IL-1β-mRNA was similar to the brain distribution of IL-1β receptors previously described (50). More recently, IL-1β-like immunoreactive neurons were identified in human basal forebrains (22).

Rabbit IL-1 obtained from peritoneal exudate cells, purified native human IL-1β obtained from macrophages, and human rIL-1β all produced similar effects on rabbit sleep. The time course of IL-1β-enhanced SWS differs from that induced by MPs in that excess SWS was observed during the first hour postinjection after IL-1β (92). This finding is consistent with the hypothesis that the somnogenic actions of MPs are mediated via enhanced production and release of IL-1 (40,83). In rabbits, IL-1β also enhances the amplitudes of EEG slow waves during SWS in a manner similar to that observed during the deep sleep following sleep deprivation (21,92,122). IL-1β also inhibits REM sleep in rabbits. Similar results were obtained by Tobler et al. (148), who injected murine astrocyte-derived IL-1 into rats; recipient animals had enhanced EEG slow-wave activity and less REM sleep than normal. Human recombinant IL-1β was also somnogenic in cats (150). Additional evidence linking IL-1 to sleep was obtained by Moldolfsky's group, who showed that IL-1-like activity peaked in human plasma (108) and in cat CSF (100) at the onset of SWS. Preliminary data from that laboratory indicate that levels of IL-1 in CSF increase after sleep deprivation (107).

IL-1α (135), TNF-β (138), and IFN-α$_2$ (82) also enhance SWS and EEG slow waves during SWS after IV or ICV injection in rabbits, although the time courses of their effects on sleep are different from that of IL-1β-enhanced SWS. Thus, enhanced SWS occurs only after about a 1-hr delay after injection of either IFN-α$_2$ or IL-1α. In contrast, TNF-β produces a biphasic effect on SWS; this effect may be related to the ability of TNF to induce IL-1 production (138). Both IL-1α and TNF-β also inhibit REM sleep in a manner similar to that observed after IL-1β treatment. In contrast, human IFN-α$_2$, when given ICV, failed to alter REM sleep (82), although it reduced latency to REM sleep when given to monkeys (125).

All of the cytokines mentioned here also are endogenous pyrogens. In rabbits, administration of an antipyretic blocked the pyrogenic action of IL-1β without affecting IL-1β-induced excess sleep (92). In agreement with this finding, Tobler et al. (148) failed to find a correlation between IL-1-induced sleep effects and IL-1-induced febrile activity. In this regard, it is important to note that in normal humans, plasma IL-1-like activity peaks at the beginning of the night (108), a time at which body temperatures are normally falling. This apparent anomaly could result from the simultaneous action of endogenous IL-1 inhibitors (127,130), perhaps acting in different physiological compartments; one of these, α-MSH, is discussed below. Another facet of temperature regulation, temperature changes that are tightly coupled to sleep states, is not affected by any of the cytokines discussed above (156).

Very little is known concerning the regulation of brain IL-1β. However, two negative feedback mechanisms for IL-1 production have been identified, and both involve substances that affect sleep. Thus, it is well known that IL-1 alters arachidonic acid metabolism, resulting in increased prostaglandin (PG) production (Fig. 10-2) (reviewed, 38). In turn, PGs can inhibit IL-1 production and release (reviewed, 37) while simultaneously enhancing IL-1 receptor synthesis (3). Indeed, IL-1-induced hypothalamic PGE_2 release may be responsible for IL-1-induced fever (reviewed, 17). In regard to sleep, PGD_2, a major PG metabolite in rats, can enhance sleep in both rats (65) and rabbits (80), whereas PGE inhibits sleep in rats (152). Whether these effects of PGs on sleep involve IL-1 and/or IL-1 receptors remains unknown. The cellular sources for brain PGs and the role of brain PGs as intracellular or intercellular messengers for sleep are also currently unclear.

Another negative feedback system involving IL-1 is the hypothalamic–adrenal neuroendocrine axis. IL-1β and IL-1α have the capacity to induce hypothalamic corticotropin-releasing factor (CRF) release (11,131). CRF in turn enhances ACTH release, which then induces glucocorticoid release from the adrenals. Glucocorticoid in turn inhibits IL-1 production (15). Of particular importance to sleep is that ACTH and α-MSH ($ACTH_{1-13}$) both inhibit sleep, and α-MSH can block IL-1β-enhanced SWS (121).

Even less information is available concerning the regulation of other cytokines, although TNF and IFN also alter arachidonic acid metabolism and TNF, IFN, and IL-1 appear to be synergistic in regard to certain immune-related activities (e.g., 119). However, indirect evidence suggests these cytokines are regulated, in part, independently of each other. For example, injection of either IL-1 (19) or MPs (136) into the brain elicits changes in certain acute-phase reactants (e.g., ceruloplasmin) by a CNS mechanism (19). In contrast, ICV injection of poly(I:C) (86), an inducer of IFN, or injection of IFN itself (18) does not alter plasma Cu levels. However, all of these substances are somnogenic after ICV administration. Thus, the somnogenic actions of these substances may be mediated differently than their actions on the acute-phase response and body temperature.

Another possible regulatory mechanism involving cytokines that is almost completely uninvestigated concerns the binding of 5HT and MPs to IFN and α-MSH. On the basis of their structures, IFN-α, ACTH, and α-MSH were predicted to contain binding sites for 5HT and MDP (128). Using nuclear magnetic resonance techniques, the interactions of these substances in solution were demonstrated (129). An interesting parallel is the observation that 5HT and MDP compete for binding sites on macrophages and glia (144). However, whether the cellular binding sites are related to either IFN-α or ACTH or whether the binding of 5HT and MPs to IFN/ACTH/α-MSH results in altered biological activity remains unknown. Such interactions, however, could be involved in the *in vivo* regulation of these substances.

Neuroendocrines: Relations to Sleep

A number of observations suggest that neuroendocrine mechanisms are involved in both sleep and immune regulation. Although the picture is far from clear, it seems that the CRF-opiomelanocortinergic system and the growth hormone-releasing factor/ vasoactive intestinal peptide/histidine-isoleucine containing peptide-growth hormone/ prolactin (GRF/VIP/PHI-GH/PRL) system represent two neuroendocrine pathways promoting wakefulness/immune suppression and sleep/immune activation, respectively. Some proposed SFs might act through the modulation of these endocrine mechanisms: for example, delta sleep-inducing peptide (DSIP) has recently been shown to promote GRF action (67) and to inhibit CRF effects (60).

CRF—Opiomelanocortins

Opiomelanocortinergic cells in the anterior pituitary, intermediate lobe, and hypothalamus produce various peptides related to ACTH and β-endorphin (118). These peptides are also synthesized by lymphocytes (157). Of the various opiomelanocortins, ACTH and α-MSH are of particular importance to the present discussion.

Immune challenges or direct administration of IL-1 elicit ACTH secretion and a subsequent rise in blood glucocorticoid levels, which inhibit further production of IL-1 (37). Another proopiomelanocortin-derived substance, α-MSH, is released in the brain in response to IL-1 (10). Acting on thermoregulatory structures in the septum and the preoptic region, α-MSH reduces body temperature and can attenuate IL-1-induced fever. α-MSH has been proposed as a physiological endogenous antipyretic controlling the central pyrogenic effect of IL-1 (99).

Previous experiments indicated that α-MSH might have an arousing action (74). The aim of our experiments was to study whether α-MSH, in fact, increases wakefulness, and whether it can decrease the somnogenic actions of IL-1 (121). ICV α-MSH (0.1–50 μg) increased wakefulness and reduced EEG slow wave activity in SWS in a dose-dependent manner; small doses (0.5–5.0 μg) were effective in attenuating IL-1-enhanced sleep. Although α-MSH also elicited specific behavioral responses such as stretching/yawning and signs of sexual excitation, the increases in wakefulness did not result from these phasic events. Instead, the number of long periods of quiet wakefulness increased. It was proposed that α-MSH might be involved in the control of sleep induced by IL-1.

IL-1β has a direct stimulatory effect on pituitary corticotropic cells *in vitro* (13). Nevertheless, this effect is weak, and IL-1 increases ACTH secretion *in vivo* dominantly (IL-1β) or exclusively (IL-1α) through the release of hypothalamic CRF. It has been suggested that release of α-MSH in the brain is also mediated through CRF (11,131). In fact, ICV CRF reduces IL-1-induced fever (12) and elicits arousal (47). Accordingly, IL-1 activates CRF-containing neurons in the supraoptic nucleus, resulting in CRF release in the median eminence and in the arcuate nucleus for stimulation of pituitary ACTH and septal α-MSH release, respectively (99). Destruction by monosodium glutamate treatment of α-MSH-containing neurons in the arcuate nucleus of neonatal rats permanently reduces wakefulness (120), thus suggesting that central α-MSH is involved in the maintenance of physiological wakefulness. α-MSH does not inhibit IL-1 binding in the CNS (50), and the site of interaction between α-MSH and IL-1 remains unknown. Finally, it is interesting to note that vasopressin, another proposed endogenous antipyretic (75), also increases wakefulness (16,95) and may elicit ACTH release (104).

In addition, two other proopiomelanocortin-derived substances, desacetyl-α-MSH (1 ng) and corticotropin-lobe intermediate peptide (CLIP) (10 ng), have recently been reported to promote selectively SWS and REM sleep when administered ICV to rats (29). Opiomelanocortins, therefore, may modulate sleep–wake activity on a broad spectrum.

GRF/VIP/PHI-GH/PRL

The major secretory peaks of two structurally related hormones that share some biological activities, GH and PRL, are temporally correlated to sleep–wake activity (132,146). The major release of GH occurs soon after sleep onset, during SWS. The first episode of PRL secretion also occurs early in sleep, though later than the GH release. Although GH secretory pulses decline and disappear as sleep continues, plasma PRL concentrations increase episodically, reaching maximum values at the end of the sleep period. PRL release shifts with changes in sleep onset time, GH secretion is suppressed during sleep deprivation, and large increases in plasma GH concentrations were reported during recovery sleep. Although the association between SWS and GH/PRL secretion is now regarded as the most well-established connection between sleep and hormones (4), dissociation may occur (102). Thus, non-REM (NREM) sleep does not induce GH or PRL secretion, and vice versa. An endogenous mechanism that simultaneously triggers both SWS and hormone secretion could explain the coupling between sleep and GH/PRL release. Hypothalamic GRF, or the structurally related peptides, VIP and PHI, could mediate such coupling.

GRF, VIP, and PHI belong to the secretin–glucagon peptide family. Each peptide can bind to the receptors of the others with varying affinities and then act as agonists or, sometimes, as partial antagonists in vitro (96,97,155). After exogenous administration in vivo, they often elicit similar effects. For example, ICV administration of VIP has been reported to elicit GH secretion in rats (20,154); endogenous VIP, however, is not considered to be involved in the regulation of GH secretion. GRF is known as the hypothalamic stimulating factor for pituitary GH release, whereas VIP and PHI may act as hypothalamic releasing factors for pituitary PRL secretion (76). Several lines of evidence indicate that GRF, VIP, and PHI also act as neurotransmitters and/or neuromodulators in the CNS (e.g., 151).

ICV administration of GRF increases EEG slow-wave activity, reduces motor activity, and increases SWS and REM sleep in rats (47,114–116). In rabbits, ICV injection of GRF (0.01–1.0 nmol/kg) promoted sleep in a dose-dependent manner. The increases in SWS were prompt, whereas REM sleep increased only after considerable latency (as long as 1 hr) (116). Increases in EEG slow-wave activity were also demonstrated during SWS for rabbits. GRF, therefore, has the capacity to increase sleep and GH secretion. It is likely that promotion of SWS and stimulation of GH release represent two parallel functions of GRF-containing neurons. If that is the case, sleep and GH secretion could be triggered independently or simultaneously; in the case of simultaneous stimulation, blockade of one output would not inhibit the manifestation of the other (i.e., dissociation may occur). GRF-containing neurons in the arcuate nucleus project mainly to the median eminence and are involved in the regulation of GH secretion (33). GRF-containing neurons around the ventromedial nucleus may also be involved in GH release (77,102); however, these neurons also project to various areas in the basal forebrain (33), and thus may provide the structural basis for synchronization of SWS and GH secretion.

Pituitary GH secretion is stimulated by GRF and inhibited by somatostatin (SOM). This regulation involves several feedback loops (58). GRF itself, and the subsequent high GH level, elicits SOM release. Both GH and SOM inhibit further GRF release, and SOM inhibits GH secretion. Although these endocrine responses are not directly involved in SWS increases elicited by GRF, they might contribute to GRF-induced REM sleep. Both ICV infusion of SOM in rats (34) and systemic administration of GH in rats (43), cats (145), and humans (106) increase REM sleep. High doses of GH inhibit NREM sleep (106), and SOM antibodies applied to the solitary nucleus increase SWS (35). These findings suggest that the increases in GH and SOM secretions elicited by GRF may provide negative feedback control of SWS and mediate the promotion of REM sleep subsequent to NREM sleep.

Increases in both SWS and REMS were reported in response to ICV administration of VIP in rats (95,117,126). VIP promoted REM sleep without significant effects on SWS in cats (42). Administration of VIP antiserum decreased REM sleep, but not SWS, in rats (126). Our preliminary studies showed increased REM sleep in rabbits after ICV VIP (0.1 nmol/kg). VIP did not increase SWS; in fact, a reduction in SWS was found after a high dose (1 nmol/kg) of VIP. Histidine/methionine-containing peptide (PHM, the human equivalent of PHI) produced effects similar to those of VIP. It seems, therefore, that the sleep-promoting action of VIP (and possibly PHI) is specific for REM sleep; the increases in SWS in rats may be attributed to a GRF-like action of VIP demonstrated previously in this species.

VIP-enhanced REM sleep may be mediated via an activation of cholinergic mechanisms in the brainstem, which was proposed as a possible site of VIP action (42,126). It is also possible, however, that VIP-altered PRL release mediates the VIP-enhanced REM sleep. PRL often has effects similar to those of GH, and GH is known to increase REM sleep. Further, the long latency (1 hr) of the increase in REM sleep after ICV injection of VIP and PHM also indicates an indirect action. To test whether PRL could promote REM sleep, PRL was subcutaneously injected into rabbits, and the sleep-wake activity was recorded for 6 hr. After a 1-hr latency, PRL (200 IU/kg) induced significant increases in REM sleep for the rest of the recording period. Jouvet also noted the sustained effect of PRL on REM sleep; after a single subcutaneous injection of PRL, REM sleep increased for several days in rats with pontine transections and hypothalamic lesions (71). In conclusion, the VIP/PHI-PRL system appears to have the capacity to promote REM sleep.

Recent observations suggest that GH (46) and PRL (14) are also involved in immune responses. Although lymphocytes produce GH/PRL-like substances (157), the pituitary-derived hormones seem essential to the normal functioning of the immune system (113). Endotoxin (54), viral infection (24), and IL-2 (7) have been shown to release GH. Endotoxin is so effective in this regard that this compound is used to assess the GH production capacity of the pituitary (54). It is not clear whether the effects of immune active substances on GH are mediated via GRF. IL-1β stimulates pituitary somatotrophs *in vitro* (13); however, this does not exclude the possibility that IL-1 acts primarily through the hypothalamus *in vivo,* as it does for its stimulatory effects on CRF/ACTH.

CONCLUSION

From the above discussion, it is clear that several immune response modifiers/ neuroendocrines have the capacity to alter sleep. We have presented two models illustrating how these substances may interact with neuronal sets and how their regulation may be related to each other. That we can now propose such models based on experimental findings emphasizes how fast this field has progressed in recent years. However, despite such advances, many fundamental questions remain unanswered.

1. Does sleep have a role in host defense?
2. Are immune mechanisms involved in normal sleep regulation?
3. Is there a normal "symbiotic" relationship between bacterial–viral products and CNS function?
4. Are "neuroendocrine" substances of immunocyte origin involved in CNS function?
5. Are cytokines of CNS origin involved in normal CNS function?
6. What is the nature of the regulatory interactions between SFs in the brain?
7. Where in the brain do sleep-regulating interactions take place?
8. What role do glia play in sleep and other CNS regulation?

Fortunately, with the identification of putative SFs and with the present and rapidly developing techniques from the fields of molecular biology and immunology, answers to these questions may be forthcoming within the next decade. Such developments will greatly change our understanding of how the brain functions. The field of sleep could play a major role in these developments.

ACKNOWLEDGMENTS

This work was supported in part by the Office of Naval Research (N00014-85-K-0773), the U.S. Army Research and Development Command (DAMD-17-86-C-6194), and the National Institutes of Health (NS-25378).

REFERENCES

1. Abreu E, Silva FA, Brezinova V, Simpson H. Sleep apnea in acute bronchiolitis. *Arch Dis Childhood* 1982; 57:467–472.
2. Adam A, Lederer E. Muramyl peptides: Immunomodulators, sleep factors, and vitamins. *Med Res Rev* 1984; 4:111–152.

3. Akahoshi T, Oppenheim JJ, Matsushima K. Induction of IL1 receptor expression on fibrocytes by glucocorticoid hormone, prostaglandins and interleukin-1 (IL1). *J Leukocyte Biol* 1987; 42:579.

4. Akerstedt T. Hormones and sleep. *Exp Brain Res* (Suppl.) 1984; 8:193–203.

5. Amsterdam JP, Winokar A, Dyson W, Herzog S, Gonzalez F, Rott R, Koprowski H. Borna disease virus: A possible etiologic factor in human affective disorders? *Arch Gen Psych* 1985; 42:1093–1096.

6. Anas N, Boettrich C, Hall CB, Brooks JG. The association of apnea and respiratory syncytial virus infection in infants. *J Pediatr* 1982; 101:65–69.

7. Atkins MB, Gould JA, Allegretta M, Li JJ, Dempsey RA, Rudders RA, Parkinson DR, Reichlin S, Mier JW. Phase I evaluation of recombinant interleukin-2 in patients with advanced malignant disease. *J Clin Oncol* 1986; 4:1380–1391.

8. Bahr GM, Chedid L. Immunological activities of muramyl peptides. *Fed Proc* 1986; 45:2541–2544.

9. Beckwith JB. The sudden infant death syndrome. *Curr Prob Pediatr* 1973; 3:3–37.

10. Bell RC, Lipton JM. Pulsatile release of antipyretic neuropeptide alpha-MSH from septum of rabbit during fever. *Am J Physiol* 1987; 252:R1152–R1157.

11. Berkenbosch F, van Oers J, Del Rey A, Tilders F, Besedovsky H. Corticotropin-releasing factor-producing neurons in the rat activated by interleukin-1. *Science* 1987; 238:524–526.

12. Bernardini GL, Richards DB, Lipton JM. Antipyretic effect of centrally administered CRF. *Peptides* 1984; 5:57–59.

13. Bernton EW, Beach JE, Holaday JW, Smallridge RC, Fein HG. Release of multiple hormones by a direct action of interleukin-1 on pituitary cells. *Science* 1987; 238:519–521.

14. Bernton EW, Meltzer MS, Holaday JW. Suppression of macrophage activation and T-lymphocyte function in hypoprolactinemic mice. *Science* 1988; 239:401–404.

15. Besedovsky H, Del Rey A, Sorkin E, Dinarello CA. Immunoregulatory feedback between interleukin-1 and glucocorticoid hormones. *Science* 1986; 233:652–654.

16. Bibene V, Arnauld E, Meynard J, Rodriguez F, Poncet C, Vincent J-D. Influence of vasopressin on circadian sleep and wakefulness. *Sleep Res* 1987; 16:43.

17. Blatteis CM. Endogenous pyrogen: Fever and associated effects. In JRS Hales (ed.), *Thermal Physiology,* Raven, New York, 1984: 539–546.

18. Blatteis CM, Ahokas RA, Dinarello CA, Ungar AL. Thermal and plasma Cu responses of guinea pigs to intrapreoptically injected rIL1, rIL2, rIFNα2 and rTNFα. *Fed Proc* 1987; 46:683.

19. Blatteis CM, Hunter WS, Llanos-Q J, Ahokas RA, Mashburn TA Jr. Activation of acute-phase responses by intrapreoptic injections of endogenous pyrogen in guinea pigs. *Brain Res Bull* 1984; 12:689–695.

20. Bluet-Pajot M-T, Mounier F, Leonard J-F, Kordon C, Durand D. Vasoactive intestinal peptide induces a transient release of growth hormone in the rat. *Peptides* 1987; 8:35–38.

21. Borbély AA. A two process model of sleep regulation. *Hum Neurobiol* 1982; 1:195–204.

22. Breder CD, Dinarello CA, Saper CB. Interleukin-1 immunoreactive innervation of human hypothalamus. *Science* 1988; 240:321–324.

23. Buchwald D, Sullivan JL, Komaroff AL. Frequency of "chronic active Epstein-Barr virus infection" in a general medical practice. *J Am Med Assoc* 1987; 257:2303–2307.

24. Bunner DL, Morris E, Smallridge RC. Circadian growth hormone and prolactin blood concentration during a self-limited viral infection and artificial hyperthermia in man. *Metabolism* 1984; 33:337–341.

25. Cady AB, Kotani S, Shiba T, Krueger JM. Somnogenic activities of synthetic lipid A. *Infection and Immunity* 1989; 57:396–403.

26. Cannon JG, Dinarello CA. Increased plasma interleukin-1 activity in women after ovulation. *Science* 1985; 227:1242–1249.

27. Cannon JG, Kluger MJ. Endogenous pyrogen activity in human plasma after exercise. *Science* 1983; 220:617–619.

28. Carter WA, DeClercq E. Viral infection and host defense. *Science* 1974; 186:1172–1178.

29. Chastrette N, Cespuglio R. Influence of proopiomelanocortin-derived peptides on the sleep-waking cycle of the rat. *Neurosci Lett* 1985; 62:365–370.

30. Chedid L. Immunopharmacology of muramyl peptides: New horizons. *Prog Immunol* 1983; 5:1349–1358.

31. Chedid L. Synthetic muramyl peptides: Their origin, present status, and future prospects. *Fed Proc* 1986; 45:2531–2533.

32. Dafny N, Lee JR, Dougherty PM. Immune response products alter CNS activity: Interferon modulates central opioid functions. *J Neurosci Res* 1988; 19:130–139.

33. Daikoku S, Kawano H, Noguchi M, Nakanishi J, Tokuzen M, Chihara K, Nagatsu I. GRF neurons in the rat hypothalamus. *Brain Res* 1986; 399:250–261.

34. Danguir J. Intracerebroventricular infusion of somatostatin selectively increases paradoxical sleep in rats. *Brain Res* 1986; 367:26–30.

35. Danguir J, De Saint-Hilaire-Kafi S. Somatostatin antiserum blocks carbachol-induced increase of paradoxical sleep in the rat. *Brain Res Bull* 1988; 20:9–12.

36. Davenne D, Krueger JM. Enhancement of quiet sleep in rabbit neonates by muramyl dipeptide. *Am J Physiol* 1987; 253:R646–R654.

37. Dinarello CA. Interleukin-1. *Rev Infect Dis* 1984; 6:51–95.

38. Dinarello CA, Bernheim HA. Ability of human leukocytic pyrogen to stimulate brain prostaglandin synthesis *in vitro*. *J Neurochem* 1981; 37:702–708.

39. Dinarello CA, Cannon JG, Mier JW, Bernheim HA, LoPreste G, Lynn DL, Love RN, Webb AC, Auron PE, Reuben RC, Rich A, Wolff SM, Putney SD. Multiple biological activities of human recombinant interleukin 1. *J Clin Invest* 1986; 77:1734–1739.

40. Dinarello CA, Krueger JM. Induction of interleukin-1 by synthetic and naturally occurring muramyl peptides. *Fed Proc* 1986; 45:2545–2548.

41. Dougherty PM, Dafny N. Central opioid systems are differentially affected by products of the immune response. *Soc Neurosci Abstr* 1987; 13:1437.

42. Drucker-Colin R, Bernal-Pedraza J, Fernandez-Cancino F, Oksenberg A. Is vasoactive intestinal polypeptide (VIP) a sleep factor? *Peptides* 1984; 5:837–840.

43. Drucker-Colin RR, Spanis CW, Hunyadi J, Sassin JF, McGaugh JL. Growth hormone effects on sleep and wakefulness in the rat. *Neuroendocrinology* 1975; 18:1–18.

44. von Economo CV. Sleep as a problem of localization. *J Nerv Mental Dis* 1930; 71:249–259.

45. Edelman GM. *Neural Darwinism*. Basic Book, New York, 1987.

46. Edwards CK III, Ghiasuddin SM, Schepper JM, Yunger LM, Kelley KW. A newly defined property of somatotropin: Priming of macrophages for production of superoxide anion. *Science* 1988; 239:769–771.

47. Ehlers CL, Reed TK, Henriksen SJ. Effects of corticotropin-releasing factor and growth hormone-releasing factor on sleep and activity in rats. *Neuroendocrinology* 1986; 42:467–474.

48. Ellouz F, Adam A, Ciorbaru R, Lederer E. Minimal structural requirements for adjuvant activity of bacterial peptidoglycan derivatives. *Biochem Biophys Res Commun* 1974; 59:1317–1325.

49. Farrar WL, Hill JM, Harel-Bellan A, Vinocour M. The immune logical brain. *Immunol Rev* 1987; 100:361–377.

50. Farrar WL, Kilian PL, Ruff MA, Hill JM, Pert CB. Visualization and characterization of interleukin-1 receptors in brain. *J Immunol* 1987; 139:459–463.

51. Fencl V, Koski G, Pappenheimer JR. Factors in cerebrospinal fluid from goats that affect sleep and activity in rats. *J Physiol* (London) 1971; 216:565–589.

52. Fontana A, Kristensen F, Dubs R, Gemsa D, Weber E. Production of prostaglandin E and an interleukin-1-like factor by cultured astrocytes and C_6 glioma cells. *J Immunol* 1982; 129:2413–2419.

53. Fontana A, Weber E, Dayer J-M. Synthesis of interleukin 1/endogenous pyrogen in the brain of endotoxin-treated mice: A step in fever induction. *J Immunol* 1984; 133:1696–1698.

54. Frohman LA, Horton ES, Lebovitz HE. Growth hormone releasing action of a pseudomonas endotoxin (Piromen). *Metab Clin Exp* 1967; 16:57–67.

55. Gahring LC, Daynes RA. The presence of functionally active ETAF/IL1 in normal human stratum corneum. In MJ Kluger, JJ Oppenheim, and MC Powanda (eds.), *The Physiologic, Metabolic and Immunologic Actions of Interleukin-1*. Liss, New York, 1985: 375–384.

56. Giulian D, Baker TJ, Young DG. Interleukin-1 as a mediator of brain cell growth. In MJ Kluger, JJ Oppenheim, and MC Powanda (eds.), *The Physiologic, Metabolic and Immunologic Actions of Interleukin-1*. Liss, New York, 1985: 133–142.

57. Goldenberg DL. Fibromyalgia syndrome: An emerging but controversial condition. *J Am Med Assoc* 1987; 257:2782–2787.

58. Gomez-Pan A, Rodriguez-Arnao MD. Somatostatin and growth hormone releasing factor: Synthesis, location, metabolism and function. *Clin Endocrin Metab* 1983; 12:469–507.

59. Gorczynski RM, Keystone EJ. Interleukin-1-like activity in human cerebrospinal fluid. *Immunol Lett* 1986; 13:231–235.

60. Graf MV, Kastin AJ, Coy DH, Fischman AJ. Delta-sleep-inducing peptide reduces CRF-induced corticosterone release. *Neuroendocrinology* 1985; 41:353–356.

61. Gouyon JB, Fantino M, Couillault G, Durand C, Pothier P, Alison M. Infections a virus respiratoire syncytial du nouveau-ne. *Arch Fr. Pediatr* 1986; 43:93–97.

62. Guilleminault G, Mondini S. Mononucleosis and chronic daytime sleepiness. *Arch Intern Med* 1986; 146:1333–1335.

63. Guntheroth WG. Sudden infant death syndrome (crib death). *Am Heart J* 1977; 93:784–793.

64. Holmes GP, Kaplan JE, Stewart JA, Hunt B, Pinsky PF, Schonberger LB. A cluster of patients with a chronic mononucleosis-like syndrome: Is Epstein-Barr virus the cause? *J Am Med Assoc* 1987; 257:2297–2302.

65. Inoue S, Honda K, Komoda Y, Uchizono K, Ueno R, Hayaishi O. Differential sleep-promoting effects of five sleep substances nocturnally infused in unrestrained rats. *Proc Natl Acad Sci USA* 1984; 81:6240–6244.

66. Ishimori K. True cause of sleep—a hynogenic substance as evidenced in the brain of sleep-deprived animals. *Tokyo Igakkai Zasshi* 1909; 23:429–459.

67. Iyer KS, McCann SM. Delta sleep-inducing peptide (DSIP) stimulates growth hormone (GH) release in the rat by hypothalamic and pituitary actions. *Peptides* 1987; 8:45–48.

68. Johanssen L, Krueger JM. Quantitation of diaminopimelic acid in human urine. *Adv Biosci* 1988; 68:445–449.

69. Johanssen L, Wecke J, Krueger JM. Macrophage processing of bacteria; CNS-active substances are produced. *Soc Neurosci Abstr* 1987; 13:261.

70. Jolles P. A possible physiological function of lysozyme. *Biomedicine* 1976; 25:275–276.

71. Jouvet M, Buda C, Cespuglio R, Chastrette N, Denoyer M, Sallanon M, Sastre JP. Hypnogenic effects of some hypothalamo-pituitary peptides. *Clin Neuropharmacol* 1986; (S4) 9:465–467.

72. Kadlecova O, Masek K. Muramyl dipeptide and sleep in rat. *Meth Find Exp Clin Pharmacol* 1986; 8:111–115.

73. Kadlecova O, Masek K, Petrovicky P. A possible site of action of bacterial peptidoglycan in the CNS. *Neuropharmacology* 1977; 16:699–702.

74. Kastin AJ, Sandman CA, Stratton LO, Schally AW, Miller LH. Behavioral and electrographic changes in rat and man after MSH. *Prog Brain Res* 1975; 42:143–150.

75. Kasting NW, Veale WL, Cooper KE. Vasopressin: A homeostatic effector in the febrile process. *Neurosci Biobehav Rev* 1982; 6:215–222.

76. Kato Y, Matsushita N, Ohta H, Tojo K, Shimatsu A, Imura H. Regulation of prolactin secretion. In H Imura (ed.), *The Pituitary Gland*. Raven, New York, 1985: 261–278.

77. Kita T, Chihara K, Kashio Y, Okimura Y, Sato M, Kitajama N, Fujita T. The effect of hypothalamic deafferentation on rat growth hormone-releasing factor (rGRF)-like immunoreactivity content in the medial basal hypothalamus of rats. *Endocrinol Jpn* 1987; 34:423–426.

78. Koella WP. The organization and regulation of sleep. *Experientia* 1984; 40:309–338.

79. Kotani S, Takada H, Tsujimoto M, Ogawa T, Mori Y, Sakuta M, Kawasaki A, Inage M, Kusumoto J, Shiba T, Kasai N. Immunobiological activities of synthetic lipid A analogs and related compounds as compared with those of bacterial lipopolysaccharide, reglycolipid, lipid A, and muramyl dipeptide. *Infect Immun* 1983; 41:758–773.

80. Krueger JM. Muramyl peptides and interleukin-1 as promoters of slow-wave sleep. In S Inoué and AA Borbély (eds.), *Endogenous Sleep Substances and Sleep Regulation*. Japan Scientific Societies Press, Tokyo, 1985: 181–192.

81. Krueger JM, Davenne D, Walter J, Shoham S, Kubillus SL, Rosenthal RS, Martin SA, Biemann K. Bacterial peptidoglycans as modulators of sleep. II. Effects of muramyl peptides on the structure of rabbit sleep. *Brain Res* 1987; 403:258–266.

82. Krueger JM, Dinarello CA, Shoham S, Davenne D, Walter J, Kubillus S. Interferon alpha-2 enhances slow-wave sleep in rabbits. *Int J Immunopharmacol* 1987; 9:23–30.

83. Krueger JM, Karnovsky ML. Sleep and the immune response. *Ann NY Acad Sci* 1987; 496:510–516.

84. Krueger JM, Karnovsky ML, Martin SA, Pappenheimer JR, Walter J, Biemann K. Peptidoglycans as promoters of slow wave sleep. II. Somnogenic and pyrogenic activities of some naturally occurring muramyl peptides: Correlations with mass spectrometric structure determination. *J Biol Chem* 1984; 259:12659–12662.

85. Krueger JM, Kubillus S, Shoham S, Davenne D. Enhancement of slow-wave sleep by endotoxin and lipid A. *Am J Physiol* 1986; 251:R591–R597.

86. Krueger JM, Majde JA, Blatteis CM, Endsley J, Ahokas RA, Cady AB. Polyriboinosinic:polyribocytidylic acid (poly I:C) enhances rabbit slow-wave sleep. *Am J Physiol* 1988; 255:R748–R755.

87. Krueger JM, Obal F Jr, Johannsen L, Cady AB, Toth L. Slow wave sleep: Physiological, pathophysiological and functional aspects. In: A Wauquier, C Dugsovic, and M Radulovacki (eds.), *Current Trends in Slow-Wave Sleep Research*. Raven, New York, 1989: 75–90.

88. Krueger JM, Pappenheimer JR, Karnovsky ML. The composition of sleep-promoting factor isolated from human urine. *J Biol Chem* 1982; 257:1664–1669.

89. Krueger JM, Pappenheimer JR, Karnovsky ML. Sleep-promoting effects of muramyl peptides. *Proc Natl Acad Sci USA* 1982; 79:6102–6106.

90. Krueger JM, Rosenthal RS, Martin SA, Walter J, Davenne D, Shoham S, Kubillus SL, Biemann K. Bacterial peptidoglycans as modulators of sleep. I. Anhydro forms of muramyl peptides enhance somnogenic potency. *Brain Res* 1987; 403:249–257.

91. Krueger JM, Toth LA, Cady AB, Johannsen L, Obal F Jr. Immunomodulation of sleep. In S. Inoué (ed.), *Sleep Regulation by Sleep Peptides*. VNU Press, Tokyo, 1988: 95–129.

92. Krueger JM, Walter J, Dinarello CA, Wolff SM, Chedid L. Sleep-promoting effects of endogenous pyrogen (interleukin-1). *Am J Physiol* 1984; 246:R994–R999.

93. Krueger JM, Walter J, Karnovsky ML, Chedid L, Choay JP, Lefrancier P, Lederer E. Muramyl peptides: Variation of somnogenic activity with structure. *J Exp Med* 1984; 159:68–76.

94. Krueger JM, Walter J, Levin C. Factor S and related somnogens: An immune theory for slow-wave sleep. In DJ McGinty, R Drucker-Colin, A Morrison, and PL Parmeggiani (eds.), *Brain Mechanisms of Sleep*, Raven, New York, 1985: 253–276.
95. Kruisbrink J, Mirmiran M, Van der Woude TP, Boer GJ. Effects of enhanced cerebrospinal fluid levels of vasopressin, vasopressin antagonist or vasoactive intestinal polypeptide on circadian sleep-wake rhythm in the rat. *Brain Res* 1987; 419:76–86.
96. Laburthe M, Amiranoff B, Boige N, Rouyer-Fessard C, Tatemoto K, Moroder L. Interaction of GRF with VIP receptors and stimulation of adenylate cyclase in rat and human intestinal epithelial membranes. *FEBS Lett* 1983; 159:89–92.
97. Laburthe M, Couvineau A, Rouyer-Fessard C, Moroder L. Interaction of PHM, PHI, and 24-glutamine PHI with human VIP receptors from colonic epithelium: Comparison with rat intestinal receptors. *Life Sci* 1985; 36:991–995.
98. Legendre R, Pieron H. Recherches sur le besoin de sommeil consecutif a une veille prolongee. *Z Allg Physiol* 1913; 14:235–262.
99. Lipton JM, Clark WC. Neurotransmitters in temperature control. *Annu Rev Physiol* 1986; 49:613–623.
100. Lue FA, Bail M, Gorczynski R, Moldofsky H. Sleep and interleukin-1-like activity in cat cerebrospinal fluid. *Sleep Res* 1987; 16:51.
101. Mandell AJ. From molecular biological simplification to more realistic central nervous system dynamics: An opinion. *Psychobiol Fdns Clin Psych* 1985; 3:1–6.
102. Martin JB. Brain regulation of growth hormone secretion. In L Martini and WG Ganong (eds.), *Frontiers in Neuroendocrinology*, Vol. 4, Raven, New York, 1976: 129–168.
103. Masek K. Immunopharmacology of muramyl peptides. *Fed Proc* 1986; 45:2549–2551.
104. McCann SM, Ono N, Khorram O, Kentrotti S, Aguila C. The role of brain peptides in neuroimmunomodulation. *Ann NY Acad Sci* 1987; 496:173–181.
105. McGinty DJ. Physiological equilibrium and the control of sleep states. In DJ McGinty, R Drucker-Colin, A Morrison, and PL Parmeggiani (eds.), *Brain Mechanisms of Sleep*, Raven, New York, 1985: 361–384.
106. Mendelson WB, Slater S, Gold P, Gillin JC. The effect of growth hormone administration on human sleep: A dose-response study. *Biol Psychiat* 1980; 15:613–618.
107. Moldofsky H, Lue F, Davidson J, Jephthah-Ochola J, Carayanniotis K, Saskin P, Gorczynski R. Sleep deprivation and plasma IL1-like activity in man. *J Leukocyte Biol* 1987; 42:602.
108. Moldofsky H, Lue FA, Eisen J, Gorczynski RM. The relationship of interleukin-1 and immune function to sleep in humans. *Psychosom Med* 1986; 48:309–318.
109. Moldofsky H, Scarisbrick P, England R, Smythe H. Musculoskeletal symptoms and non-REM sleep disturbance in patients with "fibrositis syndrome" and healthy subjects. *Psychosom Med* 1975; 37:341–351.
110. Moruzzi G. The sleep-waking cycle. *Ergebn Physiol* 1972; 64:1–165.
111. Munford RS. Enzymatic deacylation of bacterial lipopolysaccharides by human neutrophils and murine macrophages. In MA Horwitz (ed.), *Bacteria-Host Cell Interaction*. Liss, New York, 1988: 123–140.
112. Munoz C, Keusch G, Schlesinger L, Arevalo M, Arredondo S, Mendez G, Dinarello CA. Interleukin-1 in human milk. *J Leukocyte Biol* 1987; 42:604.
113. Nagy E, Berczi I, Friesen HG. Regulation of immunity in rats by lactogenic and growth hormones. *Acta Endocrinol* 1983; 102:351–357.
114. Nistico G, De Sarro GB, Bagetta G, Muller EE. Behavioural and electrocortical spectrum power effects of growth hormone releasing factor in rats. *Neuropharmacology* 1987; 26:75–78.
115. Obal F Jr. Effects of peptides (DSIP, DSIP analogues, VIP, GRF and CCK) on sleep in the rat. *Clin Neuropharmacol* 1986; (S4) 9:459–461.

116. Obal F Jr, Alfoldi P, Cady AB, Johannsen L, Sary G, Krueger JM. Growth hormone releasing factor enhances sleep in rats and rabbits. *Am J Physiol* 1988; 255:R310–R316.

117. Obal F Jr, Sary G, Alfoldi P, Rubicsek G, Obal F. Vasoactive intestinal polypeptide promotes sleep without effects on brain temperature in rats at night. *Neurosci Lett* 1986; 64:236–240.

118. O'Donohue TL, Dorsa DM. The opiomelantropinergic neuronal and endocrine system. *Peptides* 1982; 3:353–395.

119. Old LJ. Tumor necrosis factor. *Sci Am* 1988; 258:59–75.

120. Olivo M, Kitahama K, Valatx J-L, Jouvet M. Neonatal monosodium glutamate dosing alters the sleep-wake cycle of the mature rat. *Neurosci Lett* 1986; 67:186–190.

121. Opp MR, Obal F Jr, Krueger JM. Effects of αMSH on sleep, behavior and brain temperature: Interactions with IL1. *Am J Physiol* 1989; 255:R914–R922.

122. Pappenheimer JR, Koski G, Fencl V, Karnovsky ML, Krueger JM. Extraction of sleep-promoting factor S from cerebrospinal fluid and from brains of sleep deprived animals. *J Neurophysiol* 1975; 38:1299–1311.

123. Pappenheimer JR, Miller TB, Goodrich CA. Sleep-promoting effects of cerebrospinal fluid from sleep-deprived goats. *Proc Natl Acad Sci USA* 1967; 58:513–517.

124. Pappenheimer JR, Zich KE. Absorption of hydrophilic solutes from the small intestine. *J Physiol (London)* 1986; 371:138P.

125. Reite M, Laudenslager M, Jones J, Crnic C, Kaemingk K. Interferon decreases REM latency. *Biol Psychiat* 1987; 22:104–107.

126. Riou F, Cespuglio R, Jouvet M. Endogenous peptides and sleep in the rat: III. The hypnogenic properties of vasoactive intestinal polypeptide. *Neuropeptides* 1982; 2:265–277.

127. Roberts NJ, Prill AH, Mann TN. Interleukin-1 and inhibitor production by human macrophages exposed to influenza virus or respiratory syncytial virus. In MJ Kluger, JJ Oppenheim, and MC Powanda (eds.), *The Physiologic, Metabolic and Immunologic Actions of Interleukin-1*. Liss, New York, 1985: 409–418.

128. Root-Bernstein RC, Westall FC. Sleep factors: Do muramyl peptides activate serotonin binding sites? *Lancet* 1983; 1:653.

129. Root-Bernstein RC, Westall FC. Serotonin binding sites. I. Structures of sites on myelin basic protein, LHRH, MSH, ACTH, interferon, serum albumin, ovalbumin and red pigment concentrating hormone. *Brain Res Bull* 1984; 12:425–536.

130. Rosenstreich DL, Korn H, Kabir S, Brown KM. Studies on a urine-derived human interleukin-1 inhibitor. In MJ Kluger, JJ Oppenheim, and MC Powanda (eds.), *The Physiologic, Metabolic and Immunologic Actions of Interleukin-1*. Liss, New York, 1985: 419–428.

131. Sapolsky R, Rivier C, Yamamoto G, Plotsky P, Vale W. Interleukin-1 stimulates the secretion of hypothalamic corticotropin-releasing factor. *Science* 1987; 238:522–524.

132. Sassin JF. Sleep-related hormones. In R Drucker-Colin and J McGaugh (eds.), *Neurobiology of Sleep and Memory*. Academic Press, New York, 1977: 361–372.

133. Scherschlicht R, Marias J. Effects of sleep promoting 'Factor S,' muramyl dipeptide (MDP) and L-cyclserine on the sleep of rabbits. *Experientia* 1983; 39:683.

134. Schnedorf JG, Ivy AC. An examination of the hypnotoxin theory of sleep. *Am J Physiol* 1939; 125:491–505.

135. Shibata M, Blatteis CM, Krueger JM, Obal F Jr, Opp M. Pyrogenic, inflammatory and somnogenic responses to cytokines: Differential modes of action. In P Lomax and E Schönbaum (eds.), *Thermoregulation: Research and Clinical Application*. Karger, Basel, 1989: 69–73.

136. Shoham S, Ahokas RA, Blatteis CM, Krueger JM. Effects of muramyl dipeptide on sleep,

body temperature, and plasma copper after intracerebral ventricular administration. *Brain Res* 1987; 419:223–228.

137. Shoham S, Blatteis CM, Krueger JM. Effects of preoptic area lesions on MDP-induced sleep and fever responses. *Brain Res* 1989; 496:396–399.

138. Shoham S, Davenne D, Cady AB, Dinarello CA, Krueger JM. Recombinant tumor necrosis factor and interleukin-1 enhance slow-wave sleep in rabbits. *Am J Physiol* 1987; 253:R142–R149.

139. Shoham S, Krueger JM. Muramyl dipeptide-induced sleep and fever; effects of ambient temperature and time of injection. *Am J Physiol* 1988; 255:R157–R165.

140. Silva NL, Boulant JA. Effects of osmotic pressure, glucose and temperature on neurons in peroptic tissue slices. *Am J Physiol* 1984; 247:R335–R345.

141. Silva NL, Boulant JA. Effects of testosterone, estradiol and temperature on neurons in preoptic tissue slices. *Am J Physiol* 1986; 250:R625–R632.

142. Silverman DH. Specific binding and effects of muramyl peptides on some cells of the immune and nervous systems. Ph.D. Thesis, Harvard University, Cambridge, MA, 1987.

143. Silverman DHS, Krueger JM, Karnovsky ML. Specific binding sites for muramyl peptides on murine macrophages. *J Immunol* 1986; 136:2195–2201.

144. Silverman DHS, Wu, H, Karnovsky ML. Muramyl peptides and serotonin interact at specific binding sites on macrophages and enhance superoxide release. *Biochem Biophys Res Commun* 1985; 131:1160–1165.

145. Stern WC, Jalowiec JE, Shabshelowitz H, Morgane P. Effects of growth hormone on sleep-waking patterns in cats. *Horm Behav* 1975; 6:189–196.

146. Takahashi Y. Growth hormone secretion related to the sleep and waking rhythm. In R Drucker-Colin, M Shkurovich, and MB Sterman (eds.), *The Functions of Sleep.* Academic Press, New York, 1979: 113–145.

147. Tobler I, Borbély AA. Sleep regulation after reduction of brain serotonin: Effect of p-chlorophenylalanine combined with sleep deprivation in the rat. *Sleep* 1982; 5:145–153.

148. Tobler I, Borbély AA, Schwyzer M, Fontana A. Interleukin-1 derived from astrocytes enhances slow wave activity in sleep. *Eur J Pharmacol* 1984; 104:191–192.

149. Toth LA, Krueger JM. *Staphylococcus aureus* alters sleep patterns in rabbits. *Infect Immun* 1988; 56:1785–1791.

150. Totic S, Susic V. Effects of interleukin-1 on the body temperature and sleep in the cat. *Sleep Res* 1987; 16:151.

151. Twery MJ, Moss RL. Sensitivity of rat forebrain neurons to growth hormones-releasing hormone. *Peptides* 1985; 6:609–613.

152. Ueno R, Onoe H, Matsumura H, Hayaishi O, Fujita I, Nishino H, Oomura Y. Regulation of sleep by prostaglandins in conscious rhesus monkeys. *Sleep Res* 1987; 16:36.

153. Vermeulon MW, Grey GR. Processing of *Bacillus subtilis* peptidoglycan by a mouse macrophage cell line. *Infect Immun* 1984; 46:476–483.

154. Vijayan E, Samson WK, Said SI, McCann SM. Vasoactive intestinal peptide: Evidence for a hypothalamic site of action to release growth hormone, luteinizing hormone, and prolactin in conscious ovariectomized rats. *Endocrinology* 1979; 104:53–57.

155. Waelbroeck M, Robberecht P, Coy DH, Camus J-C, De Neef P, Christophe J. Interaction of growth hormone-releasing factor (GRF) and 14 GRF analogs with vasoactive intestinal peptide (VIP) receptors of rat pancreas. Discovery of (N-Ac-Tyr^1,D-Phe^2)-GRF(1-29)-NH$_2$ as a VIP antagonist. *Endocrinology* 1985; 116:2643–2649.

156. Walter J, Davenne D, Shoham S, Dinarello CA, Krueger JM. Brain temperature changes coupled to sleep states persist during interleukin-1 enhanced sleep. *Am J Physiol* 1986; 250:R96–R103.

157. Weigent DA, Blalock JE. Interactions between the neuroendocrine and immune systems: Common hormones and receptors. *Immunol Rev* 1987; 100:79–107.

158. Weiner N, Wesemann W. Receptor regulation—effect of sleep deprivation on cerebral 5-HT binding in the rat. In WP Koella (ed.), *Sleep 1982*. Karger, Basel, 1983: 261–263.

159. Wexler DB, Moore-Ede MC. Effects of a muramyl dipeptide on the temperature and sleep-wake cycles of the squirrel monkey. *Am J Physiol* 1984; 247:R672–R680.

160. White DP, Miller F, Erickson RW. Sleep apnea and nocturnal hypoventilation after western equine encephalitis. *Am Rev Resp Dis* 1983; 127:132–133.

161. Zhai S, Karnovsky ML. Qualitative detection of muramic acid in normal mammalian tissues. *Infect Immun* 1984; 43:937–941.

11

Cholinergic Mechanisms in Sleep: Basic and Clinical Applications

J. CHRISTIAN GILLIN AND P. SHIROMANI

The discovery of rapid eye movement (REM) and non-REM (NREM) sleep in 1953 by Aserinsky and Kleitman (3) opened a new field of clinical research and clinical neurophysiology. Since sleep disturbances had long been reported by patients suffering from depression, drug abuse, alcoholism, acute psychosis, mania, insomnia, hypersomnia, and so forth, it was only a matter of time before polysomnographic studies would be applied to understanding these disorders. During the past 20 years or so, these descriptive studies have identified relatively sensitive sleep abnormalities in many syndromes, although they have not yet described any specific, pathognomonic changes in sleep stages.

Of the many sleep abnormalities described, short REM latency has received perhaps the most attention. The first REM period does not usually appear until 70–90 min of NREM sleep have occurred, at least in adults. Not long after the discovery of REM sleep, however, patients with narcolepsy were found to have a very short REM latency, at times entering REM sleep from wakefulness with no intervening NREM sleep (91). Since then, short REM latency has been described in several clinical syndromes, as well as a variety of normal and abnormal situations.

Short REM latency has been particularly well documented in patients with depression (41,38,73). In general, short REM latency in depression is state related, varying roughly with severity of depression and returning toward normal with clinical recovery. It is typically associated with prolonged sleep latency, reduction in total sleep time and delta (Stages 3 and 4) sleep, and increased REM density.

Short REM latency, however, is not specific to depressive disorders. It has been reported in some but not all patients with obsessive–compulsive disorder (53), schizophrenia (65), and primary alcoholism (JC Gillin, personal observations). In addition, it is well known that REM latency is reduced following deprivation of REM sleep, whether by the awakening method in normal subjects (27), the "flower-pot" method in animals (28), or drugs such as barbiturates, amphetamine, and cocaine. Moreover, REM latency is also shortened in many normal individuals such as newborn infants (95) and "healthy insomniacs" (63,81). Finally, it is reduced in normal individuals at

186

times during the normal 24-hr day as a result of circadian influences as manifested in naps (66), in studies of people living in time-free environments (23), or acute shifts of the sleep–wake cycle (145).

The neurophysiological mechanisms controlling REM latency and other aspects of sleep are not particularly well understood, although considerable progress has been made. It is our belief that a better understanding of these fundamental physiological mechanisms will contribute considerably to the interpretation of short REM latency and other sleep abnormalities in clinical disorders and other physiological states. Since the role of the central cholinergic nervous system is one of the best understood aspects of the control of sleep states, this chapter will concentrate on reviewing our knowledge about cholinergic mechanisms and discussing certain implications for studies of depression.

Of particular importance to a discussion linking cholinergic mechanisms, short REM latency, and depression is the cholinergic–aminergic imbalance hypothesis of affective disorders, proposed by Janowsky et al. in 1972 (57). They proposed that depression results from an increased ratio of cholinergic to aminergic neurotransmission. Much of the evidence supporting this hypothesis is inferential and based on pharmacological observations of drugs that increased or decreased depression. For example, Janowsky et al. (57) originally cited studies indicating that depression resulted from drugs that had antiadrenergic or cholinomimetic properties, such as reserpine, propranolol, diisopropylfluorophosphate, or α-methyldopa. In experimental studies in normal volunteers and patients with affective disorders, Janowsky and his colleagues reported that physostigmine, a cholinesterase inhibitor, caused anergy, psychomotor retardation, drained feelings, social withdrawal, decreased thoughts, hostility, anxiety, and depression. Many of these effects could be antagonized by atropine, a muscarinic antagonist. Similarly, Nurnberger et al. (89) and Risch et al. (93) reported that arecoline, a relatively specific muscarinic agonist at the doses employed, produced somewhat similar, depression-like symptoms.

In addition, physostigmine has been reported to have antimanic effects, whereas neostigmine, which does not cross the blood–brain barrier, does not (15,24,58,84).

Since activation of the hypothalamic–pituitary–adrenal axis is another well-established sensitive but not specific finding in depression, it is relevant that physostigmine and arecoline increase serum adrenocorticotropic hormone and cortisol (56,92).

A variant on the original cholinergic–aminergic hypothesis is that patients with affective disorders have up-regulated "muscarinic receptors" at crucial central pathways. This hypothesis was inspired in part by studies in normal volunteers suggesting that scopolamine-induced muscarinic supersensitivity produced a state mimicking the sleep changes associated with depression, specifically short REM latency, increased REM density and sleep latency, and decreased total sleep time and sleep efficiency (40). Other attempts to more directly test this hypothesis by measurement of muscarinic receptors in autopsied brain tissue from suicides and skin fibroblasts have not been successful (42). Nevertheless, despite an inability to directly confirm this hypothesis, it is still a viable research strategy.

In the first part of this chapter, we will review the basic physiology of REM sleep, with particular reference to cholinergic mechanisms. In the second half we will review the Cholinergic REM Induction Test (CRIT), which has been used to test the hypothesis that a state of muscarinic supersensitivity exists in patients with affective disorder.

CHOLINERGIC MECHANISMS IN REM SLEEP: BASIC
SCIENCE MECHANISMS

The Neuroanatomical Organization of the Cholinergic System

Even though acetylcholine was the first neurotransmitter to be discovered, the lack of accurate mapping procedures comparable to those used to localize serotonin and the catecholamines has hindered progress in fully outlining the organization of the cholinergic system in the central nervous system. New procedures, such as autoradiography to locate cholinergic receptors (143), immunohistochemical labeling of the acetylcholine-synthesizing enzyme, choline-acetyltransferase (ChAT) (72), and identification of acetylcholine in neurons (36), are only now providing information on the organization of the acetylcholine system and its potential role in sleep, psychiatric and neurological disorders, and other behaviors such as information processing (6).

Earlier methods for identifying cholinergic neurons involved detection of acetylcholinesterase (AchE), the enzyme that metabolizes acetylcholine. This procedure was used by Lewis and Shute (75) to provide early maps of the cholinergic system. Conclusions from this procedure have been questioned, as this approach provides a limited, indirect method of localizing cholinergic pathways. Moreover, AchE is found in places devoid of acetylcholine, such as the zona incerta, hypothalamic arcuate and dorsomedial nuclei, lateral posterior hypothalamus, and substantia nigra (12,13). This procedure, therefore, falsely indicates many positive sites.

Recently, more direct and accurate immunohistochemical procedures have been used to label ChAT and to identify cholinergic pathways. Using this immunohistochemical technique, Mesulam and co-workers (82) have identified six major cholinergic groups. Cholinergic groups 1 and 2 (Ch1 and 2) lie within the medial septal nucleus and the vertical limb nucleus of the diagonal band, respectively. Neurons from these two groups innervate the hippocampus. Group Ch3 is partly contained in the horizontal limb nucleus of the diagonal band and innervates the olfactory bulb. The largest collection of cholinergic cells is located within the nucleus basalis of Meynert and in the nucleus of the ansa lenticularis, in the nucleus of the ansa peduncularis, and in the medullary laminae of the globus pallidus and substantia inominata. Collectively, these cholinergic neurons are referred to as the Ch4 group, and they are the principal cause of the cholinergic innervation of amygdala and neocortex. Loss of these cholinergic neurons has been hypothesized to cause the cognitive deterioration observed in Alzheimer's disease (22).

In the brainstem the largest collection of cholinergic cells occurs in the pedunculopontine nucleus (Ch5), which borders the brachium conjunctivum, and the lateral dorsal tegmental nucleus (Ch6), which is medial to the locus coeruleus. These two groups, which form the ascending cholinergic pathway of Lewis and Shute (75,146), innervate the thalamus, hippocampus, hypothalamus, and cingulate cortex (82,101, 122,146). In the brainstem, cholinergic neurons are also found in the cranial motor nerve nuclei.

We will refer to the medial pontine reticular formation (PRF) as the region between the locus coeruleus and the abducens and from the midline to the motor trigeminal nucleus. In the cat, using Berman's terminology, this region refers to the rostral portion of the gigantocellular tegmental field (FTG) and portions of the lateral and central tegmental fields. In the rat, this region comprises the pontis caudalis and oralis regions. In our terminology the medial PRF is ventral to the locus coeruleus and the dorsal tegmental cholinergic groups.

Transection and Lesion Studies

Transections provide a quick way of determining the brain structure important for REM sleep. Jouvet initially showed that transections at the midbrain level did not interfere with REM sleep in areas caudal to the cut (64). Behind the cut the animal's sleep, which could be identified by the occurrence of spindles at the pontine level, was interrupted often by episodes of REM sleep. These episodes are characterized by complete disappearance of muscle activity (loss of decerebrate rigidity). Jouvet argues that these episodes were indeed REM sleep since the duration of atonia was similar to intact animals and each episode was marked by irregular respiration and relaxed nictating membrane. Therefore, structures rostral to the cut are not required for the generation of REM sleep (48,64,142). Moreover, cerebellectomy or decortication do not eliminate REM sleep (25,64,90). Recently, Siegel et al. (116) showed, in cats with transection at the pontomedullary level, that REM sleep was absent in the medullary portions but present in forebrain and attached pons. However, the timing was different in that REM sleep occurred sooner and lasted longer. This suggests that the medullary reticular formation may play a role in the timing of REM sleep. Webster et al. (144) used a retractable wire knife to make cuts and noted that transections through the entire brainstem at the pontomedullary level eliminated REM sleep. Transection of the dorsal half of the reticular formation did not reduce REM sleep, but PGO waves were diminished slightly. Muscle atonia was not disturbed. Ventral transections, however, eliminated atonia and REM sleep was greatly disturbed. They suggest that descending tegmentoreticular pathways that course ventrally are needed for atonia and are important for REM sleep.

Lesions have been made in pontine regions to further isolate the regions involved in REM sleep generation. Jouvet initially showed that large electrolytic lesions of the pontine reticular formation eliminated REM sleep. Jones (61) confirmed this observation with smaller lesions of the pons. Moreover, Jones' group has found that when electrolytic lesions are made in the medial and lateral portions of the FTG, only the lateral portions eliminated REM sleep (34). Lavie et al. (74), in a case report, noted that a man with a localized pontine lesion inflicted by a shrapnel fragment had virtually no REM sleep even though NREM sleep was not disturbed. In sharp contrast to the above findings, it has been determined that injection of the neurotoxin kainic acid, which destroys cell bodies without affecting fibers of passage, into the medial PRF, does not eliminate REM sleep (31,102). In the study by Drucker-Colin et al. (31) it was shown that in kainic acid-lesioned animals carbachol did not trigger REM sleep. In nonlesioned animal carbachol has been shown to trigger REM sleep. This suggests that kainic acid may have destroyed a large percentage of neurons involved in the cholinergic induction of REM sleep without affecting the main group of cells necessary for REM sleep. The differing effects on REM sleep produced by kainic acid and electrolytic lesions suggest that electrolytic lesions may impair REM sleep by destroying fibers of passage.

Other pontine structures that are the source of major ascending and descending neurotransmitter systems have been lesioned. For example, Jones et al. have shown that, in cats, electrolytic lesions of the locus coeruleus (LC) produced no changes in REM sleep even though forebrain noradrenaline levels were severely depleted (60). This finding has been confirmed in the rat (85). However, Braun and Pivik (11) showed that in rabbits, electrolytic lesions of the LC eliminate REM sleep and fragment sleep. Caballero et al. (14) noted that unilateral lesions of the LC increase REM sleep. Cespuglio et al. (17) showed that bilateral cooling of LC promotes NREM and REM sleep in cats.

Thus, even though transection studies show that REM sleep originates from the pons, the lesion studies have not been able to unequivocally pinpoint the pontine structure(s) responsible for REM sleep generation. Like others, we argue that no single anatomic region is solely responsible for REM sleep generation. Rather, several regions interact to produce this state.

Neuronal Activity in the Pontine Reticular Formation (PRF)

Investigators have examined the firing patterns of pontine neurons in an effort to identify a group of neurons that shows a pattern of firing directly related to REM sleep. A number of neurons within the pontine tegmentum (as elsewhere in the brain) markedly increase their firing rates during REM sleep compared to NREM sleep. Data derived from unanesthetized, head-restrained cats indicate that the discharge rate of medial PRF cells is highest during REM sleep (49,50), and that the increase occurs as much as several minutes before each REM sleep episode (49). However, evidence derived from freely moving cats (113–115), and rats (140,141) shows that although medial PRF cells increase their output during PS, the unit discharge rate is comparable to that obtained during waking with movement. As such, it has been suggested that activity of the medial PRF neurons may reflect motor activity instead of being specific to a particular sleep state (112).

Nevertheless, Shiromani et al. (108) along with Sakai (99) found some neurons in the medial PRF and the locus subcoeruleus region that increase discharge selectively from waking-to-NREM-to-REM sleep. These cells represent about 8–10% of the recorded cells in the medial pons. Moreover, we have shown that some medial PRF neurons are activated before and during cholinergic-induced REM sleep (109). Thus, these neurons must be considered as possible generators of REM sleep. Intracellular studies by McCarley and his group (78) showed that some medial PRF neurons depolarize well before REM sleep onset and maintain a tonic level of depolarization during the REM episode (see chapter 8, this volume).

In sharp contrast to the medial PRF neurons, there are cells in the dorsal raphe and LC that slow their rate or cease firing during REM sleep (18,19,79,105). The inverse relationship in firing rates between LC, dorsal raphe, and medial PRF neurons led to the formulation of the reciprocal-interaction model of REM sleep generation (77). This model, based on the Lotka–Volterra equations, relates the time course and rate of timing of "on" and "off" cells and accounts for the oscillation between REM and NREM sleep. The recent revision of the model postulates that REM sleep is initiated when some pontine cells (such as those in the locus coeruleus and dorsal raphe) cease firing and, thereby, allow other pontine cells (such as those in the medial PRF) to assume high discharge rates (52). It has been suggested that those neurons that increase discharge during REM sleep are cholinergic or cholinoceptive. This part of the model is amply supported by studies where cholinergic stimulation of the medial PRF readily triggers REM sleep.

Thus, single-unit studies that at best provide correlational data show that some pontine cells selectively increase or decrease firing in conjunction with REM sleep. That these neurons interact reciprocally is an attractive hypothesis.

Acetylcholine and REM Sleep Generation

Of all the neurotransmitter or peptidergic systems, the evidence supporting the role of acetylcholine in triggering REM sleep is the strongest.

Increase in Acetylcholine Availability

Firm evidence that acetylcholine may be involved in arousal and REM sleep is provided by studies that show alterations in acetylcholine levels as a function of electroencephalogram (EEG) activation. For instance, cortical desynchronization induced by stimulation of the mesencephalic reticular formation releases acetylcholine into the cortex (16,20,133). During REM sleep, increased acetylcholine is found during REM sleep in cortex (16) and striatum of normal cats (35), and in ventricular perfusates of conscious dogs (45).

Additional evidence linking acetylcholine with cortical activity is provided from studies in which administration of acetylcholine into the carotid artery induces a state of cortical desynchronization (86). This effect can also be elicited by administration of the acetylcholinesterase inhibitor, physostigmine (30). Aside from their effects in initiating arousal, acetylcholine-potentiating agents also increase REM sleep. For example, in chronic pontile or reserpinized cats physostigmine significantly increases REM sleep (64,67). The REM sleep facilitory effect is also seen in humans (118,119), and normal cats (30). In fact, in humans physostigmine decreases the latency of both the first and second REM sleep periods without altering their duration (39). This latter finding is particularly interesting since it suggests that cholinergic mechanisms may control the periodicity of REM sleep rather than its duration. Similar effects are also seen with arecoline, a muscarinic receptor agonist (68). In human subjects, intravenous infusions of physostigmine or arecoline during NREM sleep decrease the latency to REM sleep, although infusion during or immediately after REM sleep produces arousal (118–120). In normal humans, a three consecutive morning treatment with scopolamine decreases the latency to REM sleep at night and also potentiates the REM-inducing effect of arecoline at night (122). In addition, an orally active muscarinic agonist (RS-86) shortens REM latency in normal volunteers (128). Finally, there have been reports of farmers exposed to anticholinesterase insecticides who have increased amounts and early onset of REM sleep (131).

The possibility that brainstem cholinergic mechanisms may be responsible for the REM sleep augmentation is suggested by studies in which application of cholinergic-potentiating agents directly into the pontine reticular formation in cats and rat, or intravenously in pontile cats, elicits both the tonic and phasic components of REM sleep.

In 1963 Cordeau et al. (21), noticed that injections of acetylcholine into the cat brainstem were followed by periods in which the cat was "motionless." In this study the EMG was not recorded. However, the authors noted that injections into the rostral portions of the pontine reticular formation produced periods of "activated sleep." George et al. (37) injected oxotremorine or carbachol directly into the nucleus reticularis pontis oralis and caudalis (i.e., the medial PRF area). The cats displayed all the characteristic signs of REM sleep, viz. rapid eye relaxation and miosis of the pupils. These episodes lasted up to 60 min and were usually followed by awakening during which the animals were atonic. Administration of atropine was able to block the development of the drug-induced REM sleep.

Khazan et al. (70) showed, in rats, that intraperitoneal injections of eserine or neostigmine reversed the REM blocking effects of chlorpromazine and imipramine. Baxter (7) placed carbachol crystals in the mesencephalic gray area, not the medial PRF, and obtained a behavioral pattern that can be characterized only as intensely emotional in that the animals hissed and growled. When the carbachol was placed in or near the ventricles, however, the EEG as well as the behavioral signs of REM sleep were obtained. Van Dongen (139) confirmed the behavioral observation of Baxter and found that carbachol injection into the pontis oralis area elicited emotional reaction similar to that obtained by Baxter. Van Dongen also found that carbachol injection into the LC and pontis caudalis produced atonia comparable to that seen during REM sleep (138). Mitler and Dement (83) injected carbachol into the LC area and obtained atonia, increased pontogeniculooccipital (PGO) waves, and REM. Atropine was able to reverse the carbachol-induced behavior.

Perhaps the most detailed study of the effects due to cholinergic stimulation has been made by Alan Hobson's group at Harvard. They have injected a variety of cholinergic agonists such as carbachol, bethanechol, and neostigmine into various brainstem regions and found that there is a localized region within the medial PRF from which REM sleep can be most readily triggered following drug infusion (1,4,5, 51,117).

We have also sought to determine how REM sleep is generated and have relied on the cholinergic-REM induction model to provide some answers. Initially, we showed, in rats, that long-term cholinergic stimulation of the medial PRF via an Alzet osmotic minipump augmented REM sleep during the 5-day period of drug infusion (110). In the same study we also determined that similar continuous infusions of scopolamine blocked physiological REM sleep for the period of drug infusion. The carbachol-induced REM sleep augmentation was a result of an increase in the number of REM sleep bouts and not the result of lengthening the REM sleep bouts. This is a very important finding because it indicates that cholinergic mechanisms trigger REM sleep. Recently, Gnadt and Pegram (43) have also shown increased REM sleep following pontine carbachol administration in rats.

In another study we determined that the cholinergic-induced REM sleep was similar to physiologic REM sleep in that there was an REM sleep-related decrease in blood pressure during both drug and physiologic REM sleep (106). We have also examined the firing pattern of pontine neurons before and after infusion of carbachol and found that a majority of medial PRF neurons showed either a decrease (55%) or no change (17%) in activity during carbachol-induced REM sleep (109). During physiological REM sleep these neurons had increased discharge, which is typical of most medial PRF neurons. This finding was important because it indicated, for the first time, that a majority of medial PRF neurons were not responsible for REM sleep but subserved other functions as suggested by Siegel (112). Even though most medial PRF neurons were either inhibited or showed no change following carbachol, we did find that a small percentage of neurons (28%) increased firing in conjunction with carbachol-induced REM sleep. The change in activity of these neurons was temporally related to the emergence of the carbachol-induced REM sleep. This suggests that only a small percentage of neurons is responsible for REM sleep.

Recently, we began to focus on the relationship between central muscarinic receptors and REM sleep and found that, in rats, REM sleep augmentation occurred in conjunction with muscarinic receptor up-regulation during withdrawal from a 7-day chronic scopolamine treatment (132). In this study increased muscarinic density was found in the caudate and hippocampus but unchanged density was observed in the cortex, brainstem, and cerebellum. Finally, we began to study the sleep pattern in a strain of rats genetically bred for increased numbers of central cholinergic receptors. We found that these rats have normally elevated levels of REM sleep (+35%) compared to randomly bred rats (111). The increased levels of REM sleep are the result of an increased number of REM sleep bouts and not of change in the duration of REM sleep bouts. Moreover, we found that the cholinergic hyperactive rats entered into REM sleep more often from a drowsy state and that REM–REM cycle length (i.e., time from the end of the REM bout to the beginning of the next REM bout) was about 2 min faster compared to controls. Therefore, the REM sleep pattern seen in the cholinergic hyperactive rats is similar to that obtained following cholinergic drug infusion.

Another good animal model that displays aberrant REM sleep patterns is the narcoleptic dog. In narcoleptic dogs, muscarinic receptor agonists readily trigger cataplexy, whereas nicotinic agonists have no effect (26). In narcoleptic dogs, increased muscarinic receptors are located in the medial PRF regions implicated in REM sleep generation (10,71).

Decrease in Acetylcholine Availability

Acetylcholine can be depleted by hemicholinium-3, which blocks choline reuptake. Consistent with the hypothesis that acetylcholine is required to initiate REM sleep, hemicholinium-3, administered intraventricularly, abolishes REM sleep (29,46).

The muscarinic effects of acetylcholine can be blocked by scopolamine and atropine. Both drugs selectively suppress REM sleep in animals and humans. This is seen even in REM sleep-deprived cats (47). Administration of scopolamine or atropine decreases physiologic REM sleep and blocks the cholinergic-induced REM sleep in cats and rats (5,110). In humans, administration of scopolamine delays onset of REM sleep and lengthens the interval between REM sleep episodes (96,120). Further, scopolamine also blocks the REM sleep-potentiating effects of arecoline (120).

Thus, the data from pharmacological studies show very convincingly that acetylcholine is involved in triggering REM sleep.

Neuronal Network Involved in REM Sleep Generation

Even though numerous pharmacological studies implicate cholinergic mechanisms in REM sleep generation, these studies indicate that neurons sensitive to acetylcholine can generate REM sleep, but do not specify which cholinergic neurons are responsible. Indeed, we find no cholinergic cell bodies in the medial PRF, an area from where REM sleep is readily triggered by the application of cholinergic agonists. Also, we show that those neurons in the medial PRF that show a progressive increase in discharge from waking to REM sleep are not located near cholinergic cells (107). Previously, Sakai (98) identified some "REM-on" neurons and suggested that they are important for REM sleep generation, since they show a unique firing increase related to REM sleep.

Since no cholinergic cell bodies are located in the medial PRF, as an alternate hypotheses, we suggest that a cholinergic input depolarizes and "primes" the cholinoceptive neurons in the medial PRF. Thus, the medial PRF may actually represent a common path in a sequence of events originating elsewhere, which eventuates in the initiation and maintenance of REM sleep. Since REM sleep originates from within the isolated pons we have to look in the pons for the source of cholinergic afferents to the medial PRF. There are two groups of cholinergic cells in the pons that may innervate the medial PRF. These two groups correspond to the pedunculopontine (PPT) and laterodorsal tegmental (LDT) groups. These cells form the largest collection of cholinergic cells in the PRF (2,72,82,103), and they form the ascending cholinergic pathway of Shute and Lewis (146), which innervates the thalamus, hippocampus, hypothalamus, and cingulate cortex (82,127). The PPT and LDT may also be a component of the ascending reticular activating system described by Moruzzi and Magoun (88).

Much evidence indicates that cholinergic cells in the PPT and LDT play a very important role in some tonic and phasic components of REM sleep. For example, Steriade et al. (129) suggest that EEG activation during waking and REM sleep may be result from a tonic activation of an ascending cholinergic system in the rostral reticular core. Steriade et al. (129) suggest that midbrain–subthalamic–thalamic–cortical loops underlie the ascending activating reticular influences. The PPT and LDT innervate the thalamus (for review see 146), and microinfusion of carbachol into the rostral portions of the PPT induces a sustained behavioral arousal characterized by EEG desynchronization (5,106). Indeed, acetylcholine is released from the cerebral cortex during REM sleep (59). PGO activity is another component of REM sleep hypothesized to be under the control of cholinergic cells in the PPT and LDT (98,99). PGO waves are a phasic component of REM sleep, and they occur just before and during REM sleep. The PPT and LDT project to the lateral geniculate nuclei (where PGO waves are recorded easily) (69,98,99,137). Some neurons in the PPT and LDT fire before and with PGO, leading some investigators to suggest that these are PGO executive neurons (87,98,99). Finally, the muscle atonia that accompanies REM sleep may be a result of descending cholinergic neurons in the more mediocaudal portions of the PPT located in the nucleus locus subcoeruleus and LC alpha (97–99).

We have begun a series of studies to determine whether the cholinergic neurons from the LDT and PPT innervate the medial PRF. We injected wheat germ agglutinin–horseradish peroxidase (WGA–HRP) (5%, 0.1–0.05 μl) unilaterally into the medial PRF region from which REM sleep can be most readily triggered following cholinergic stimulation. We found that some neurons from the LDT and PPT do project to the medial PRF and they are cholinergic. We are currently determining whether the LDT–PPT cholinergic neurons may project to both the medial PRF and medial thalamus. There is considerable evidence that the LDT and PPT cholinergic neurons innervate the medial thalamus (100,127,146). If we find that these neurons also innervate the medial PRF, then we may be able to suggest that cortical desynchrony during waking and

REM sleep is generated by the LDT–PPT cholinergic neurons. Thus, these cholinergic neurons influence the medial PRF during waking and REM sleep. In waking, however, the medial PRF neurons are inhibited by the LC and dorsal raphe neurons, and when this inhibition is lifted than REM sleep is generated.

Thus, we tentatively suggest that REM sleep results from the interaction of at least three cell groups: (a) the LC and dorsal raphe cells, which decrease firing during REM sleep, (b) the LDT and PPT cholinergic cells, which provide the cholinergic input to the medial PRF, and (c) some medial PRF cholinoceptive cells. We believe that this network within the pons accounts for many of the individual components of REM sleep as well as the unified REM sleep state. Further studies must be performed to test the implications of this model.

Like others, including Hobson and McCarley, we agree that wakefulness, NREM sleep, and REM sleep states result from reciprocal interaction between various cell groups. We suggest that cholinergic cells, probably located within the PPT and LDT, interact with cholinoceptive, catecholaminergic, and indoleaminergic cells to produce the regular transition between waking, NREM sleep, and REM sleep. Obviously, other neuronal systems are also involved in the regulation and initiation of these complex behavioral states.

In our model we can account for some of the inconsistencies in lesion data. For example, kainic acid lesions in medial PRF do not alter physiologic REM sleep even though cholinergic-induced REM sleep is impaired (31). In this case we suggest that the kainic acid may have destroyed the cholinoceptive medial PRF cells that in our model are one of the three neural groups responsible for REM sleep. Since the kainic acid was not placed in the cholinergic cell population, which is a second group important for REM sleep, physiologic REM sleep was unchanged.

Recently, Webster and Jones (144) showed that kainic acid lesions of the cholinergic cell population abolishes physiologic REM sleep. Our model predicts that this should happen. We, however, also predict that if the cholinergic cells are eliminated, REM sleep can still be triggered with cholinergic drugs into the medial PRF. Our model also predicts that the cholinergic cells should not show a pattern of activity unique to REM sleep because these cells also subserve other tonic and phasic components of REM sleep such as EEG desynchronization, PGO waves, and muscle atonia. Thus, groups of these cells should be active during both waking and REM sleep, or during periods of atonia or PGO activity.

We also suggest that treatments that increase activity of the LDT and PPG cholinergic neurons should accelerate REM sleep. Frederickson and Hobson (33) showed that electrical stimulation of the parabrachial region, where the cholinergic cells are located, decreased REM latency and increased REM sleep. They also showed that tectal stimulation was ineffective.

We also suggest that another input from the basal forebrain may be responsible for the orderly transition from waking to non-REM sleep to REM sleep. We suggest that since rostral transections do not eliminate REM like states in the isolated pons, the cholinergic input from the basal forebrain or other rostral sites might exert modulation control over REM sleep rather than be the sole regulation of REM sleep. The basal forebrain region along with the raphe is considered to be one of the somnogenic sites (80). Electrolytic (80,136) and kainic acid (134) lesions of the basal forebrain produce long-lasting insomnia, and electric stimulation produces sleep (130). Diathermic warming in this region also produces sleep (94). More importantly, Szymusiak and McGinty (135) found that some basal forebrain neurons discharge only during sleep. The chemical identity of this type of basal forebrain neuron is unknown, but since these cells are localized in areas found to contain cholinergic cells (72), the cells causing sleep may be cholinergic.

Most studies have examined the ascending projections of the cholinergic neurons. The descending projections of the basal forebrain have not been thoroughly examined. Recently, retrograde studies demonstrated that there is a descending projection from the basal forebrain to the PRF in rats (104). We have preliminary evidence in cats to support the findings in the rats. However, we have not yet determined whether cholinergic neurons innervate the PRF. This determination is vitally important considering that the basal forebrain represents a somnogenic center whereas the PRF is important for arousal and REM sleep. The interplay between cholinergic basal forebrain cells and cholinoceptive medial PRF cells may be responsible for the regular transition from waking to sleep to REM sleep. For example, we noted earlier that some basal forebrain neurons discharge selectively during NREM sleep. If these neurons are cholinergic, then increased discharge during NREM sleep could release acetylcholine in the medial PRF and prime the medial PRF cholinoceptive neurons responsible for REM sleep. Subsequent interplay between acetylcholine, catecholamine, and indoleamine neuronal systems, and other chemically unidentified neurons in the pons, may then be responsible for the initiation and maintenance of REM sleep (52,77).

Even though we suggest that a cholinergic input primes the cholinoceptive medial PRF, the medial PRF neurons may have an intrinsic property to exhibit a tonic or bursting firing pattern similar to that seen in thalamic neurons (54,55,76). Indeed, Greene and McCarley (44) have begun to examine, in pontine slices, the firing pattern of medial PRF neurons, and they find similarities with thalamic neurons (see chapter 8, this volume).

THE CHOLINERGIC REM INDUCTION TEST: MUSCARINIC SUPERSENSITIVITY IN DEPRESSION?

As mentioned above, short REM latency is commonly found in patients with moderate to severe depression. Since cholinergic mechanisms have been shown to play an important role in initiating REM sleep, we have been interested for some time in the hypothesis that functionally increased cholinergic neurotransmission may account for short REM latency and other signs and symptoms of depression (41). As a result of our earlier studies on scopolamine-induced apparent muscarinic supersensitivity in normal subjects (123), we postulated that muscarinic supersensitivity might be involved in the pathophysiology of depression.

In the original development of the CRIT, we infused arecoline (0.5 and 1.0 mg) intravenously during the second NREM period (25 min following the end of the first REM period) and measured the latency to the second REM period (123). In later modifications of this strategy, M. Berger and his colleagues in Germany have infused physostigmine (0.5 mg) shortly after sleep onset or administered RS-86, an experimental muscarinic agonist, by mouth at bedtime. The results of these studies in depression are shown in Table 11-1. As shown, three studies with arecoline indicate that patients

Table 11-1 Previous Studies of the Cholinergic REM Induction Test[a]

Authors	Measure	Drug	Normals (N)	Response (min)	Patients	N	Response (min)
Sitaram et al.	REMP #2	Placebo	16	54 ± 14	1° short-term	11	50 ± 18
(123, 125)	latency	A 0.5 mg	12	38 ± 22	drug-free	9	11 ± 68
		A 1.0 mg	10	19 ± 12	Euthymic	9	7 ± 4
		Placebo			Long-term drug-	8	48 ± 13
		A 0.5 mg			free	8	14 ± 8
		A 0.5 mg			Depressed	7	11 ± 11
					In-patients		
Jones et al.	REMP #2	Placebo	19	55 ± 12	MDD-End	24	46 ± 15
(62)	latency	A 0.5 mg	20	42 ± 12		25	15 ± 15
		Placebo			MDD-NonE	26	54 ± 9
		A 0.5 mg				28	36 ± 13
		Placebo			Nonaffective	16	54 ± 9
		A 0.5 mg			patients	16	44 ± 15
Dube et al.	REMP #2	A 0.5 mg	26	42 ± 20	MDD-End	20	14 ± 11
(32)	latency				1° MDD + Anx	19	24 ± 19
					1° Anx	18	42 ± 17
					1° Anx + 2°	14	34 ± 13
					MDD		
Sitaram et al.	REMP #2	Placebo			MDD probands	34	56 ± 23
(126)	latency	A 0.5 mg			(responders)	34	11 ± 6
		Placebo			Ill 1° relatives	35	51 ± 27
		A 0.5 mg				35	25 ± 21
		Placebo			Well relatives	31	56 ± 13
		A 0.5 mg				31	41 ± 20
Berger et al.	Awakening REM	P 0.5 mg	8	1 ± 1	Depressives	45	13 ± 29
(8)	latency	P 0.5 mg	8	54 ± 10	Sleeping depres-	19	37 ± 29
					sives		
Berger et al.	REM latency	Placebo	16	74 ± 25	Acute depression	16	70 ± 33
(9)		RS86	16	50 ± 29		16	15 ± 21
		Placebo			Other psychiatric	20	74 ± 21
		RS 86			patients	20	57 ± 19
		Placebo			Remitted	8	74 ± 38
		RS 86				8	65 ± 49

[a]A, arecoline; P, physostigmine; MDD, major depressive disorder; End, endogenous; 1°, primary; 2°, secondary; Anx, anxiety disorder.

with either primary depression or endogenous depression enter REM sleep signifi-cantly faster than normal controls following the active drug infusion (31,62,124,125). Both patients and controls have similar responses after placebo infusion and both show a dose dependent shortening of the infusion-to-REM period (REMP) #2 latency fol-lowing arecoline (0.5 and 1.0 mg). In the first study, the response appeared to be state independent, that is, the faster response latency appeared in currently ill patients, as well as in recently drug-free euthymic patients (2 weeks or more), and in euthymic patients who were either drug free for at least 4 months or who had never received somatic therapy (124,125). In the second series of studies conducted at the Lafayette

Clinic in Detroit, Dr. Sitaram's group showed that the positive response was found in endogenous patients with major depressive disorder (MDD), whether or not they had concurrent secondary anxiety disorder but not in patients with nonendogenous depression, nonaffective patients, or in patients with primary anxiety disorders whether or not they had concurrent secondary depression (31,62).

In an effort to determine whether or not the CRIT might be a genetic marker for endogenous depression, Sitaram et al. (126) undertook a family study. The index case was chosen to be a patient with an endogenous MDD who was a positive responder on the CRIT. As predicted, first degree relatives who also suffered from affective illness showed a faster response than relatives who were well. Although the results are not strikingly robust, they do suggest that muscarinic supersensitivity might be a genetically influenced marker for endogenous depression.

In variants of these studies, Berger et al. (8) infused physostigmine (0.5 mg) 5 min after the onset of NREM sleep in both normal controls and patients with depression. Overall, the patients were more likely than the controls to wake up. Since we had previously shown that physostigmine exerted a dose-dependent alerting effect in normal volunteers (123), these findings by Berger et al. (8) could be interpreted as being consistent with muscarinic receptor supersensitivity in depression. On the other hand, even in patients who remained asleep, physostigmine-induced shortening of REM latency was not apparently different compared with baseline (47 min on baseline, 37 min on physostigmine); in normal controls, however, physostigmine did shorten REM latency (from 78 min to 56 min, $p < .01$). The effect of physostigmine on REM latency has previously been shown to be dose and time dependent in normal volunteers (123), thereby, possibly, it may be more difficult to interpret the results from subjects whose baseline REM latencies differed so much between controls and patients.

Using the long acting, orally active muscarinic agonist RS-86, Berger et al. (9) showed that depressed patients entered REM sleep significantly faster than normal controls. Patients with other psychiatric diagnoses behaved like normal controls. In contrast to the original study with arecoline (124),125), Berger et al. did not find a positive effect in remitted patients.

Although there are differences in technique between these studies, they do support the hypothesis that patients with endogenous or primary depression show an enhanced sleep response to cholinergic agonists. In the following sections, we will present our preliminary results from studies conducted in San Diego attempting to replicate the original CRIT with two doses of arecoline.

Preliminary Results from Current Studies with the CRIT

The patients in this study were admitted for the treatment of depression to the Special Treatment and Evaluation Unit (UCSD Mental Health Clinical Research Center) in the San Diego Veterans Administration Medical Center. Both patients and controls underwent a comprehensive diagnostic evaluation prior to entry into the study, including physical examination, laboratory tests, a seasonal affective disorder symptoms interview, and consensus conference diagnosis. All subjects were drug free for at least 2 weeks and had two to three nights of adaptation to the sleep laboratory before study. Infusions were administered by a physician who was blind to whether placebo or arecoline was given. Sleep records were scored by a technician who was also unaware of drug status.

Table 11-2 Baseline Sleep Measures in Controls and Depressives

Sleep measure	Controls	Depressives	F-ratio	p
Sleep latency (min)	12 ± 10	27 ± 24	12.25	.0008
REM latency (min)	76 ± 33	53 ± 34	8.00	.006
Delta sleep, first NREMP	23 ± 21	11 ± 15	7.42	.008
REM%	23.0 ± 5.4	27.0 ± 18	8.17	.006
REMP #1 (min)	19 ± 8	27 ± 18	7.15	.009
REM density	1.5 ± 1.0	1.8 ± 1.0	2.16	NS
Stage 3%	4.7 ± 3.9	4.7 ± 4.2	0.00	NS
Stage 4%	7.2 ± 10.2	5.6 ± 6.9	0.512	NS
REM density	1.9 ± 0.9	2.0 ± 0.8	0.113	NS
Sleep efficiency (%)	91.3 ± 4.6	86.2 ± 7.7	11.69	.001

$df = 1,69$

As shown in Table 11-2, during the baseline night before inserting intravenous canulae or administering drugs, depressive patients took significantly longer to fall asleep, showed shorter REM latency, less delta (Stage 3 and 4) sleep during the first NREM period, and lower sleep efficiency, and had greater REM% than normal controls.

As shown in Table 11-3, we obtained acceptable or successful data on 173 of the 271 attempted subject-study-nights (63.8%). Awakenings (defined as equal to or greater than 4 min) prior to, during, or after the infusion constituted one reason for excluding data; awakenings during or after the infusion occurred significantly more often following arecoline 1.0 mg compared with either placebo or arecoline 0.5 mg (33.3% compared with 2.1%, $p < .001$, Fisher exact probability test). At the arecoline 1.0 mg dose only, normal controls awakened significantly more often than patients during or after the infusion (48.8% compared with 17.5%, $p < .001$, chi square test corrected for continuity).

Of the 16 patients and 17 controls on whom we attempted to establish the reliability of the effect of arecoline 0.5 mg on REM induction, 6 patients and 7 controls were successfully studied on two nights. The reliability between the first and second infu-

Table 11-3 Successful and Unsuccessful Attempts to Conduct the CRIT

	Attempts	Awakenings			Misscellaneous	
		Prior	During	Post	Failures[a]	Success
Placebo						
Patients	47	0	0	0	14	33
Controls	33	0	0	0	9	24
0.5 mg						
Patients	61	0	0	1	20	40
Controls	49	1	2	1	16	29
1.0 mg						
Patients	40	1	2	5	5	27
Controls	41	5	2	18	15	20

[a]Miscellaneous problems: no infusion given, 14; IV problems, 17; REM sleep identification problems, 20; no second REM period, 9; minor medical problems (colds, fever, etc.), 11; positive toxicology screen, 5; other, 13.

sion was statistically significant (ρ = .734, p < .05, Spearman rank correlation coefficient). In addition, the average infusion-to-REMP #2 latency was significantly shorter on the second night than on the first (first night 51 ± 22 min, second night 34 ± 23 min, p < .05, Wilcoxon matched pairs signed ranks test, two-tailed).

Of the 7 patients and 14 controls in whom we attempted on two separate nights with a dose of arecoline 1.0 mg, we obtained two successful nights in only 5 subjects, 3 patients and 2 controls (p = NS, Fisher exact probability test). The Spearman rank correlation coefficient was statistically significant (ρ = .95, p < .05). The mean infusion-to-REMP #2 latency was not significantly different on the two nights.

The infusion-to-REMP #2 latencies differed significantly between patients and controls only after the arecoline 1.0 mg infusion (patients: mean ± SD = 14 ± 22 min; controls: 31 ± 34 min, p < .05, Mann–Whitney U test). The two groups did not differ significantly following either placebo or 0.5 mg arecoline.

When we examined the data from the 1.0 mg arecoline study more carefully, it appeared that there was a bimodal response, with some subjects showing an increased latency following arecoline rather than a shortening. Furthermore, the controls were statistically more likely to show an arecoline-induced increase in latency than the patients: for subjects on whom we had both a placebo night and a successful 1.0 mg arecoline night, 3 of 7 controls had an increased latency on arecoline compared with placebo whereas only 2 of 15 patients did (p < .05, Fisher exact probability test). For the three controls who showed an increase, the mean latency increased from 53 to 78 min; for the 2 patients, the mean latency increased from 50 to 75 min. This analysis was confirmed when we examined the length of the second NREM period (excluding those nights with awake > 5 min). Compared with that on the baseline night, duration of the second NREM period increased in 5 of 14 controls and 3 of 16 patients (p < .02, Fisher exact probability test).

In contrast to 1.0 mg arecoline, 0.5 mg arecoline did not differentially increase or decrease latency to the second REM period in patients as compared to controls. Both groups showed an increase in about one-third of subjects following arecoline.

DISCUSSION

As the basic science review indicates, cholinergic mechanisms play an important role in the initiation and maintenance of REM sleep. As a result of new techniques, a better understanding of the anatomic pathways involved is beginning to emerge. Preliminary data indicate that cholinergic neurons originating in the LDT and PPT terminate in the medial PRF and the cholinergic and cholinoceptive groups play an important part in this complex process.

The role of cholinergic mechanisms in the sleep disturbances of depression remains largely speculative at this time. The ability to mimic the short REM latency by cholinergic pharmacological manipulation is suggestive but hardly conclusive. Likewise, the muscarinic supersensitivity hypothesis remains interesting but unproven. Although the earlier studies, outlined in Table 1, suggest that depressives show a brisker response to a cholinergic agonist than controls, with arecoline, physostigmine, and RS-86, the preliminary results of our own study offer only weak confirmation. Although we did report a statistically significant response to arecoline, it is only at the upper dose (1.0 mg), not the lower dose (0.5 mg), which has been more commonly used (32,62,124,125). Furthermore, our results also indicate that the differential response to arecoline in patients compared with controls may result from a greater tendency of normals to increase latency more than a faster response by patients. This result might be interpreted as follows. If arecoline acts on both presynaptic and postsynaptic receptors, it is possible that patients are more likely to respond postsynaptically and controls presynaptically.

Further studies are needed both at the preclinical and clinical level. Whether or not patients with depression do exhibit a muscarinic supersensitivity, cholinergic mechanisms must be viewed as part of the physiological control system responsible for the physiological and pathophysiological mechanism involved in short REM latency and other sleep abnormalities.

ACKNOWLEDGMENTS

Supported by the San Diego Veterans Administration Medical Center, MH 30914, MH 38738, AGO 5131, NS25212 (PJS) and a grant from American Narcolepsy Association.

REFERENCES

1. Amatruda TT, Black DA, McKenna TM, McCarley RW, Hobson JA. Sleep cycle control and cholinergic mechanisms: Differential effects of carbachol at pontine brainstem sites. *Brain Res* 1975; 98:501–515.
2. Armstrong D, Saper C, Levey A, Wainer B, Terry R. Distribution of cholinergic neurons in the rat brain: Demonstrated by the immunocytochemical localization of choline acetyltransferase. *J Comp Neurol* 1983; 216:53–68.
3. Aserinsky E, Kleitman N. Regularly occurring periods of eye motility and concomitant phenomenon during sleep. *Science* 1953; 118:273–274.
4. Baghdoyan HA, Rodrigo-Angula ML, McCarley RW, Hobson JA. Site-specific enhancement and suppression of desynchronized sleep signs following cholinergic stimulation of three brainstem sites. *Brain Res* 1984; 306:39–52.
5. Baghdoyan HA, Monaco AP, Rodrigo-Angula ML, Assens F, McCarley RW, Hobson JA. Microinjection of neostigmine into the pontine reticular formation of cats enhances desynchronized sleep signs. *J Pharmacol Exp Ther* 1984; 321:173–180.
6. Bartus RT, Dean RL, Beer B, Lippa AS. The cholinergic hypothesis of geriatric memory dysfunction. *Science* 1982; 217:408–417.
7. Baxter BL. Induction of both emotional behavior and a novel form of REM sleep by chemical stimulation applied to cat mesencephalon. *Exp Neurol* 1969; 23:220–230.
8. Berger M, Lund R, Bronisch T, von Zerrsen D. REM latency in neurotic and endogenous depression and the cholinergic REM induction test. *Psychiat Res* 1983; 10:113–123.
9. Berger M, Riemann D, Hoechi D, Spiegel R. The cholinergic REM induction test with RS 86: State or trait marker for depression. *Arch Gen Psychiat* 1989; 46:421–428.
10. Boehme RE, Baker TL, Mefford IN, Barchas JD, Dement WC, Ciaranello RD. Narcolepsy: Cholinergic receptor changes in an animal model. *Life Sci* 1984; 34:1825–1828.
11. Braun CMJ, Pivik RT. Effects of locus coeruleus lesions upon sleeping and waking in the rabbit. *Brain Res* 1981; 230:133–151.
12. Brushart TM, Mesulam MM. Transganglionic demonstration of central sensory projections from skin and muscle with HRP-lectin conjugates. *Neurosci Lett* 1980; 17:1–6.

13. Butcher LL, Talbot K, Bilezikjian L. Acetylcholinesterase neurons in dopamine-containing regions of the brain. *J Neural Transm* 1975; 37:127–153.

14. Caballero A, De Andres I. Unilateral lesions in locus coeruleus area enhance paradoxical sleep. *Electroenceph Clin Neurophysiol* 1986; 64:339–346.

15. Carroll BJ, Frazer A, Schless A, Mendels J. Cholinergic reversal of manic symptoms. *Lancet* 1973; 1:427.

16. Celesia GG, Jasper HH. Acetylcholine released from cerebral cortex in relation to state of activation. *Neurology (Minneap)* 1966; 16:1053–1064.

17. Cespuglio R, Gomez ME, Faradji H, Jouvet M. Alterations in the sleep-waking cycle induced by cooling of the locus coeruleus area. *Electroenceph Clin Neurophysiol* 1982; 54:570–578.

18. Chu NS, Bloom FE. Norepinephrine containing neurons: Changes in spontaneous discharge patterns during sleeping and waking. *Science* 1973; 179:908–910.

19. Chu NS, Bloom FE. Activity patterns of catecholamine pontineneurons in the dorso-lateral tegmentum of unrestrained cat. *J Neurobiol* 1974; 5:527–544.

20. Collier B, Mitchell JF. The central release of acetylcholine during consciousness and after brain lesions. *J Physiol (London)* 1967; 188:83–99.

21. Cordeau JP, Moreau A, Beaulnes A, Laurin C. EEG and behavioral changes following microinjections of acetylcholine and adrenaline in the brain stem of cats. *Arch Ital Biol* 1963; 101:30–47.

22. Coyle J, Price DL, DeLong MR. Alzheimer's disease: A disorder of cortical cholinergic innervation. *Science* 1983; 219:1184–1190.

23. Czeisler CA, Weitzman ED, Moore-Ede WC. Human sleep: Its duration and organization depend on its circadian phase. *Science* 1980; 210:1264–1267.

24. Davis KL, Berger PA, Hollister LE, Defraites E. Physostigmine in man. *Arch Gen Psychiat* 1978; 136:1581–1584.

25. De Andres I, Reinoso-Suarez F. Participation of the cerebellum in the regulation of the sleep-wakefulness cycle through the superior cerebellar peduncle. *Arch Ital Biol* 1979; 117:140–163.

26. Delashaw JB, Foutz AS, Guilleminault C, Dement WC. Cholinergic mechanisms and cataplexy in dogs. *Exp Neurol* 1979; 66:745–757.

27. Dement WC. The effect of dream deprivation. *Science* 1960; 131:1705–1707.

28. Dement WC, Ferguson J, Cohen H, Barchas J. Non-chemical methods and data using a biochemical method: The REM quanta. In A Mandell (ed.), *Some Current Issues in Psychochemical Research Strategies in Man.* Academic Press, New York, 1970: 275–325.

29. Domino EF, Stawiski M. Effects of the cholinergic antisynthesis agent HC-3 on the awake-sleep cycle of cat. *Psychophysiology* 1971; 7:315–316.

30. Domino EF, Yamamoto K, Dren AT. Role of cholinergic mechanisms in states of wakefulness and sleep. *Prog Brain Res* 1968; 28:113–133.

31. Drucker-Colin R, Bernal-Pedraza JG. Kainic acid lesions of gigantocellular tegmental field (FTG) neurons does not abolish REM sleep. *Brain Res* 1983; 272:387–391.

32. Dube S, Kumar N, Etledgui E, Pohl R, Jones D, Sitaram N. Colinergic REM induction response: Separation of anxiety and depression. *Biol Psychiat* 1985; 20:208–418.

33. Frederickson CJ, Hobson JA. Electrical stimulation of the brain stem and subsequent sleep. *Arch Ital Biol* 1970; 108:564–576.

34. Friedman L, Jones BE. Computer graphic analysis of sleep-wakefulness state changes after pontine lesions. *Brain Res Bull* 1984; 13:53–68.

35. Gadea-Ciria M, Stadler H, Lloyd KG, Bartholini G. Acetylcholine release within the cat striatum during the sleep-wakefulness cycle. *Nature (London)* 1973; 243:518–519.

36. Geffard M, McRae-Degueurce A, Souan ML. Immunocytochemical detection of acetylcholine in the rat central nervous system. *Science* 1985; 229:77–79.

37. George R, Haslett WL, Jenden DJ. A cholinergic mechanism in the pontine reticular formation: Induction of paradoxical sleep. *J Neuropharmacol* 1964; 3:541–552.
38. Gillin JC, Borbely AA. Sleep: A neurobiological window on affective disorders. *Trends Neurosci* 1985; 8:537–542.
39. Gillin JC, Sitaram N, Duncan WC. Physostigmine alters onset but not duration of REM sleep in man. *Psychopharmacology* 1978; 58:111–114.
40. Gillin JC, Duncan WC, Pettigrew KD, Frankel BL, Snyder F. Successful separation of depressed, normal, and insomniac subjects by EEG sleep data. *Arch Gen Psychiat* 1979; 36:85–90.
41. Gillin JC, Sitaram N, Wehr T, Duncan W, Post R, Murphy DL, Mendelson WB, Wyatt RJ, Bunney WE. Sleep and affective illness. In RM Post and J Ballenger (eds.), *Neurobiology of Mood Disorders.* William & Wilkins, Baltimore, 1984: 157–189.
42. Gillin JC, Sitaram N, Janowsky DS, Risch C, Storch FI. Cholinergic mechanisms in REM sleep. In A Wauquier et al. (eds.), *Sleep: Neurotransmitters and Neuromodulators.* Raven, New York, 1985: 153–164.
43. Gnadt JW, Pegram GV. Cholinergic brainstem mechanisms of REM sleep in the rat. *Brain Res* 1986; 384:29–41.
44. Greene RW, Haas HL, McCarley RW. A low threshold calcium spike mediates firing pattern alterations in pontine reticular neurons. *Science* 1986; 234:738–740.
45. Haranath PS, Venkatakrishna-Bhatt H. Release of acetylcholine from perfused cerebral ventricles in unanesthetized dogs during waking and sleep. *Jpn J Physiol* 1973; 23:241–250.
46. Hazra J. The effect of hemicholinium-3 on slow wave and paradoxical sleep of cat. *Eur J Pharmacol* 1970; 11:395–397.
47. Henriksen SJ, Dement WC. Effects of chronic intravenous administration of alpha-methyl paratyrosine on sleep in the cat. *Sleep Res* 1972; 1:55.
48. Hobson JA. The effects of chronic brain-stem lesions on cortical and muscular activity during sleep and waking in the cat. *Electroenceph Clin Neurophysiol* 1965; 19:41–62.
49. Hobson JA, McCarley RW, Freedman R, Pivik RT. Time course of discharge rate changes by cat pontine brainstem neurons during the sleep cycle. *J Neurophysiol* 1974; 37:1297–1309.
50. Hobson JA, McCarley RW, Pivik RT, Freedman R. Selective firing by cat pontine brain stem neurons in desynchronized sleep. *J Neurophysiol* 1974; 37:497–511.
51. Hobson JA, Goldberg M, Vivaldi E, Riew D. Enhancement of desynchronized sleep signs after pontine microinjection of the muscarinic agonist bethanechol. *Brain Res* 1983; 275:127–136.
52. Hobson JA, Lydic R, Baghdoyan H. Evolving concepts of sleep cycle generation: From brain centers to neuronal populations. *Behav Brain Sci* 1986; 9:371–448.
53. Insel TR, Gillin JC, Moore A, Mendelson WB, Loewenstein RJ, Murphy DL. The sleep of patients with obsessive-compulsive disorder. *Arch Gen Psychiat* 1982; 39:1371–1377.
54. Jahnsen H, Llinas R. Electrophysiological properties of guinea-pig, thalamic neurones: An in vitro study. *J Physiol* 1984; 349:205–226.
55. Jahnsen H, Llinas R. Ionic bases for the electroresponsiveness and oscillatory properties of guinea-pig thalamic neurones in vitro. *J Physiol* 1984; 349:227–247.
56. Janowsky D, Risch SC. Cholinomimetic and anticholinergic drugs to investigate an acetylcholine hypothesis of stress. *Drug Dev Res* 1984; 4:125–142.
57. Janowsky DS, El-Youseff MK, Davis JM. A cholinergic-adrenergic hypothesis of mania and depression. *Lancet* 1972; 2:632–635.
58. Janowsky DS, Risch SC, Parker D, Huey LY, Judd LL. Increased vulnerability to cholinergic stimulation in affect disorder patients. *Psychopharmacol Bull* 1980; 16:29–31.

59. Jasper HH, Tessier J. Acetylcholine liberation from cerebral cortex during paradoxical (REM) sleep. *Science* 1971; 172:601–602.

60. Jones BE, Harper ST, Halaris A. Effects of locus coeruleus lesions upon cerebral monoamine content, sleep-wakefulness states and the response to amphetamine in the cat. *Brain Res* 1977; 124:473–496.

61. Jones BE. Elimination of paradoxical sleep by lesions of the pontine gigantocellular tegmental field in the cat. *Neurosci Lett* 1979; 13:285–293.

62. Jones D, Kelwala S, Bell J, Dube S, Jackson E, Sitaram N. Cholinergic REM sleep induction response correlation with endo genous depressive subtype. *Psychiat Res* 1985; 14:99–110.

63. Jones HS, Oswald I. Two cases of healthy insomnia. *Electroenceph Clin Neurophysiol* 1968; 24:378–380.

64. Jouvet M. Recherches sur les structures nerveuses et les mechanismes responsales des differentes du sommeil physiologique. *Arch Ital Biol* 1962; 100:125–206.

65. Jus K, Bouchard M, Jus AK, Villeneuve A, Lachance R. Sleep EEG studies in untreated, long-term schizophrenic patients. *Arch Gen Psychiat* 1973; 29:386–390.

66. Karacan I, Williams NL, Finley WW, Hursch CJ. The effects of naps on nocturnal sleep: Influence on the need for stage-1 REM and stage-4 sleep. *Biol Psychiat* 1970; 2:391–399.

67. Karczmar AG, Longo VG, Scotti de Carolis A. A pharmacological model of paradoxical sleep: The role of cholinergic and monoamine systems. *Physiol Behav* 1970; 5:175–182.

68. Katayama Y, DeWitt DS, Becker DP, Hayes RL. Behavioral evidence for cholinoceptive pontine inhibitory area: Descending control of spinal motor output and sensory input. *Brain Res* 1984; 296:241–262.

69. Kayama Y. Ascending, descending and local control of neuronal activity in the rat lateral geniculate nucleus. *Vision Res* 1985; 25:339–347.

70. Khazan N, Bar R, Sulman FG. The effect of cholinergic drugs on paradoxical sleep in the rat. *Int J Neuropharmacol* 1967; 6:279–282.

71. Kilduff TS, Bowersox S, Kaitin K, Baker T, Ciaranello R, Dement W. Muscarinic cholinergic receptors and the canine model of narcolepsy. *Sleep* 1986; 9:102–106.

72. Kimura H, McGeer PL, Peng JH, McGeer EG. The central cholinergic system studied by choline acetyltransferase immunohistochemistry in the cat. *J Comp Neurol* 1981; 200:151–201.

73. Kupfer DJ, Thace ME. The use of the sleep laboratory in the diagnosis of affective disorders. *Psychiat Clin North Am* 1983; 6:3–25.

74. Lavie P, Pratt H, Scharf B, Peled R, Brown J. Localized pontine lesion: Nearly total absence of REM sleep. *Neurology* 1984; 34:118–120.

75. Lewis PR, Shute CCD. Cholinergic pathways in CNS. In LL Iversen, SD Iversen, and SH Snyder (eds.), *Handbook of Psychopharmacology,* Vol. 9. Plenum, New York, 1978: 315–355.

76. Llinas R, Jahnsen H. Electrophysiology of mammalian thalamic neurones in vitro. *Nature (London)* 1982; 297:406–408.

77. McCarley RW, Hobson JA. Neuronal excitability modulation over the sleep cycle: A structural and mathematical model. *Science* 1975; 189:58–60.

78. McCarley RW, Ito K. Desynchronized sleep-specific changes in membrane potential and excitability in medial pontine reticular formation neurons: Implications for concepts and mechanisms of behavioral state control. In DJ McGinty, R Drucker-Colin, A Morrison, and PL Parmeggiani (eds.), *Brain Mechanisms of Sleep,* Raven, New York, 1985: 63–80.

79. McGinty DJ, Harper RM. Dorsal raphe neurons: Depression of firing during sleep in cats. *Brain Res* 1976; 101:569–575.

80. McGinty DJ, Sterman MB. Sleep suppression after basal forebrain lesions in the cat. *Science* 1968; 160:1253–1255.

81. Meddis R, Pearson A, Langford G. An extreme case of healthy insomnia. *Electroencep Clin Neurophysiol* 1973; 35:213–214.

82. Mesulam MM, Mufson EJ, Wainer BH, Levey AI. Central cholinergic pathways in the rat: An overview based on an alternative nomenclature. *Neuroscience* 1983; 10:1185–1201.

83. Mitler M, Dement WC. Cataplectic-like behavior in cats after microinjection of carbachol in pontine reticular formation. *Brain Res* 1974; 68:335–343.

84. Modestin JJ, Hunger J, Schwartz RB. Uber die depressogene wirkum on physostigmine. *Arch Psychiat Nervenkrankheiten* 1973; 218:67–77.

85. Monmaur P, Delacour J. Effects de la lesion bilaterale du tegmentum pontique dorsolateral sur l'activite theta hippocampigue au cours du sommeil paradoxal ches le rat. *CR Acad Sci* 1978; 286:761–764.

86. Monneir M, Romanowski W. Les systemes cholinoceptifs cerebraux-actions de l'acetylcholine, de la physostigmine, pilocarpine et de GABA. *Electroenceph Clin Neurophysiol* 1962; 14:486–500.

87. Nelson JP, McCarley RW, Hobson JA. REM sleep burst neurons, PGO waves, and eye movement information. *J Neurophysiol* 1983; 50:784–797.

88. Moruzzi G, Magoun HW. Brainstem reticular formation and the activation of the EEG. *Electroenceph Clin Neurophysiol* 1949; 1:544–473.

89. Nurnburger J Jr, Sitaram N, Gerson ES, Gillin JC. A twin study of cholinergic REM induction. *Biol Psychiat* 1983; 18:1161–1165.

90. Paz C, Reygadas E, Fernandez-Guardiola A. Sleep alterations following total cerebellectomy in cats. *Sleep* 1982; 3:218–226.

91. Rechtschaffen A, Wolpert W, Dement WC, Mitchell S, Fisher C. Nocturnal sleep of narcoleptics. *Electroenceph Clin Neurophysiol* 1963; 15:599–609.

92. Risch C, Cohen RM, Janowsky DS, Kalin NH, Murphy DL. Plasma beta-endorphin and cortisol elevations accompany the mood and behavioral effects of physostigmine in man. *Science* 1980; 209:1545–1546.

93. Risch C, Janowsky DS, Gillin JC, Rausch J, Loevinger BL, Huey LY. Muscarinic supersensitivity of anterior pituitary ACTH release in major depressive illness, adrenal cortical dissociation. *Psychopharmacol Bull* 1983; 19:343–346.

94. Roberts W, Robinson TC. Relaxation and sleep induced by warming of preoptic region and anterior hypothalamus in cats. *Exp Neurol* 1969; 25:282–294.

95. Roffwarg HP, Muzio JM, Dement WC. Ontogenetic development of the human sleep-dream cycle. *Science* 1966; 152:604–619.

96. Sagales T, Erill S, Domino EF. Effects of repeated doses of scopolamine on the electroencephalographic stages of sleep in normal volunteers. *Clin Pharmacol Ther* 1975; 18:727–732.

97. Sakai K, Sastre JP, Salvert D, Touret M, Tohyama M, Jouvet M. Tegmentoreticular projections with special reference to the muscular atonia during paradoxical sleep in the cat: An HRP study. *Brain Res* 1979; 176:233–254.

98. Sakai K. Some anatomical and physiological properties of ponto-mesencephalic tegmental neurons with special reference to the PGO waves and postural atonia during paradoxical sleep in the cat. In JA Hobson and MB Brazier (eds.), *The Reticular Formation Revisited*. Raven, New York, 1980: 427–447.

99. Sakai K. Anatomical and physiological basis of paradoxical sleep. In D McGinty, A Morrison, RR Drucker-Colin, and PL Parmeggiani (eds.), *Brain Mechanisms of Sleep*. Spectrum, New York, 1984: 111–137.

100. Saper CB, Loewy AD. Projections of the pedunculopontine tegmental nucleus in the rat: Evidence for additional extrapyramidal circuitry. *Brain Res* 1982; 252:367–372.

101. Saper CB, Loewy AD. Projections of the pedunculopontine tegmental nucleus in the rat: Evidence for additional extrapyramidal circuitry. *Brain Res* 1982; 252:367–372.

102. Sastre JP, Sakai K, Jouvet M. Persistance du sommeil paradoxal chez le Chat apres desturction de l'aire gigantocellulaire du tegmentum pontique par l'acide kainique. *CR Acad Sci* 1979; 289:959–964.

103. Satoh K, Armstrong DM, Fibiger HC. A comparison of the distribution of central cholinergic neurons as demonstrated by acetylcholinesterase pharmacohistochemistry and choline acetyltransferase immunohistochemistry. *Brain Res Bull* 1983; 11:693–720.

104. Shammah-Lagnado SJ, Negrao N, Silva BA, Silva JA, Ricardo JA. Afferent connections of the magnocellular reticular formation: A horseradish peroxidase study in the rat. *Soc Neurosci Abstr* 1985; 11:1026.

105. Sheu YS, Nelson JP, Bloom FE. Discharge patterns of cat raphe neurons during sleep and waking. *Brain Res* 1974; 73:263–276.

106. Shiromani P, Siegel JM, Tomaszewski K, McGinty DJ. Alterations in blood pressure and REM sleep after pontine carbachol microinfusion. *Exp Neurol* 1986; 91:285–292.

107. Shiromani P, Armstrong DM, Groves PM, Gillin JC. Combined neurophysiological and immunohistochemical mapping of the medial-lateral pontine reticular formation: Relation of REM-on cells with cells containing choline acetyltransferase. *Sleep Res* 1986; 15:12.

108. Shiromani P, Armstrong DM, Bruce G, Hersh LB, Groves PM, Gillin JC. Relation of choline acetyltransferase immunoreactive neurons with cells which increase discharge during REM sleep. *Brain Res Bull* 1987; 18:447–455.

109. Shiromani P, McGinty DJ. Pontine neuronal response to local cholinergic microinfusion: Relation to REM sleep. *Brain Res* 1986; 386:20–31.

110. Shiromani P, Fishbein W. Continuous pontine cholinergic microinfusion via mini-pump induces sustained alteration in rapid eye movement sleep. *Pharmacol, Biochem Behav* 1986; 25:1253–1261.

111. Shiromani PJ, Overstreet D, Levy D, Goodrich C, Campbell SS, Gillin JC. Increased REM sleep in rats genetically bred for cholinergic hyperactivity. *Neuropsychopharmacology* 1988; 1:127–133.

112. Siegel JM. Behavioral functions of the reticular formation. *Brain Res Rev* 1979; 1:69–105.

113. Siegel JM, McGinty DJ, Breedlove SM. Sleep and waking activity of pontine gigantocellular field neurons. *Exp Neurol* 1977; 56:553–573.

114. Siegel JM, McGinty DJ. Pontine reticular formation neurons: Relationship of discharge to motor activity. *Science* 1977; 196:678–680.

115. Siegel JM, Wheeler RL, McGinty DJ. Activity of reticular formation neurons in the unrestrained cat during waking and sleep. *Brain Res* 1979; 179:49–60.

116. Siegel JM, Nienhuis R, Tomaszewski KS. REM sleep signs rostral to chronic transections at the pontomedullary junction. *Neurosci Lett* 1984; 45:241–246.

117. Silberman E, Vivaldi E, Garfield J, McCarley RW, Hobson JA. Carbachol triggering of desynchronized sleep phenomena: Enhancement via small volume infusions. *Brain Res* 1980; 191:215–224.

118. Sitaram N, Wyatt RJ, Dawson S, Gillin JC. REM sleep induction by physostigmine infusion during sleep in normal volunteers. *Science* 1976; 191:1281–1283.

119. Sitaram N, Mendelson WB, Wyatt RJ, Gillin JC. Time dependent induction of REM sleep and arousal by physostigmine infusion during normal human sleep. *Brain Res* 1977; 122:565–567.

120. Sitaram N, Moore AM, Gillin JC. Experimental acceleration and slowing of REM ultradian rhythm by cholinergic agonist and antagonist. *Nature (London)* 1978; 274:490–492.

121. Sitaram N, Moore AM, Gillin JC. Induction and resetting of REM sleep rhythm in normal man by arecoline: Blockade by scopolamine. *Sleep* 1978; 1:83–90.

122. Sitaram N, Moore AM, Gillin JC. Scopolamine-induced muscarinic supersensitivity in normal man: Changes in sleep. *Psychiat Res* 1979; 1:9–16.

123. Sitaram N, Gillin JC. Development and use of pharmacological probes of the CNS in man:

Evidence for cholinergic abnormality in primary affective illness. *Biol Psychiat* 1980; 15:925–955.

124. Sitaram N, Nurnberger J, Gershon E, Gillin JC. Faster cholinergic REM sleep induction in euthymic patients with primary affective illness. *Science* 1980; 208:200–202.

125. Sitaram N, Nurnberger J, Gershon ES, Gillin JC. Cholinergic regulation of mood and REM sleep: A potential model and marker vulnerability to affective disorder. *Am J Psychiat* 1982; 139:571–576.

126. Sitaram N, Dube S, Keshovan M. The association of super-sensitive cholinergic REM induction and affective illness within pedigrees. *J Psychiat Res* 1987; 21:487–97.

127. Sofroniew MV, Priestley JV, Consolazione A, Eckenstein F, Cuello AC. Cholinergic projections from the midbrain and pons to the thalamus in the rat, identified by combined retrograde tracing and choline acetyltransferase immunohistochemistry. *Brain Res* 1985; 329:213–223.

128. Spiegel R. Effects of RS-86, an orally active cholinergic agonist, on sleep in man. *Psychiat Res* 1984; 11:1–13.

129. Steriade M, Ropert N, Kitsikis A, Oakson G. Ascending activating neuronal networks in midbrain reticular core and related rostral systems. In JA Hobson and M Brazier (eds.), *The Reticular Formation Revisited*. Raven, New York, 1980: 125–167.

130. Sterman MB, Clemente C. Forebrain inhibitory mechanisms: Sleep patterns induced by basal forebrain stimulation in the behaving cat. *Exp Neurol* 1962; 6:103–117.

131. Stoyva J, Metcalf D. Sleep patterns following chronic exposure to cholinesterase inhibiting organophosphate compounds. *Psychophysiology* 1968; 5:206.

132. Sutin E, Shiromani P, Kelsoe J, Storch F, Gillin JC. Chronic scopolamine treatment increases REM sleep and muscarinic receptor binding during withdrawal. *Life Sci* 1986; 39:2419–2427.

133. Szerb JC. Cortical acetylcholine release and electroencephalographic arousal. *J Physiol (London)* 1967; 192:329–345.

134. Szymusiak R, McGinty DJ. Sleep-suppression after kainic acid-induced lesions of the basal forebrain in cats. *Sleep Res* 1985; 14:2.

135. Szymusiak R, McGinty DJ. Sleep-related neuronal discharge in the basal forebrain damage of cats. *Brain Res* 1986; 370:82–92.

136. Szymusiak R, Satinoff E. Ambient temperature-dependence of sleep disturbances produced by basal forebrain damage in rats. *Brain Res Bull* 1984; 12:295–305.

137. Tohyama M, Satoh K, Sakumoto T, Kimoto Y, Takahashi Y, Yamamoto K, Itakura T. Organization and projections of the neurons in the dorsal tegmental area of the rat. *J Hirnforsch* 1977; 19:165–176.

138. Van Dongen PA, Broekamp LE, Coola AR. Atonia after carbachol microinjections near the locus coeruleus in cats. *Pharmacol Biochem Behav* 1978; 8:527–532.

139. Van Dongen PAM. Locus ceruleus region: Effects on behavior of cholinergic, noradrenergic and opiate drugs injected intracerebrally into freely moving cats. *Exp Neurol* 1980; 67:52–78.

140. Vertes RP. Selective firing of rat pontine gigantocellular neurons during movement of REM sleep. *Brain Res* 1977; 128:146–152.

141. Vertes RP. Brainstem gigantocellular neurons: Patterns of activity during behavior and sleep in the freely moving rat. *J Neurophysiol* 1979; 42:224–228.

142. Villablanca J. Behavioral and polygraphic study of sleep and wakefulness in chronic decerebrate cats. *Electroenceph Clin Neurophysiol* 1966; 21:562–577.

143. Wamsley JK, Lewis MS, Young WS 3d, Kuhar MJ. Autoradiographic localization of muscarinic cholinergic receptors in rat brainstem. *J Neurosci* 1981; 1:176–191.

144. Webster HH, Friedman L, Jones BE. Modification of paradoxical sleep following transections of the reticular formation at the pontomedullary junction. *Sleep* 1986; 9:1–23.

145. Weitzman ED, Kripke DF, Goldmacher D, McGregor P, Nogeire C. Acute reversal of the sleep-waking cycle in man. *Arch Neurol* 1970; 22:483–489.

146. Wilson PM. A photographic perspective on the origins, form, course and relations of the acetylcholinesterase containing fibres of the dorsal tegmental pathway in the rat brain. *Brain Res Rev* 1985; 10:85–118.

12

Do Studies of Sedative/Hypnotics Suggest the Nature of Chronic Insomnia?

WALLACE B. MENDELSON

It is becoming increasingly evident that insomnia is a much more complex problem than may originally have been supposed. The most fundamental—and probably mistaken—view is that insomnia is a condition characterized primarily by lack of sleep. This was phrased most eloquently, perhaps, by W. C. Fields, who remarked that the only thing wrong with insomniacs is that they don't get enough sleep. In this chapter we will review data suggesting that a much more complex process is involved. In parallel, we will examine clinical studies of hypnotics and indicate that, similarly, the benefits of hypnotics may not merely be a matter of increasing polygraphically measured sleep. The intention is to show that there are some similarities between the anomalies that appear in observations of insomniacs and reports of actions of hypnotics, and that these might suggest some fruitful areas for future research. First, however, it might be well to briefly define insomnia as discussed here, and to review reports of alterations in physiological and psychophysiological measures in insomniacs.

DESCRIPTION OF INSOMNIA

Insomnia refers to the subjective sensation of inadequate quality or quantity of sleep. Obviously, difficulty sleeping may be of very brief duration—in which case it is often related to specific upsetting life events—or may be a chronic problem that has lasted for months. In the more chronic situation there are often specific pathophysiologic or psychiatric disorders that result in the complaint of insomnia. Among these, for instance, are the sleep apnea syndromes, nocturnal myoclonus, and major depressions (1). When these conditions have been ruled out, however, there remains an interesting group whose difficulties are at this time best described in psychological terms. In the terminology of the Association of Sleep Disorders Centers nosology (1) these include "persistent psychophysiological Disorders of Initiating and Maintaining Sleep (DIMS)" (A.1.b.) and "subjective DIMS complaint without objective findings" (A.9.b.). The former is a conditioned state in which internal cues (the worry about having poor sleep) and external cues (the bedroom environment) become associated with insomnia (13). In general, during laboratory studies sleep is relatively normal, but whether it is disturbed or not, the patient's subjective retrospective report on his sleep is fairly accurate. In subjective DIMS without objective findings, polysomnograms reveal relatively normal sleep, but the patient's subjective report in the morning is of poor quality, unrefreshing sleep. In contrast to persistent psychophysiological DIMS, then, the patient with subjective DIMS is a poor judge of his own physiological sleep. In this chapter we will focus on insomniacs with these two conditions. The effort is to deal with subjective insomnia; unfortunately, many research reports do not always define their subjects well. The distinction between these forms is also sometimes blurred because conditioned factors may develop in subjective—and all other forms— of chronic sleep disturbance.

SLEEP IN CHRONIC INSOMNIA

There have been many studies of sleep in insomniacs. Earlier ones have been reported in detail by the Institute of Medicine (10). Interpretation is difficult, however, because many studies were done on the basis of clinical history, without the benefit of polysomnography to rule out disorders such as sleep apnea. In general, the reports seem to indicate relatively small changes in sleep. In a study that did include polysomnographic screening, 10 insomniacs were found to have more intermittent waking time and lower sleep efficiency than controls (15). In a later study, insomniacs differed from controls

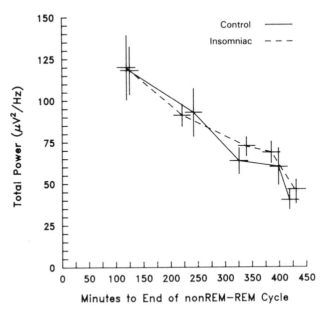

Figure 12-1 Total power (expressed as $\mu V^2/Hz$) in the EEG (0.23–25 Hz) during sleep in 10 insomniacs and age- and sex-matched controls. Methodology and presentation are the same as those used by Mendelson et al. (16).

only in having more early morning awakening time, although there was a trend toward shorter sleep and lower sleep efficiency (17). Reynolds et al. (25) found that in persistent psychophysiological DIMS sleep efficiency was 81.5% and total sleep was 359.8 min. These values are only slightly shorter than control measures in the previously mentioned studies (389 and 383 min, respectively). A review of 25 hypnotic efficacy studies found mean total sleep baseline values of 383 min in insomniacs (6). There have also been reports of decreased delta sleep (5), and some authors have stressed the possible importance of this in insomnia (4). On the other hand, a recent study employing electronic analysis of the electroencephalogram (EEG) found no difference in power in either the delta or entire EEG band between groups of insomniacs and controls (Fig. 12-1). Certainly there are individual patients with greatly decreased slow-wave sleep, and it may be that with time these will turn out to be a special subgroup.

In summary, then, the usual measures of polygraphic sleep show relatively mild, nonspecific changes compared to normal sleepers. As we will see later, it is possible that more subtle measures of sleep continuity may turn out to be critical in understanding disturbed sleep. Another implication may be that the sleep disturbance in chronic insomnia is not something that is measured by present technology. Alternatively, it may be that among insomniacs there is some dysfunction in perception of the experience of sleep. Now, though, let us turn to the question of whether insomniacs differ from normal sleepers in other physiological measures.

PHYSIOLOGICAL ALTERATIONS IN INSOMNIACS

Temperature

One of the classical studies of poor sleepers, performed by Monroe in 1967 (20), found that they maintained a significantly higher rectal temperature throughout sleep compared to good sleepers. Other differences included higher mean number of phasic vasoconstrictions and body movements, and trends toward higher heart rate and pulse volume. Mendelson et al. (16) found increased rectal temperature throughout the night in 10 insomniacs compared to controls (Fig. 12-2). There was no evidence of a phase shift in their temperature rhythm as reflected in these nighttime recordings. One possible interpretation might have been that the increased temperature was a reflection of hightened awakening time after sleep onset. As can be seen in the bottom of Figure 12-2, this did not appear to be the case; in the first 2 hr after the insomniacs did fall asleep, they had the same or less wakefulness than controls, yet temperatures remained higher. Another view of these findings might be that insomniacs have some form of autonomic hyperarousal associated with subjectively poor sleep. On the other hand, at least one finding of Monroe's would be difficult to interpret in that manner. As Rechtschaffen (24) pointed out, the poor sleepers in the Monroe study (20) had higher skin resistance, which is usually considered to be a sign of more relaxation. Thus, although heightened autonomic arousal remains a consideration, this is clearly a complex, polyfaceted process. It has also been speculated that it is the lack of a temperature drop associated with sleep onset that results in possibly decreased slow-wave sleep in insomniacs (32).

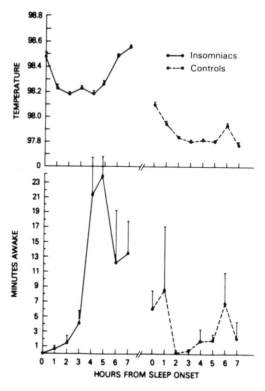

Figure 12-2 Core temperature in the 7 hr after sleep onset (upper panel) and waking time after sleep onset (lower panel) in 10 insomniacs (solid lines) and age- and sex-matched controls (dashed lines). From Mendelson et al. (13).

Responsiveness to External Environment

Another way in which insomniacs might differ from normals could conceivably be in their responsiveness to the environment during sleep. It might be speculated, for instance, that insomniacs are more disturbed by external stimuli during sleep. One type of measure of this is the auditory evoked response (AER). Surprisingly, at least one study has suggested that insomniacs might be sensory reducers, that is, display *lower* amplitude EEG responses to auditory stimuli (3). The authors argued that having a reduced responsivity to the environment might contribute to poor sleep in another way—it might allow insomniacs to continue to be disturbed by the anxious ruminative worrying that is often associated with the disorder.

Another approach to the issue of responsiveness to external stimulation is to examine auditory arousal thresholds. Mendelson et al. (17) found that 10 insomniacs did not differ from controls in the amplitude of an auditory tone necessary to induce an arousal response from five points in sleep. This suggests that poor sleep is not necessarily the same as "light" sleep. The AER finding of course measures a somewhat different process, and whether this indeed indicates another physiological difference between insomniacs and controls awaits further study.

Association of Nighttime Sleep Disturbance and Daytime Wakefulness

It is intuitive that the degree of disturbance of nighttime sleep might be positively associated with daytime sleepiness. There is some suggestion that although this may be true for some sleep disorders, it may not be so for insomnia. Stepanski et al. (35) reported that among patients complaining of daytime sleepiness associated with sleep apnea or nocturnal myoclonus the total number of nocturnal arousals was positively associated with objective measures of daytime sleepiness (the degree of sleepiness was assessed by the Multiple Sleep Latency Test or MSLT). In contrast, there was no significant association between these two variables among controls. Insomniacs were found to have a significant *inverse* correlation—the more arousals during the night, the more awake the patients were the next day. More detailed analysis showed that the type of arousal was also important; very modest arousals (increases in EEG frequency and electromyogram (EMG) amplitude) were inversely associated with sleepiness, whereas full awakenings from sleep were positively associated with sleepiness. In a later study, Stepanski et al. (34) reported that shorter total nocturnal sleep time was associated with increased objective measures of wakefulness the next day. As in other studies, they found that insomniacs were actually more alert during the daytime than controls. Taken together, these data may suggest that insomniacs respond to sleep disturbance in a manner different from noncomplaining subjects.

PSYCHOPHYSIOLOGICAL DIFFERENCES BETWEEN INSOMNIACS AND CONTROLS

Belief about the Depth of REM Sleep

It is also possible that insomniacs perceive different stages of sleep—and the experience of being asleep—differently than controls. Mendelson et al. (16) awakened insomniacs with an electronic tone at five points during the night (5 min after "lights out," 10 min after the onset of stage 2, during stage 4, rapid eye movement (REM) sleep, and intermittent waking time), and questioned subjects about their experience before being awakened. Among those subjects who believed that they had been sleeping, insomniacs were more likely than controls to describe REM sleep as "light" sleep.

The Perception of Being Awake

Rechtschaffen (24) found that when an investigator entered a subject's room 10 min after the first sleep spindle, the poor sleepers were more likely to report that they had been awake. Coates et al. (2) had similar findings at the time of the first sleep spindle and 10 min after the second spindle. Mendelson et al. (16) did not observe this when insomniacs were awakened by a loud (80-dB) tone, but did find the same phenomenon when subjects were awakened by a tone of gradually increasing intensity (17). In the intervals between testing, both insomniacs and controls fell asleep with equal rapidity, and had approximately the same amounts of EEG-defined sleep. The retrospective impression of the insomniacs, however, was that they had slept only half as much. These observations suggest that insomniacs may somehow misperceive the experience of being asleep. If such a process were important in the pathogenesis of insomnia, it might explain why there are relatively small alterations in polysomnographically defined sleep—it might be that the "lesion" in chronic insomnia involves something that is not currently measured electrophysiologically. There are other tools available, however. An additional source of information could conceivably come from studies of hypnotics, the compounds that offer some relief to insomniacs.

HYPNOTICS

The hypnotics are a heterogeneous group of drugs comprised of a variety of pharmacologic classes. Indeed, one of the mysteries about them is how drugs of such greatly differing structures may induce a relatively similar effect—improvement in sleep as determined by polysomnographic measures and subjective reports. One possibility, which is beyond the scope of this review, is that a number of different substances that induce sleep may act at various subcomponents of the benzodiazepine receptor complex (12). If such a view were to continue to be fruitful, it might help bring some common theme to our understanding of how drugs enhance sleep. For the purposes of this review, however, we will focus on the benzodiazepines, both because they are the most widely prescribed hypnotics and because their mechanism of action is more clearly elucidated at this time.

Effects on Sleep Stages

One of the puzzles about the effects of benzodiazepines on sleep is that these compounds, which enhance the subjective quality of sleep, are potent suppressors of slow-wave sleep, which has traditionally been considered to be deep or restful. This is particularly difficult to understand insofar as sleep studies of insomniacs have tended to show that amounts of slow-wave sleep are normal or slightly reduced. One possibility might be that the interpretation of the nature of slow-wave sleep needs to be reconsidered. It is clearly the stage in which auditory arousal thresholds to meaningless stimuli are highest, and in this sense is "deep." On the other hand, in normal volunteers the amount of stage 4 has been associated with retrospective reports the next morning of "light" sleep (30). Sewitch (31) found that subjects believed themselves to have previously been awake after 56% of forced awakenings from stage 2 and 77% of awakenings from slow-wave sleep. Mendelson et al. (17) found that both insomniacs and normal volunteers tended to associate various measures of slow-wave sleep with lower scores on a scale of quality of sleep retrospectively assessed the following morning. Obviously there are some data in the other direction as well. A study of cancer patients, for instance, found that those who considered themselves to sleep well had a small but significantly greater (3.4 min) amount of slow-wave sleep than those who slept poorly (33). In healthy older women, but not men, reports of soundness of sleep was positively associated with amounts of slow-wave sleep (8). This suggests that gender and age need also be considered in evaluating the relation of subjective and objective measures of sleep. Nonetheless, these studies leave open the possibility that although slow-wave sleep is clearly the "deepest" in terms of auditory arousal threshold, the subjective experience of slow-wave sleep continues to need to be explored.

Effects on Total Sleep

Obviously, clinically used hypnotics enhance total sleep as defined by polysomnography. It is less clear, however, whether increased total sleep can explain all of their therapeutic actions. One review of hypnotic efficacy studies meeting basic standards of quality found that hypnotics increased total sleep only by a mean of 35 min (6). One of the studies most often cited as showing the efficacy of 30 mg flurazepam reported an increase in total sleep of only 6–8% during a 1 month trial; sleep latency was decreased significantly only on nights 11–13 (11). A 5-week study indicated that 30 mg flurazepam given to insomniacs increased total sleep by a mean of 21 min (19). A 1-week study indicated that 15 mg flurazepam given to insomniacs increased total sleep by 29 min (28). Although this degree of improvement in total sleep seems modest, roughly 20 million prescriptions for benzodiazepine hypnotics including flurazepam are written each year. Patients clearly feel helped by them. In one review, patients reported that total sleep time had been significantly enhanced compared to placebo in six of seven studies (26). In five of the studies they believed their sleep quality to have been significantly improved. One possible interpretation of such reports is that this small increase in sleep is sufficient to make insomniacs feel substantially better. Alternatively, one might argue that the subjective benefits of hypnotics seem disproportionately greater than the improvement in polysomnographic measures of sleep. (In a way, this view is complementary to the observation that the subjective distress experienced by insomniacs if often disproportionately greater than the decrements in polysomnographically measured sleep.) Obviously we do not have very precise ways of assessing the subjective benefits of hypnotics. On the other hand, there are some indications that there may be a disparity between subjective and polysomnographic benefits. If one accepts for argument's sake that subjective benefits from hypnotics may often exceed polysomnographically measured changes in sleep, then several interesting possibilities might be considered:

1. The benefits of hypnotics at least partially involve some other (perhaps more subtle) polysomnographically measured process. This might include improvements in sleep continuity rather than total sleep. There is some reason to suggest that we will continue to find more and more importance in the issue of sleep continuity. On the other hand, authors such as Stepanski et al. (35) did not find that the sleep of insomniacs was excessively disrupted. In three of four measures of arousal (increases in EEG frequency and EMG amplitude, alpha bursts, and awakenings of at least 30 seconds), insomniacs had less arousals than patients with sleep apnea or nocturnal myoclonus and had values similar to controls. Only one category of arousals—stage shifts to a lighter stage—occurred more frequently in insomniacs. If their sleep is not greatly more disrupted than controls, it is difficult to argue that hypnotics act by enhancing continuity. Obviously such a view awaits further studies using a variety of possible measures of sleep continuity.

2. Hypnotics affect some other physiological process not typically measured by polysomnography. Certainly one possibility is that alterations in core temperature by hypnotics indirectly affect both sleep staging and the perception of sleep. We have previously described studies suggesting that insomniacs may have higher core temperatures throughout sleep, and there are data indicating

that hypnotics lower body temperature (23). As slow-wave sleep is altered by changes in core temperature (9), one might speculate that the decrease in slow-wave sleep induced by benzodiazepines is at least partially associated with drug-induced alterations in temperature. Obviously this is a complex issue, as slow-wave sleep is also sensitive to ambient temperature (7,21) and other factors, but it is certainly a possibility to be considered.

3. Hypnotics alter some process that at this time is not available to physiological measurement. Certainly one candidate for this might be drug-induced changes in cognitive function. Benzodiazepines clearly alter various cognitive processes such as episodic memory, the ability to learn new verbal information (18) and perhaps other aspects of memory (29). In addition to being assessed in the hours after administration in waking subjects, cognitive changes have also often been examined as a type of residual daytime effect of hypnotics (22,27). In one study, memory decrements observed the day after flurazepam administration were very significant, and comparable to those seen after agents such as ethanol (14). One could argue that there are few or no clinically used hypnotics that do not alter cognitive function. Could it be, then, that alterations in memory or perception are an inherent part of the action of hypnotics in improving subjective reports of sleep? Perhaps in addition to enhancing polysomnographic measures of sleep, hypnotics alter the perception and experience of sleeping. If that were the case, then the cognitive changes that we measure after hypnotic administration might not be "side effects"—rather, they might be manifestations of the mechanism by which hypnotics improve the insomniac's experience of sleep.

Finally, it is well worth considering how hypnotic-induced cognitive changes might relate to what is known about the molecular actions of these compounds. In the last decade, interest has focused on the benzodiazepine receptor complex, a macromolecular structure that includes recognition sites for benzodiazepines and GABA as well as a chloride ionophore (12). In addition to benzodiazepines, which bind in a stereospecific, saturable manner, other sedatives such as barbiturates and ethanol may influence ion channel function of this complex. This may suggest that in the future we will find that effects on this receptor complex are the common link in sedative properties of disparate classes of pharmacologic agents. It is not yet clear how this bears on the question of insomnia. One might speculate that insomniacs are deficient in a hypothetical endogenous ligand for the benzodiazepine receptor. On the other hand, we have mentioned earlier that insomnia is not a simple matter of decrements in currently available physiological measures of sleep. If there is an endogenous ligand for the benzodiazepine receptor, and if it is deficient in insomniacs, one would have to speculate that it—like hypnotic medications—might also affect the perception of sleep.

REFERENCES

1. Association of Sleep Disorders Centers. Diagnostic classification of sleep and arousal disorders. *Sleep* 1979; 1:1–137.

2. Coates TJ, Killen JD, Silberman S, Marchini J, Hamilton S, Thoresen CE. Cognitive activity, sleep disturbance, and stage specific differences between recorded and reported sleep. *Psychopharmacology* 1983; 20:243.

3. Coursey RD, Buchsbaum M, Frankel BL. Personality measures and evoked responses in chronic insomniacs. *J Abnorm Psychol* 1975; 84:239–249.

4. Gaillard JM. Chronic primary insomnia: Possible physiopathological involvement of slow wave sleep deficiency. *Sleep* 1978; 1:133–147.

5. Gillin JC, Duncan W, Pettigrew KD, Frankel BL, Snyder F. Successful separation of depressed, normal, and insomniac subjects by EEG sleep data. *Arch Gen Psychiat* 1979; 36:85–90.

6. Gillin JC, Mendelson WB. Sleeping pills: For Whom? When? How long? In GC Palmer (ed.), *Neuropharmacology of Central Nervous System and Behavioral Disorders*. Academic Press, New York, 1981: 285–316.

7. Haskell EH, Palca JW, Walker JM, Berger RJ, Heller HC. The effects of high and low ambient temperature on human sleep stages. *Electroenceph Clin Neurophysiol* 1981; 51:494–501.

8. Hoch CC, Reynolds CF, Kupfer DJ, Berman SR, Houck PR, Stack JA. Empirical note: Self-report versus recorded sleep in healthy seniors. *Psychophysiology* 1987; 24(3):293–299.

9. Horne JA, Moore VJ, Reid AJ, Shackell BS. Waking body temperature manipulation and subsequent sleep (SWS). *Sleep Res* 1985; 14:15.

10. Institute of Medicine. *Sleeping Pills, Insomnia, and Medical Practice*. National Academy of Sciences, Washington, D.C., 1979: 1–46.

11. Kales A, Kales JD, Bixler EO, Scharf MB. Effectiveness of hypnotic drugs with prolonged use: Flurazepam and pentobarbital. *Clin Pharmacol Ther* 1975; 18(3):356–363.

12. Mendelson WB, Sack DA, James SP, Martin JV, Wagner R, Garnett D, Milton J, Wehr TA. *Psychiat Res* 1987; 21:89–94.

13. Mendelson WB. *Human Sleep: Research and Clinical Care*. Plenum, New York, 1987: 1–436.

14. Mendelson WB, Weingartner H, Greenblatt DJ, Garnett D, Gillin JC. A clinical study of flurazepam. *Sleep* 1982; 5:350–360.

15. Mendelson WB, Garnett D, Gillin JC, Weingartner H. The experience of insomnia and daytime and nighttime functioning. *Psychiat Res* 1984; 12:235–250.

16. Mendelson WB, Garnett D, Linnoila M. Do insomniacs have impaired daytime functioning? *Biol Psychiat* 1984; 19(8):1261–1262.

17. Mendelson WB, James SP, Garnett D, Sack DA, Rosenthal NE. A psychophysiological study of insomnia. *Psychiat Res* 1986; 19:267–284.

18. Mendelson WB, Martin JV, Wagner RR, Hommer DW, Weingartner H. Effects of benzodiazepine hypnotics on memory and EEG. *Sleep Res* 1987; 16:107.

19. Mitler MM, Seidel WF, Van Den Hoed J, Greenblatt DJ, Dement WC. Comparative hypnotic effects of flurazepam, triazolam and placebo: A long-term simultaneous nighttime and daytime study. *J Clin Psychopharmacol* 1984; 4(1):2–13.

20. Monroe LJ. Psychological and physiological differences between good and poor sleepers. *J Abnorm Psychol* 1967; 72:255–264.

21. Muzet A, Libert J-P, Candas V. Ambient temperature and human sleep. *Experientia* 1984; 40:425–429.

22. Pishkin V, Lovallo WR, Fishkin SM, Shurley JT. Residual effects of temazepam and other hypnotic compounds on cognitive function. *J Clin Psychiat* 1980; 41:358–364.

23. Pleuvry BJ, Maddison SE, Odeh RB, Dodson ME. Respiratory and psychological effects of oral temazepam in volunteers. *Br J Anaesth* 1980; 52:901.

24. Rechtschaffen A. Polygraphic aspects of insomnia. In H Gastaut, E Lugaresi, and G Berti-Ceroni (eds.), *The Abnormalities of Sleep in Man*. Gaggi, Bologna, 1968: 109–125.

25. Reynolds CF, Taska LS, Sewitch DE, Restifo K, Coble PA, Kupfer DJ. Persistent psychophysiologic insomnia: Preliminary research diagnostic criteria and EEG sleep data. *Am J Psychiat* 1984; 141:804–805.

26. Rickels K. Clinical trials of hypnotics. *J Clin Psychopharmacol* 1983; 3(2):133–142.

27. Roehrs T, Kribbs N, Zorick F, Roth T. Hypnotic residual effects of benzodiazepines with repeated administration. *Sleep* 1986; 9:194–199.

28. Roehrs T, Zorick F, Kaffeman M, Sicklesteel BA, Roth T. Flurazepam for short-term treatment of complaints of insomnia. *J Clin Pharmacol* 1982; 22:290–296.

29. Roth T, Roehrs T, Wittig R, Zorick F. Benzodiazepines and memory. *Br J Pharmacol* 1984; 18:458–498.

30. Saletu B. Is the subjectively experienced quality of sleep related to objective sleep parameters? *Behav Biol* 1975; 13:433.

31. Sewitch DE. NREM sleep continuity and the sense of having slept in normal sleepers. *Sleep* 1984; 7:147.

32. Sewitch DE. Slow wave sleep deficiency insomnia: A problem in thermo-downregulation at sleep onset. *Psychophysiology* 1987; 24(2):200–215.

33. Silberfarb PM, Hauri PJ, Oxman TE, Lash S. Insomnia in cancer patients. *Soc Sci Med* 1985; 20:849–850.

34. Stepanski E, Zorick F, Roehrs T, Young D, Roth T. Daytime alertness in patients with chronic insomnia compared with asymptomatic control subjects. *Sleep* 1988; 11(1):54–60.

35. Stepanski E, Lamphere J, Badia P, Zorick F, Roth T. Sleep fragmentation and daytime sleepiness. *Sleep* 1984; 7(1):18–26.

13

Fundamental and Clinical Neuropharmacology of Sleep Disorders: Restless Legs Syndrome with Periodic Movements in Sleep and Narcolepsy

ROGER GODBOUT, JACQUES MONTPLAISIR,
MARC-ANDRÉ BÉDARD, DIANE BOIVIN, AND ODILE LAPIERRE

Sleep disturbance is a major complaint in health care practice, and surveys show that among the medical specialties, psychiatry is the one in which sleep complaints are the most frequently reported (13). A major step in the management of sleep difficulties was taken 10 years ago with the publication, by the Association of Sleep Disorders Centers (6), of a nosology for the classification of sleep and arousal disorders. Basically, this classification includes four main categories: (a) disorders of initiating and maintaining sleep (the insomnias), (b) disorders of excessive somnolence (the hypersomnias), (c) disorders of the sleep–wake schedule, and (d) dysfunctions associated with sleep, sleep stages, or partial arousals (the parasomnias). The most prevalent disorders are insomnia and hypersomnia. Of patients attending sleep disorder clinics, 31.2% complain of the former condition and 15.8% of the latter (25). Such a nosology is of major importance not only for clinicians but also for sleep researchers who use it as a guide for selecting homogeneous patient populations.

More recently, mechanisms governing the action of several drugs effective in the treatment of sleep disorders have been elucidated, and more specific treatments have been developed. The aim of this chapter is to review some of the recent advances in the pharmacology of sleep disorders and to discuss results in terms of physiopathology. We will focus on two syndromes: one associated with insomnia (the restless legs syndrome with periodic movements in sleep) and one associated with hypersomnia (narcolepsy).

RESTLESS LEGS SYNDROME AND PERIODIC MOVEMENTS IN SLEEP

Description

The restless legs syndrome (RLS) with periodic movements during sleep (PMS) (24,81) is the fourth most frequent diagnosis in insomniac patients, and represents approximately 12% of insomniacs investigated at the sleep disorders center (25). RLS can be described as an irresistible urge to keep the limbs in motion, usually accompanied by paresthesia, that appears at rest and delays sleep onset. Symptoms often appear at puberty and the condition is thought to be familial in a large percentage of cases (40,78). RLS is exacerbated by heat, fatigue, and stress. The serious discomfort it creates often triggers psychological distress. RLS may be secondary to various medial conditions, but primary (essential) RLS is free of significant psychiatric or neurological findings.

PMS are found in almost every RLS patient subjected to a polysomnographic evaluation. PMS are brief, rhythmic, and stereotyped movements, affecting mostly the legs and appearing during sleep. Leg movements can be noted on visual monitoring, but they are best documented with appropriate surface electromyograms (EMG) of the anterior tibialis muscles. Leg muscle bursts can be unilateral or bilateral, synchronous or asynchronous, and they appear mostly in the first half of the sleep period, during non-rapid eye movement (NREM) sleep (39). Patients with RLS/PMS may report one or more of the following sleep symptoms: delayed sleep onset, frequent nocturnal awakenings, shallow sleep, restless sleep, and excessive daytime fatigue. There is an increased prevalence of PMS with age and in various sleep disorders, especially narcolepsy.

The diagnosis of RLS is mainly clinical and based on characteristic complaints of delayed sleep onset associated with creeping or crawling sensations deep in the legs (35,81). The diagnosis of PMS has to be confirmed by the polygraphic recording of at least five periodic leg movements per hour of sleep. The criteria used to score PMS are usually derived from those of Coleman (24) and include the following: EMG bursts last between 0.5 and 5 sec, they occur in clusters of at least four consecutive movements separated by 4 to 90 sec, and leg EMG bursts are not followed by a prolonged (>10–15 sec) awakening.

RLS and PMS are often considered two manifestations of a common central nervous system (CNS) disorder (65,78). Indeed, almost all patients with RLS also show PMS during their sleep, although the reverse is not necessarily true. RLS can accordingly be viewed as a prolongation of PMS activity extending to daytime. A rhythmicity can also be shown in leg movements associated with RLS if they are scored with the same criteria used for PMS (21,78). Finally, medications that are effective in treating PMS also suppress RLS in patients with both conditions. This last item will be reviewed in more detail.

Several classes of CNS-active drugs have been investigated in recent years, especially benzodiazepines, γ-aminobutyric acid (GABA) agonist, and drugs acting on opioid or dopamine (DA) mechanisms in the CNS.

Treatments

Benzodiazepines

The most common treatment of RLS/PMS is the benzodiazepines, clonazepam being the most frequently prescribed. However, experimental evaluations of clonazepam's efficacy are scarce and sometimes yield contradictory results. It was found effective in treating RLS in open clinical trials (16,67,78,85), but in a more controlled study (17) it was not found to be superior to a placebo. In our clinical experience, the therapeutic response of RLS to clonazepam shows major individual differences. There is little doubt that clonazepam is helpful in treating RLS in a subgroup of patients, but there is no criteria to predict the outcome of treatment.

In two studies involving polysomnographic recordings, benzodiazepines were found effective in treating 30 patients with primary PMS. In one study (85), clonazepam administered at bedtime reduced significantly the number of leg movements per hour of sleep and the number of PMS clusters per night. The mean duration of movements and the duration of intermovement intervals remained unchanged. These results were confirmed by others (71) for clonazepam and were extended to temazepam. However, in both studies, the number of leg movements per hour of sleep (PMS index) remained pathological (PMS index >5) after treatment. In a third study (73), involving 13 patients with PMS secondary to various medical conditions, another benzodiazepine, nitrazepam, also improved PMS.

Benzodiazepines not only reduce PMS but also consolidate sleep in patients with PMS. These drugs reduce the number of arousals associated with leg movements, increase sleep efficiency, and shorten sleep latency. Mechanisms by which benzodiazepines suppress PMS and improve sleep are largely unknown. Clonazepam does not influence the duration of intervals between successive movements (85), suggesting that benzodiazepines do not affect the PMS "rhythm generator."

GABA Agonist

Baclofen is a GABA-II agonist, depressing spinal excitatory transmission through hyperpolarization of the primary afferent terminals. Since sedative benzodiazepines are known to influence GABEergic transmission, it would be interesting to know whether baclofen can affect RLS and/or PMS. Only one study has addressed this question (46). It is reported that 20–40 mg of baclofen at bedtime increases the number of leg movements in patients with PMS, shortens the intermovement intervals, and leaves the duration of movements unchanged. This shows the possible effect of baclofen on a hypothetical "pacemaker" of PMS activity, a mode of action not shared by the benzodiazepines or by any other treatment of PMS. On the other hand, baclofen decreases the amplitude of anterior tibialis potential and improves sleep organization, increasing total sleep time and slow wave sleep and decreasing awakenings associated with leg jerks (46).

Results obtained with baclofen and the benzodiazepines in the treatment of RLS/PMS show that it is possible to control independently various aspects of this condition, namely, the number of leg movements, their rhythmicity, the amplitude of leg EMG discharges, and sleep architecture.

Opioids

Opioids have specific and potent therapeutic effects on RLS/PMS, although no controlled study has been performed yet. The therapeutic effect of codeine and opium in RLS was actually reported as early as in 1960 (18) but the risk of addiction kept their use for highly selected and severe cases. Since then, several opioids, such as morphine (3), codeine sulfate (2,53), oxycodone (111,113), propoxyphene (53,113) and methadone (51,53,111,113), have been used to treat RLS. Polysomnographic recordings reveal that PMS also decrease markedly after opioid treatment (53). Trzepacz et al. (111) suggested that the efficacy of opioids may be restricted to low doses. In our laboratory, however, one patient showing severe RLS and 986 movements per night (PMS index = 88.8) was treated with codeine sulfate administered 1 hr before bedtime. This resulted in a dose-response curve, and a complete suppression of symptoms was obtained only at doses between 120 and 180 mg (unpublished data), which is more than 10 times the therapeutic dose reported by Akpinar (2).

Effects of the opioids on RLS/PMS can be reversed by naloxone, an opioid receptor blocker that has no effects of its own (3,52,53). Moreover, meperidine, a κ opioid receptor agonist, has no therapeutic effect (3). Now the κ subtype is the most prominent among the opioid receptors in the spinal cord, and it is less sensitive to naloxone than μ receptors (96,110). These observations suggest that spinal cord opioid receptors are not involved in the physiopathology of RLS/PMS and raise the possibility that more rostral structures containing μ, σ, or δ binding sites may be involved. Further studies should examine the effect of opioids not only on the severity of RLS/PMS, but also on other aspects of this syndrome such as the amplitude, duration and periodicity of movements, daytime vigilance, and nocturnal sleep organization.

L-Dopa

Many observations support the hypothesis that primary PMS/RLS result from a decreased DA transmission in the CNS. Clinical reports show that L-dopa administered with a decarboxylase inhibitor is indeed helpful in treating the subjective complaints of RLS (2,3,21) and PMS (21,80). In these patients, L-dopa also improves sleep quality and daytime vigilance. The effect of L-dopa on RLS can also be objectively demonstrated with a special procedure called the "Suggested Immobilization Test," intended to evoke symptoms of RLS by requiring the patient to remain motionless with his legs outstretched while an electromyogram is recorded. This method has been described in detail elsewhere (21). A variant of this technique, called the "Forced Immobilization Test" is currently being developed in our laboratory (63a).

Nocturnal polygraphic recordings performed in patients with both RLS and PMS showed that single does of L-dopa (80) at bedtime improves sleep: it decreases sleep latency and the number of awakenings and therefore increases sleep efficiency. Leg movement clusters are shifted after treatment from the first to the last third of the night, a time course compatible with the pharmacokinetics of L-dopa (80). In a controlled study using repeated dosage, RLS improved and PMS activity decreased throughout the night (21), along with subjective and objective decreases of awakenings associated with leg jerks. Intermovement intervals and amplitude of leg movements are not affected by L-dopa. Bromocriptine mesylate, a DA postsynaptic D_2 receptor agonist, suppresses both RLS (59) and PMS, whereas pimozide, a D_2 receptor antagonist, worsens RLS (3).

Other observations suggest an involvement of DA in RLS/PMS. For example, increased concentration and decreased turnover of homovanillic acid (107) as well as decreased DA binding sites (101) are found in normal aging, whereas the prevalence of PMS increases with age (14). Finally, it was hypothesized that DA transmission is reduced in narcolepsy (17), a disease in which pathological PMS are found in approximately 50% of cases (112). PMS observed in narcolepsy are also responsive to L-dopa therapy (10). These observations led to the hypothesis that RLS and/or PMS result from a decrease of DA neurotransmission in the CNS. The basic mechanism of impaired central DA transmission is unknown, and may vary for RLS/PMS associated with different conditions (80).

Table 13-1 summarizes the therapeutic effect of drugs most commonly used to treat RLS/PMS. Other treatments are proposed in the literature, namely carbamazepine (109), serotoninergic agents such as trazodone and methysergide (32), and adrenergic drugs such as clonidine (49), propranolol (108), phenoxybenzamine (114), and imipramine (102). In most cases, however, treatments either lacked specificity regarding the neurotransmitter involved, or were not properly evaluated in primary RLS/PMS.

The Pathophysiology of RLS and PMS

Opioid and DA systems are most likely involved in the physiopathology of RLS/PMS. Both systems interact in many CNS areas, including basal ganglia, brainstem, and spinal cord, and some of the units identified in DA/opioid colocalization studies are implicated in motor output (63,104). It is known, for example, that naloxone can inhibit the therapeutic effect of opioids in RLS/PMS but cannot reverse the therapeutic effect of L-dopa (3). Moreover, L-dopa is immediately effective in treating RLS/PMS, whereas prolonged exposure to opioids may be necessary before a therapeutic effect is observed (58). It is then possible that DA and opioids interact in a hierarchical manner in which the DA element constitutes the final common pathway. It still remains to be proven, however, that a DA antagonist, such as pimozide, can block the effect of opioids as well as it counteracts L-dopa in RLS/PMS (2,3,80a).

In addition to pharmacological studies, other approaches have raised the question of the localization of CNS processes involved in the genesis of RLS/PMS. Spinal, truncular, and telencephalic loci are all potential candidates. For example, there are spinal and truncular rhythmic activities that share a comparable period to that of PMS (reviewed in 66), but there is no direct evidence of a dysfunction at these levels in RLS/PMS. However, it is known that spinal reflexes, motor nerve conduction, and muscle biopsies are normal in primary RLS/PMS (51,78). At the brainstem level, Wechsler et al. (115) have shown abnormalities of the blink reflex in RLS/PMS patients, but we could not duplicate this finding in our laboratory and neither could we observe changes in blink reflex responses after treatment with L-dopa in spite of a marked reduction of RLS and PMS (unpublished observations). At the cortical level, finally, leg movements associated with PMS are accompanied, and even preceded, by EEG signs of arousal such as K complexes and low-voltage fast activity. However, using EEG back-averaging techniques, Lugaresi et al. (64) were unable to identify a particular cortical event preceding leg movements in sleeping PMS patients.

Vascular or metabolic factors may also play a role in the etiology of RLS/PMS. Factors such as low ambiant temperature, hypoglycemia, changes in hormonal levels

Table 13-1 Effect of Pharmacological Bedtime
Treatment on RLS/PMS Symptomatology

Benzodiazepines
  Improve sleep quality
  Decrease leg movements (RLS + PMS)
  Do not affect leg EMG amplitude
  Do not affect rhythmicity
  Improve daytime vigilance

Baclofen
  Improves sleep quality
  Increases leg movements (PMS index)
  Effect on RLS is unknown
  Decreases leg EMG amplitude
  Accelerates the "rhythm generator"
  Effect on daytime vigilance is unknown

Opioids
  Variable effects on sleep organization
  Decrease leg movements (RLS + PMS)
  Do not affect PMS "rhythmicity"
  Effect on leg EMG amplitude is unknown
  Effect on daytime vigilance is unknown

L-Dopa
  Improves sleep quality
  Decreases leg movements (RLS + PMS)
  Does not affect leg EMG amplitude
  Does not affect rhythmicity
  Improves daytime vigilance

RLS = restless legs syndrome; PMS = periodic movements
during sleep.

(e.g., those related to puberty, menses, or pregnancy), renal insufficiency, and varicose veins are sometimes associated with onset or worsening of RLS/PMS symptoms. Some of these factors are related to vasoconstriction, and it is known that fever and vasodilators are effective in reducing RLS/PMS symptoms (30). This mode of action may explain, in part, the therapeutic effect of some adrenergic drugs (48,112) or of peripheral cholinomimetic agents (30). In addition, behavioral treatments involving vasodilation, such as thermal biofeedback, may be effective in treating RLS/PMS (4). Vasodilation may also be the active ingredient of some of the behaviors associated with the syndrome, namely moving or rubbing the legs. However, these movements may also increase DA release in the CNS.

NARCOLEPSY: THE TREATMENT OF EXCESSIVE DAYTIME SOMNOLENCE AND CATAPLEXY

Description

Narcolepsy is characterized by three groups of symptoms: excessive daytime somnolence (EDS), REM sleep-related events, and disrupted sleep.

EDS in narcolepsy is most often the first symptom to appear (11,81). Its severity waxes and wanes throughout the day, often culminating in irresistible and recuperative sleep attacks, usually of short durations (26). The REM sleep-related symptoms of narcolepsy include cataplexy, sleep paralysis, and hypnagogic hallucinations. Cataplexy is a reversible loss of muscle tone without alteration of consciousness and it is triggered by emotions such as sadness or anger, or by emotion-charged events such as laughing or competing. Cataplexy is thought to be induced by an inappropriate triggering of the muscle atonia normally prevailing during REM sleep (45). Sleep paralysis takes place while the patient is waking up or falling asleep, and it probably involves the same mechanism as cataplexy. Hypnagogic hallucinations are mainly vivid auditory or visual hallucinations most often experienced at sleep onset. They are most likely related to REM-sleep dream activity.

Narcoleptic patients also complain of poor sleep, with frequent awakenings throughout the night and vivid unpleasant dreams. Polysomnographic recordings performed in narcoleptic patients (74) show excessively short sleep latencies, an elevated proportion of time spent in the waking state and in stage 1, and numerous sleep stage shifts, especially shifts from REM sleep to waking and stage 1. As a result, REM sleep is frequently interrupted, a phenomenon known as REM sleep fragmentation. This fragmentation is related in time to the onset of cataplexy (76). In approximately 50% of the sleep recordings, REM sleep appears within 10 min of sleep onset, a phenomenon called "sleep onset REM periods" (SOREMPs). These observations have led some authors to consider narcolepsy a disease of REM sleep (90).

The diagnosis of narcolepsy is based on a clear history of EDS and cataplexy, but this clinical diagnosis must to be confirmed by polysomnographic recordings (70). One all-night sleep recording is necessary to rule out other causes of EDS, such as the sleep apnea syndrome. Then, on the following day, the Multiple Sleep Latency Test (MSLT) must demonstrate the presence of two SOREMPs to confirm the diagnosis. In patients presenting a diagnosis dilemma, human leukocyte antigens (HLA) determination may help, as nearly all narcoleptic patients carry HLA-DR2 antigen (56).

The treatment of narcolepsy is pharmacological, and most medications effective in treating EDS have only a slight effect on cataplexy and vice versa. This observation suggests that the symptoms are under different control mechanisms (1).

EDS is most commonly treated with psychostimulants such as methylphenidate and *d*-amphetamine, drugs known as potent catecholaminergic agonists. Several clinical trials suggest that treatment with selective DA agonists may be effective against EDS (47,72,103). This and other evidence support the view that DA may be specifically involved in the physiopathology of EDS. For instance, decreased levels and increased turnover of DA (30,77) and decreased levels of its extracellular metabolite, homovanillic acid (87), were found in the cerebrospinal fluid (CSF) of narcoleptic and idiopathic hypersomniac patients.

Cataplexy is best treated with tricyclic antidepressants (TADs) (44). Most TADs block the central reuptake of both norepinephrine (NE) and serotonin (5HT), therefore increasing their bioavailability. Both neurotransmitter systems are thought to take part in REM-off mechanisms (68). Indeed, most TADs are potent REM sleep inhibitors. TADs also block muscarinic cholinergic receptors, believed to be involved in REM-on mechanisms (68). Therefore, all three neurotransmitters systems possibly take part in the treatment of cataplexy.

Many questions remain unresolved with regard to the physiopathology of narcolepsy. In this part of the chapter, issues related to the role of DA in EDS and to the contribution of NE and 5HT in the physiopathology of cataplexy will be raised. Several selective monoamine agonists were recently tested in our laboratory and evaluations of four experimental treatments of narcolepsy will be described, namely L-dopa (a direct precursor of DA synthesis), γ-hydroxybutyric acid (GHB: a DA antagonist with DA synthesis stimulation properties), viloxazine (an NE reuptake blocker), and zimelidine (a 5HT reuptake blocker) (Table 13-2).

Drugs were tested on patients with a clear clinical and polysomnographic diagnosis of narcolepsy. All patients were free of psychostimulants for at least 1 week and of TADs for at least 2 weeks before entering the study. Patients taking other CNS-active drugs or suffering from other conditions associated with EDS were excluded.

Table 13-2 Effect of Experimental Pharmacological Treatments on Narcoleptic Symptomatology

L-Dopa (multiple daily doses)
    Decreases sleepiness (AVS)
    Increases psychomotor performance (4CRTT)
    No change in sleep latency (MSLT)
    Nonsignificant improvement of cataplexy
    No change in sleep stages
    Increases wake time after sleep onset
    Marked reduction of PMS

γ-Hydroxybutyrate (administered at night)
    Decreases subjective sleepiness
    Psychomotor performance not tested
    No change in sleep latency (MSLT)
    Improvement of cataplexy
    Decreases REM sleep latency and fragmentation
    Increases stages 3 and 4
    No change in PMS

Viloxazine (multiple daily doses)
    Decreases number of sleep attacks and sleepiness (AVS)
    Psychomotor performance not tested
    No change in sleep latency (MSLT and MWT)
    Improvement of cataplexy
    Decreases number of SOREMPs
    No change in sleep stages
    Effect on PMS not tested

Zimelidine (single morning administration)
    No change in daytime sleepiness
    No change in psychomotor peformance (4CRTT)
    No change in sleep latency (MSLT)
    Improvement of cataplexy
    Decreases number of SOREMPs (morning nap)
    No change in nocturnal sleep architecture
    Effect on PMS not tested

AVS = analog vigilance scale; 4CRTT = four choice reaction time test; MSLT = multiple sleep latency test; MWT = maintenance of wakefulness test.

Treatments

L-*Dopa*

As stated above, DA mechanisms are thought to play a role in EDS found in narcolepsy. Early support for this hypothesis comes from a study by Gunne et al. (48) who, on the basis of the catecholaminergic-releasing property of the *d*-amphetamines, decided to treat six narcoleptic patients with L-dopa. Within 2–3 weeks, three patients reported improved "mental alertness" at least comparable to what they experienced with amphetamines; one of these patients also reported a decrease of cataplexy and sleep paralysis. A fourth patient did not notice any change in symptomatology and two others could not tolerate the treatment even at low dosage. A brief clinical note (43) supports these observations. Both studies, however, showed the presence of severe side-effects preventing use of L-dopa. At the same time, Kendel et al. (60) reported that L-dopa (200 mg) with benserazide (50 mg) improved vigilance deficit in 11 of 13 patients, and no side-effects were noted at this dosage. More recently, a double-blind crossover study was conducted in our laboratory and we used a multiple dosage regimen of L-dopa in order to maintain a steady level of the drug throughout the day (18,19).

Treatment consisted of a placebo or L-dopa with benserazide administered orally five times per day at 9:00, 13:00, 17:00, 21:00, and 03:00 hr for two consecutive weeks. On the first week of treatment, 50 mg of L-dopa was given five times a day, and on the second week the dose was doubled for a total daily dosage of 500 mg. A 1-week washout period separated the two treatments, and the order of administration was reversed for half the subjects. Patients filled a daily questionnaire reporting the frequency of EDS and cataplexy; they were also evaluated at the sleep laboratory for 36 consecutive hours at the end of each treatment period. Daytime vigilance was measured at the laboratory by the Four Choice Reaction Time Test (4CRTT) (118) and by an analog vigilance scale (AVS).

L-Dopa led to a significant improvement of EDS as measured by the AVS and the 4CRTT (18), and to a nonsignificant decrease of cataplexy. No changes relative to placebo were seen in nocturnal or diurnal (MLST) sleep recordings performed after treatment with L-dopa except for a marked reduction of PMS (18,19). These results suggest that drugs increasing DA transmission improve daytime vigilance and further suggest that such drugs may reduce cataplexy. This suggestion is congruent with recent studies reporting that impaired DA release in the mesolimbic system may play a role in animal narcolepsy (19).

γ-Hydroxybutyrate (GHB)

GHB decreases the firing rate of DA neurons and stimulates DA synthesis (94). Animal studies suggest that on cessation of the effect of GHB, the release of accumulated DA facilitates DA-related behaviors (91). Consequently, it was hypothesized that GHB administered at night may improve daytime vigilance in narcoleptic patients. Open clinical trials and patients' observations indicate that GHB administered at night has alerting effects the next day in narcoleptic and idiopathic CNS hypersomniac patients (22,75,98). This hypothesis was further tested in six narcoleptic patients studied for 36 hr before and after 1 month of treatment with 2.25 g of GHB taken at bedtime (9). As reported previously by others (22), we found that GHB facilitated REM sleep and shortened REM latency. However, GHB did not decrease sleepiness since it did not lead to longer sleep latencies during the MSLT performed the next day. However, one may question the sensitivity of the MSLT in evaluating improvement of vigilance in narcoleptic patients. In our study with L-dopa (19), no change in sleep latency was seen during the MSLT, although performance tests showed significant improvement. To further elucidate this point, measures of the capacity to resist to sleep onset such as the MWT (69) or performance tests like the 4CRTT should be studied in a double-blind fashion with repeated doses of GHB and placebo.

The neural basis of this anticataplectic effect of GHB is not known. Since GHB taken at bedtime facilitates REM sleep at night, it may reduce REM pressure during the daytime and consequently improve cataplexy. Alternatively, it is the diurnal release of accumulated DA that may have an anticataplectic effect. Confirmation of the anti-cataplectic effect of L-dopa would support this last hypothesis.

The facilitation of REM sleep by GHB is also an unresolved question. There is evidence of species specificity for this response to GHB. For instance, GHB is a potent REM sleep inducer in the cat (28), but this effect was not seen in the rat or in the rabbit (36,41). In humans, GHB is very potent to trigger REM sleep in narcoleptic subjects. Recently, facilitation of REM sleep by GHB was also seen in depressed patients and in normal subjects with advancing age, two conditions in which REM sleep latency is already short before GHB administration. Consequently, GHB seems to facilitate REM sleep when the propensity for REM sleep is already high (62). The neural mechanism for this effect of GHB is unknown. It may be postulated that GHB facilitates REM sleep by suppressing its inhibition normally conveyed by DA neuronal systems. This hypothesis will need further experimental support.

Viloxazine

Some of the evidence supporting the hypothesis of DA involvement in the physiopathology of EDS is nonspecific and may result from an impairment of NE mechanisms. For example, biochemical study of the CSF showed a decreased utilization of NE in narcoleptic patients (12). Psychostimulants are known to be NE agonists (7), and part of L-dopa administered orally is converted into NE in the CNS.

Viloxazine was originally derived from the β-adrenoreceptor blocker propranolol in an attempt to develop a nontricyclic antidepressant. It is a selective NE reuptake blocker (42), and its therapeutic effect on cataplexy is described in the preliminary report of a multicenter evaluation program (47).

Patients were treated for six consecutive weeks with 50 mg viloxazine, taken orally twice a day. Active treatment was preceded by 1 week of placebo and followed by 2 weeks of progressive withdrawal. Objective evaluation of symptoms was performed during 48 hr spent at the sleep laboratory at the end of each treatment period. Vigilance was measured by the Wilkinson Addition Test (WAT) (114), the MSLT, and the MWT.

Clinically, all patients reported an improvement of cataplexy and no anticholinergic side-effects during treatment with viloxazine. Daytime polysomnographic recordings showed that REM sleep was decreased during the MSLT and the MWT. This is in agreement with the hypothesis that daytime REM sleep suppression is needed to control cataplexy. Patients reported fewer sleep attacks after treatment and a nonsignificant increase in sleep latency was also noted on the MWT. However, the MSLT and the WAT did not show evidence of increased vigilance with viloxazine.

These results suggest that increasing NE bioavailibility without presumably affecting 5HT or acetylcholine (ACh) activity is associated with a decrease of REM sleep symptomatology. This is in concordance with previous studies of other NE reuptake blockers, such as desipramine (1,55). The present results also suggest that viloxazine may decrease subjective sleepiness in narcoleptic patients. This effect can be related to the role of NE in the control of cortical arousal (57). The effect of viloxazine on vigilance should be further investigated using higher dosages administered to a large group of narcoleptic patients.

Zimelidine

Like viloxazine, zimelidine is a nontricyclic antidepressant free of anticholinergic activity. However, it is a specific 5HT reuptake blocker in the CNS (84). Since 5HT neuronal systems in the raphé nuclei exert an REM-off influence, zimelidine was seen as a potential anticataplectic agent. Other evidence suggests that increased 5HT bioavailibility may be linked to anticataplectic action. For example, clomipramine, probably the most effective anticataplectic drug (88), is also one of the most potent 5HT reuptake blockers (93). There are also reports of successful clinical trials with fluoxetine (61) and fluvoxamine (97), both selective central 5HT reuptake blockers.

There is also evidence that 5HT reuptake blockers may improve EDS in narcoleptic patients. Zimelidine administration is followed by EEG signs of alertness (99) and elevated thresholds on the critical flicker frequency fusion test (54). Trazodone, a nonselective 5HT reuptake blocker, was also reported to decrease EDS in a single-case study of narcolepsy (95).

The effect of zimelidine on nocturnal and diurnal manifestation in narcolepsy was studied in 10 patients. Nocturnal sleep was evaluated for three consecutive nights before and after 4 weeks of treatment with 100 mg zimelidine administered orally in the morning. Daytime vigilance was evaluated by the MSLT and the 4CRTT. The inhibition of 5HT reuptake was controlled by measuring 5HT concentration in the platelets before and during treatment. This measure is a good index of central 5HT reuptake activity (105). Anticholinergic side-effects were evaluated with a standard questionnaire.

A drop of approximately 80% in platelet 5HT levels was seen 24 hr after the last administration of zimelidine, attesting that the dosage used in the study was sufficient to block 5HT reuptake. No anticholinergic side-effects were reported. It was shown that zimelidine had a potent anticataplectic effect (37,79) but had no effect on EDS, both evaluated subjectively and objectively. Results of the MSLT remained unchanged after treatment with zimelidine, except for a significant increase in REM latency during the first morning nap (approximately 2 hours after the zimelidine intake). In addition, results of the 4CRTT showed that psychomotor performance was not affected by zimelidine (38). Zimelidine had little effect on sleep architecture except for a slight decrease in the percentage of stages 3 and 4. These results show that a selective increase of 5HT bioavailability, without affecting NE or cholinergic activity, is sufficient to control cataplexy.

The Physiopathology of Narcolepsy

Results obtained recently with L-tyrosine (83) and our observations with L-dopa support the hypothesis that central DA mechanisms are involved in the physiopathology of

EDS. Since viloxazine also leads to some improvement of EDS, it is suggested that NE may also play a role. In that respect, modafinil, an α_1-adrenoreceptor agonist, was recently used in humans and showed an alerting effect both in narcolepsy and idiopathic CNS hypersomnia (8). However, this effect was not reported with clonidine, an α_2-receptor agonist (89).

It is possible that a catecholaminergic/opiate coactivation is involved in the physiopathology of EDS. Two studies have shown a decrease in EDS following treatment of narcoleptic patients with pentazocine and codeine (34,50) and this was thought to be related to a facilitating effect of opiates on NE neurotransmission. However, naloxone does not seem to have a major effect on daytime vigilance in narcoleptic patients (34) and further studies are required in order to clarify the role of opiates in EDS.

Regarding the physiopathology of cataplexy, there is a certain amount of evidence relating this symptom to REM sleep atonia (45). For example, most drugs effective in treating cataplexy also suppress REM sleep. Furthermore, narcoleptic patients have frequently been observed to go directly from cataplexy into REM sleep. Brainstem cholinergic neurons are thought to control the organization of REM sleep and this system is under the inhibitory influence of 5HT and NE ("REM-off") brainstem nuclei (68) (see Chapter 8, 9, and 11 in this book). There is strong evidence that brainstem cholinergic neurons are involved in the physiopathology of canine narcolepsy (27) but there is no clear indication that these neurons are responsible for cataplexy or for any other symptom of human narcolepsy. There is also no direct evidence that NE or 5HT neurons are primarily affected in narcoleptic patients although drugs effective in blocking NE or 5HT reuptake are effective in treating cataplexy. This effect may be secondary to the increased activity of "REM-off" neurons.

The neuronal network involved in human cataplexy possibly extends more rostrally than the brainstem generator of REM sleep atonia. Anticataplectic agents such as TADs and GHB may well be acting on rostral limbic and hypothalamic structures involved in the control of emotions leading to attacks of cataplexy (29). The role of the forebrain in the physiopathology of human narcolepsy is also supported by the study of secondary narcolepsies. In all typical cases in which the syndrome was associated with a localized brain lesion, the basal forebrain region was always affected (5,92,100,106).

The primary involvement of the basal forebrain in human narcolepsy may explain some of the differences between the therapeutic responses noted in human and animal narcolepsy. For instance, the oral administration of GHB or clomipramine, potent anticataplectic agents in humans (22,88,97) has little effect in narcoleptic dogs (33). Conversely, anticholinergic drugs that effectively control cataplexy in animals (27) have little effect on human narcolepsy (45,55).

GENERAL CONCLUSION

Recent advances in the treatment of RLS/PMS and narcolepsy were reviewed. It is interesting to note that PMS are reported to be found approximately 10 times more frequently in narcoleptic patients than in the general population (112). It is also striking that RLS/PMS and narcolepsy are both associated with a very high familial prevalence, although pedigrees suggest different modes of transmission. The data presented here suggests that the catecholaminergic systems, and particularly DA, are involved in both syndromes. In that respect, it has been shown that variations in the function of the catecholaminergic system can be inherited and participate in the physiopathology of some diseases (116). Thus, it is possible that RLS/PMS and narcolepsy are related to one another by means that lie outside the immediate boundaries of sleep control mechanisms. Some of the future research efforts should therefore attempt to understand the implications of these observations for the field of sleep disorders medicine.

ACKNOWLEDGMENTS

This work was supported by grants from the "Fonds de la recherche en santé du Québec" and the Medical Research Council of Canada.

REFERENCES

1. Akimoto H, Honda Y, Takahashi Y. Pharmacotherapy in narcolepsy. *Dis Nerv Sys* 1960; 21:704–706.
2. Akpinar S. Treatment of restless legs syndrome with levodopa plus benserazide. *Arch Neurol* 1982; 39:739.
3. Akpinar S. Restless legs syndrome treatment with dopaminergic drugs. *Clin Neurophar-macol* 1987; 10:69–79.
4. Ancoli-Israel S, Seifert AR, Lemon M. Thermal biofeedback and periodic movements in sleep: Patients' subjective reports and a case study. *Biofeedback Self Regul* 1986; 11:177–188.
5. Anderson M, Salomon MV. Symptomatic cataplexy. *J Neurol Neurosurg Psychiatr* 1977; 40:186–191.
6. Association of Sleep Disorders Centers. Diagnostic classification of sleep and arousal disorders. *Sleep* 1979; 1:1–137.
7. Axelrod J. Amphetamines: Metabolism, physiological disposition and its effect on cate-cholamine storage. In E Casta and S Garattini (eds.), *Amphetamine and Related Com-pounds*. Raven, New York, 1970: 207.
8. Bastuji H, Jouvet M. Traitement des hypersomnies par le modafinil. *Presse Méd* 1986; 15:1330–1331.
9. Bédard MA, Montplaisir J, Godbout R, Lapierre O. Nocturnal γ-hydroxybutyrate: Effect of periodic leg movements and sleep organization of narcoleptic patients. *Clin Neurophar-macol* 1989; 12:29–36.
10. Bédard MA, Montplaisir J, Godbout R. Effect of L-dopa on periodic movements in sleep in narcolepsy. *Eur Neurol* 1987; 27:35–38.
11. Billiard M. Narcolepsy. Clinical features and aetiology. *Ann Clin Res* 1985; 17:220–226.
12. Billiard M, Joanny P. Stenberg P, Tognetti P, Pavy A, Brissaud L, Besset A. Nightime and daytime urinary excretion of MHPG-SO4 in narcoleptic subjects and controls. *Sleep Res* 1987; 16:61.
13. Bixler EO, Kales A, Soldatos CR. Sleep disorders encountered in medical practice: a national survey of physicians. *Behav Med* 1979; 6:1–6.
14. Bixler EO, Kales A, Vela-Bueno A, Jacoby JA, Scarone JS, Soldatos CR. Nocturnal myoclonus and nocturnal myoclonic activity in a normal population. *Res Commun Chem Pathol Pharmacol* 1982; 36:129–140.
15. Boehme RE, Baker TL, Mefford IN, Barchas JD, Dement WC, Ciaranello RD. Narcolep-sy: cholinergic receptor changes in an animal model. *Life Sci* 1984; 34:1825–1828.

16. Boghen D. Successful treatment of restless legs with clonazepam. *Ann Neurol* 1980; 8:341.

17. Boghen D, Lamothe L, Elie R, Godbout R, Montplaisir J. The treatment of restless legs syndrome with clonazepam: A prospective controlled study. *Can J Neurol Sci* 1986; 13:245–247.

18. Boivin DB, Montplaisir J, Poirier G. Effects of L-dopa on daytime vigilance in narcolepsy. *Sleep Res* 1989; 18:204.

19. Boivin DB, Montplaisir J, Poirier G. The effects of L-dopa on periodic leg movements and sleep organization in narcolepsy. *Clin Neuropharmacol* 1989; 12:339–345.

20. Bowersox SS, Kilduff TS, Faull KF, Zeller-De Amicis L, Dement WC, Ciaranello RD. Brain dopamine receptor levels elevated in canine narcolepsy. *Brain Res* 1987; 402:44–48.

21. Brodeur C, Montplaisir J, Godbout R, Marinier R. Treatment of restless legs syndrome and periodic movements during sleep with L-dopa: A double-blind controlled study. *Neurology* 1988; 38:1845–1848.

22. Broughton R, Mamelak M. Treatment of narcolepsy-cataplexy with nocturnal gamma-hydroxybutyrate. *Can J Neurol Sci* 1979; 6:1–6.

23. Broughton R, Mamelak M. Effects of nocturnal gamma-hydroxybutyrate on sleep/waking patterns in narcolepsy-cataplexy. *Can J Neurol Sci* 1980; 7:23–31.

24. Coleman RM. Periodic movements in sleep (nocturnal myoclonus) and restless legs syndrome. In: C Guilleminault, (ed.), *Sleeping and Waking Disorders: Indications and Techniques*. Addison-Wesley, Menlo Park, CA 1982: 265–295.

25. Coleman RM, Roffwarg HP, Kennedy SJ, Guilleminault C, Cinque J, Cohn MA, Karacan I, Kupfer DJ, Lemni H, Miles LE, Orr WC, Phillips ER, Roth T, Sassin JF, Schmidt HS, Weitzman ED, Dement WC. Sleep-wake disorders based on a polysomnographic diagnosis. *J Am Med Assoc* 1982; 247:997–1003.

26. Daly DD, Yoss RE. Narcolepsy. *Med Clin North Am* 1960; 44:953–968.

27. Delashaw JB, Foutz AS, Guilleminault C, Dement WC. Cholinergic mechanisms and cataplexy in dogs. *Exp Neurol* 1979; 66:745–757.

28. Delorme F, Riotte M, Jouvet M. Conditions de déclenchement du sommeil paradoxal par les acides gras à chaîne courte chez le chat pontique chronique chronique. *CR Soc Biol* 1966; 160:1457–1460.

29. Doherty JD, Mattox SE, Snead OC, Roth RH. Identification of endogenous γ-hydroxybutyrate in human and bovine brain and its regional distribution in human, guinea-pig and rhesus monkey brain. *J Pharmacol Exp Ther* 1978; 207:130–139.

30. Ekbom KA. Restless legs syndrome. *Neurology* 1960; 10:868–873.

31. Faull KF, Guilleminault C, Berger PA, Barchas JD. Cerebrospinal fluid metabolites in narcolepsy and hypersomnia. *Ann Neurol* 1983; 13:258–263.

32. Fleming JAE, Isomura T, Rungta KM. The effects of trazodone hydrochloride on periodic legs movements. *Sleep Res* 1988; 17:39.

33. Foutz AS, Delashaw JB, Guilleminault C, Dement WC. Monoaminergic mechanisms and experimental cataplexy. *Ann Neurol* 1981; 10:369–376.

34. Fry J, Pressmann MR, DiPhillipo MA, Forst-Paulus M. Treatment of narcolepsy with codeine. *Sleep* 1986; 9:269–74.

35. Gibb WRG, Lees AJ. The restless legs syndrome. *Postgrad Med J* 1986; 62:329–333.

36. Godbout R, Pivik RT. EEG and behavioral effects of gamma-hydroxybutyrate in the rabbit. *Life Sci* 1982; 31:739–748.

37. Godbout R, Montplaisir J. The effect of zimelidine, a serotonin-reuptake blocker, on cataplexy and daytime sleepiness of narcoleptic patients. *Clin Neuropharmacol* 1986; 9:46–51.

38. Godbout R, Montplaisir J. Psychomotor performance in narcoleptic patients after serotoninergic control of cataplexy. *Sleep Res* 1987; 16:203.

39. Godbout R, Montplaisir J, Poirier G, Bédard MA. Distinctive electrographic manifestations of periodic leg movements during sleep in narcoleptic vs insomniac patients. *Sleep Res* 1988; 17:182.
40. Godbout R, Montplaisir J, Poirier G. Epidemiological data in familial restless legs syndrome. *Sleep Res* 1987; 16:338.
41. Godschalk M, Dzoljic MR, Bonta IL. Slow wave sleep and a state resembling absence epilepsy induced in the rat by gamma-hydroxybutyrate. *Eur J Pharmacol* 1977; 44:105–111.
42. Greenwood DT. Viloxazine and neurotransmitter function. In: Costa E, Racagni G, eds. *Typical and atypical antidepressants: molecular mechanisms.* New York: Raven, 1982: 287–300.
43. Guilleminault C, Castaigne P, Cathala PH. Observations on the effectiveness of amantadine, L-dopa, L-dopa plus dopa decarboxylase inhibitor, and dopa decarboxylase inhibitor in the treatment of narcolepsy. *Sleep Res* 1972; 1:150.
44. Guilleminault C, Carskadon M, Dement WC. On the treatment of rapid eye movement narcolepsy. *Arch Neurol* 1974; 30:90–93.
45. Guilleminault C. Cataplexy. In C Guilleminault, WC Dement, and P Passouant (eds.), *Narcolepsy.* Spectrum, New York, 1976: 125–143.
46. Guilleminault C, Flagg W. Effect of baclofen on sleep-related periodic leg movements. *Ann Neurol* 1984; 15:234–239.
47. Guilleminault C, Mancuso J, Quera Salva MA, Hayes B, Mitler M, Poirier G, Montplaisir J. Viloxazine hydrochloride in narcolepsy: A preliminary report. *Sleep* 1986; 9:275–279.
48. Gunne LM, Lindvall HF, Widén L. Preliminary clinical trial with L-dopa in narcolepsy. *Psychopharmacologia* 1971; 19:204–206.
49. Handwerker JV, Palmer RF. Clonidine in the treatment of "restless leg" syndrome. *N Engl J Med* 1985; 313:1228–1229.
50. Harper JM. Gelineau's narcolepsy relieved by opiates. *Lancet* 1981; 1:92.
51. Harriman D, Taverner D, Woolf A. Ekbom's syndrome and burning paresthesia. *Brain* 1970; 93:393–406.
52. Hening W, Walters A, Coté L, Fahn S. Opiate responsive myoclonus. *Ann Neurol* 1983; 14:112.
53. Hening WA, Walters A, Kavey N, Gidro-Franck S, Coté L, Fahn S. Dyskinesias while awake and periodic movements in sleep in restless legs syndrome: Treatment with opioids. *Neurology* 1986; 1363–1366.
54. Hindmarch I, Subhan Z, Stoker MJ. The effects of zimelidine and amitriptyline on car driving and psychomotor performance. *Acta Psychiatr Scand* 1983; 68(Suppl. 308):141–146.
55. Hishikawa Y, Ida H, Nakai K, Kaneko Z. Treatment of narcolepsy with imipramine (Tofranil) and desmethylimipramine (Pertofran). *J Neurol Sci* 1966; 3:453–461.
56. Honda Y, Juji T (eds.). *HLA in Narcolepsy.* Berlin, Springer-Verlag, 1988.
57. Iversen SD. Cortical monoamines and behavior. In L Descarries, TR Reader, and HH Jasper (eds.), *Monoamine Innervation of Cerebral Cortex.* Liss, New York, 1984: 321–344.
58. Kavey N, Walters AS, Hening W, Gidro-Frank S. Opioid treatment of periodic movements in sleep in patients without restless legs. *Neuropeptides* 1988; 11:181–184.
59. Kavey NB, Walters AS, Hening WA, Whyte J, Gidro-Frank S, Chikroverty S. Treatment of the restless legs syndrome with bromocriptine. *Sleep Res* 1988; 17:46.
60. Kendel K, Rüther E, Beck U, Meier-Ewert K. Zur behandlung der narkolepsie mit L-dopa. *Nervenarzt* 1973; 44:434–436.
61. Langdon N, Shindler J, Parkes JD, Bandack S. Fluoxetine in the treatment of cataplexy. *Sleep* 1986; 9:371–373.

62. Lapierre O, Lamarre M, Montplaisir J, Lapierre G. The effects of gamma-hydroxybutyrate: A double-blind study of normal subjects. *Sleep Res* 1988; 17:99.

63. Lindvall O, Bjorklund A, Skagerberg G. Dopamine-containing neurons in the spinal cord: anatomy and some functional aspects. *Ann Neurol* 1983; 14:255–260.

63a. Lorrain D, Montplaisir J. The forced immobilization test: An objective method of quantifying severity of the restless legs syndrome. *Sleep Research* 1990; 19:247.

64. Lugaresi E, Cirignotta F, Coccagna G, Montagna P. Nocturnal myoclonus and restless legs syndrome. In S Fahn, CD Marsden, and MH Van Woert (eds.), *Advances in Neurology, Vol. 43: Myoclonus.* Raven, New York, 1986: 295–307.

65. Lugaresi E, Coccagna G, Berti-Ceroni G, Ambrosetto C. Restless legs syndrome and nocturnal myoclonus. In H Gastaut, E Lugaresi, and G Berti-Ceroni (eds.), *The Abnormalities of Sleep in Man.* Aulo Gaggi, Bologna, 1968: 285–294.

66. Lugaresi E, Coccagna G, Mantovani M, Lebrun R. Some periodic phenomena arising during drowsiness and sleep in man. *Electroenceph Clin Neurophysiol* 1972; 32:701–705.

67. Matthews WB. Treatment of the restless legs syndrome with clonazepam. *Br Med J* 1979; 281:751.

68. McCarley RW. Mechanisms and models of behavioral state control. In JA Hobson, MAB Brazier, (eds.), *The reticular formation revisited.* Raven Press, New York, 1980: 375–403.

69. Mitler M, Gujavarty K, Browman C. Maintenance of wakefulness test: A polysomnographic technique for evaluating treatment in patients with excessive somnolence. *Electroenceph Clin Neurophysiol* 1982; 53:658–661.

70. Mitler MM. The multiple sleep latency test as an evaluation for excessive somnolence. In C Guilleminault (ed.), *Sleeping and Waking Disorders. Indications and Techniques.* Addison-Wesley, Menlo Park, CA, 1983: 145–153.

71. Mitler MM, Browman CF, Menn SJ, Gujavarty K, Timms RM. Nocturnal myoclonus: Treatment efficacy of clonazepam and temazepam. *Sleep* 1986; 9:385–392.

72. Mitler MM, Shafor R, Hajdukovitch R, Timms RM, Browman CP. Treatment of narcolepsy: Objective studies on methylphenidate, pemoline, and protriptyline. *Sleep* 1986; 9:260–264.

73. Moldofsky H, Tullis C, Quance G, Lue FA. Nitrazepam for periodic movements in sleep (sleep-related myoclonus). *Can J Neurol Sci* 1986; 13:52–54.

74. Montplaisir J, Billiard M, Takahashi S, Bell IR, Guilleminault C, Dement WC. Twenty-four-hour recording in REM-narcoleptics with special reference to nocturnal sleep disruption. *Biol Psychiat* 1978; 13:73–89.

75. Montplaisir J, Barbezieux M. Le gamma-hydroxybutyrate de sodium (GHB) dans le traitement de l'hypersomnie essentielle. *Can J Psychiat* 1981; 26:162–166.

76. Montplaisir J, Walsh J, Lapierre G. Nocturnal sleep of hypersomniacs: a positive correlation between REM fragmentation and cataplexy. *Sleep Res* 1981; 10:218.

77. Montplaisir J, De Champlain J, Young SN, Missala K, Sourkes TL, Walsh J, Rémillard G. Narcolepsy and idiopathic hypersomnia: Biogenic amines and related compounds in the CSF. *Neurology* 1982; 32:1299–1302.

78. Montplaisir J, Godbout R, Boghen D, De Champlain J, Young SN, Lapierre G. Familial restless legs with periodic movements in sleep: Electrophysiologic, biochemical and pharmacological study. *Neurology* 1985; 35:130–134.

79. Montplaisir J, Godbout R. Serotoninergic reuptake mechanisms in the control of cataplexy. *Sleep* 1986; 9:280–284.

80. Montplaisir J, Godbout R, Poirier G, Bédard MA. Restless legs syndrome and periodic movements in sleep: Physiopathology and treatment with L-dopa. *Clin Neuropharmacol* 1986; 9:456–463.

80a. Montplaisir J, Lorrain D, Godbout R. Restless legs syndrome and periodic movements in sleep: the primary role of dopaminergic mechanisms. *Eur Neurol* 1990 (in press).

81. Montplaisir J, Poirier G, Godbout R, Marinier R. La narcolepsie: Un modèle d'étiologie multifactorielle. *Médecine Sciences* 1988; 4:239–244.

82. Montplaisir J, Godbout R. Restless legs syndrome and periodic movements during sleep. In MH Kryger, T Roth, and WC Dement (eds.), *Principles and Practice of Sleep Medicine*. Saunders, Philadelphia, 1989: 402–409.

83. Mouret J, Lemoine P, Sanchez P, Robelin N, Taillard J, Canini F. Treatment of narcolepsy with L-tyrosine. *Lancet* 1988; 2:1458–1459.

84. Ogren SO, Ross SB, Hall H, Holm AC, Renyi AL. The pharmacology of zimelidine: a 5-HT selective reuptake inhibitor. *Acta Psychiatr Scand* 1981; 63 (Suppl 290):127–151.

85. Ohanna N, Peled R, Rubin AHE, Zomer Z, Lavie P. Periodic leg movements in sleep: effect of clonazepam treatment. *Neurology* 1985; 35:408–411.

86. Oshtory MA, Vijayan N. Clonazepam treatment of insomnia due to sleep myoclonus. *Arch Neurol* 1980; 37:119–120.

87. Parkes JD, Fenton C, Struthers G, Curzon G, Kantamanemi BK, Buxton BH, Record C. Narcolepsy and cataplexy. Clinical features, treatment and cerebrospinal fluid findings. *Q J Med* 1974; 43:525–536.

88. Passouant P, Baldy-Moulinier M, Aussilioux C. Etat de mal cataplectique au cours d'une maladie de Gélineau: Influence de la chlorimipramine. *Rev Neurol (Paris)* 1970; 123:56–60.

89. Putkonen PT, Bergstroen L. Inhibition of cataplectic attacks of narcolepsy by clonidine. *Neurosci Lett* 1979; 3 (Suppl):S270.

90. Rechtschaffen A, Dement WC. Studies on the relation of narcolepsy, cataplexy, and sleep with low voltage random EEG activity. In: SS Kety, EV Evarts, and HL Williams (eds.), *Sleep and Altered States of Consciousness*. Williams & Wilkins, Baltimore, 1963: 488–498.

91. Redgrave P, Taha EB, White L, Dean P. Increased food intake following the manipulation of intracerebral dopamine levels with gamma-hydroxybutyrate. *Psychopharmacology* 1982; 76:273–277.

92. Rivera VM, Meyer JS, Hata T, Ishikawa Y, Imai A. Narcolepsy following cerebral hypoxic ischemia. *Ann Neurol* 1986; 19:505–508.

93. Ross SB, Renyi AL. Tricyclic antidepressant agents: 2. Effects of oral administration on the uptake of 3H-noradrenaline and 14C-5-hydroxytriptamine in slices of the midbrain-hypothalamus region of the rat. *Acta Pharmacol Toxicol* 1975; 36:395–408.

94. Roth RH, Doherty JD, Walters JR. Gamma-hydroxybutyrate: A role in the regulation of central dopaminergic neurons? *Brain Res* 1980; 189:556–560.

95. Sandyk R. Efficacy of trazodone in narcolepsy. *Eur Neurol* 1985; 24:335–337.

96. Sawynok J, Pinsky C, LaBella FA. Mini review on the specificity of naloxone as an opiate antagonist. *Life Sci* 1979; 25:1631–1632.

97. Schachter M, Parkes JD. Fluvoxamine and clomipramine in the treatment of cataplexy. *J Neurol Neurosurg Psychiatry* 1980; 43:171–174.

98. Scharf MB, Brown D, Woods M, Brown L, Hirschowitz J. The effects and effectiveness of gamma-hydroxybutyrate in patients with narcolepsy. *J Clin Psychiat* 1985; 46:222–225.

99. Schenk GK, Filler W, Ranft W, Zerbin D. Double-blind comparisons of a selective serotonin reuptake inhibitor, zimelidine, and placebo on quantified EEG parameters and psychological variables. *Acta Psychiatr Scand* 1981; 290:303–313.

100. Schwartz WJ, Stakes JW, Hobson JA. Transient cataplexy after removal of a craniopharyngioma. *Neurology* 1984; 34:1372–1375.

101. Severson JA, Marcusson J, Winbald B, Finch CE. Age-correlated loss of binding sites in human basal ganglia. *J Neurochem* 1982; 39:1623–1631.

102. Sewitch B, Liebman KO. Treatment of periodic movements in sleep "nocturnal myoclonus" with a low dosage of the tricyclic antidepressant imipramine. *Sleep Res* 1988; 17:256.

103. Shindler J, Schachter M, Brincat S, Parkes JD. Amphetamine, mazindol, and fencam-famin in narcolepsy. *Br Med J* 1985; 290:1167–1170.
104. Skirboll LR, Grace AA, Hommer DW, Rehfeld J, Goldstein M, Hokfelt T, Bunney BS. Peptide-monoamine coexistence: studies of the action of cholecystokinin-like peptides on the electrical activity of midbrain dopamine neurons. *Neuroscience* 1981; 6:2111–2124.
105. Stahl SM, Meltzer HY. A kinetic and pharmacological analysis of 5-hydroxytryptamine transport by human platelets and platelet storage granules: Comparison with central sero-toninergic neurons. *J Pharmacol Exp Ther* 1978; 205:118–132.
106. Stahl SM, Layzer RB, Aminoff MJ, Townsend JJ, Feldon S. Continuous cataplexy in a patient with a midbrain tumor: The limp man syndrome. *Neurology* 1980; 30:1115–1118.
107. Stahl SM, Faull KF, Barchas JD, Berger PA. CSF monoamine metabolites in movement disorders and normal aging. *Arch Neurol* 1985; 42:166–169.
108. Strang RR. The symptoms of restless legs. *Med J Aust* 1969; 1:1211–1213.
109. Telstad W, Sorensen O, Larsen S, Lillevold PE, Stensrud P, Nyberg-Hansen R. The treatment of restless legs syndrome with carbamazepine: A double blind study. *Br Med J* 1984; 89:1–7.
110. Traynor JR, Kelley PD, Rance MJ. Multiple opiate binding sites in rat spinal cord. *Life Sci* 1982; 31:1377–1380.
111. Trzepacz PT, Violette EJ, Sateia MJ. Response to opioids in three patients with restless legs syndrome. *Am J Psychiat* 1984; 141:993–995.
112. Van den Hoed J, Kraemer M, Guilleminault C, Zarcone Jr VP, Miles LE, Dement WC, Mitler MM. Disorders of excessive daytime somnolence: Polygraphic and clinical data for 100 patients. *Sleep* 1981; 4:23–37.
113. Walters A, Hening W, Coté L, Fahn S. Dominantly inherited restless legs with myoclonus and periodic movements of sleep: A syndrome related to the endogenous opiates? In S Fahn, CD Marsden, and MH Van Woert (eds.), *Advances in Neurology, Vol. 43: Myo-clonus*. Raven, New York, 1986: 309–319.
114. Ware JC, Pittard JT, Blumoff RL. Treatment of sleep-related myoclonus with an alpha-receptor blocker. *Sleep Res* 1981; 10:242.
115. Wechsler LR, Stakes JW, Shahani BT, Busis NA. Periodic leg movements of sleep (noctur-nal myoclonus): An electrophysiological study. *Ann Neurol* 1986; 19:168–173.
116. Weinshilboum RM. Biochemical genetics of catecholamines in humans. *Mayo Clin Proc* 1983; 58:319–330.
117. Wilkinson RT. Methods for research on sleep deprivation and sleep function. In E Hartmann (ed.), *Sleep and Dreaming*. Little Brown, Boston, 1970: 369–381.
118. Wilkinson RT, Houghton D. Portable four-choice reaction time test with magnetic tape memory. *Behav Res Methods Instrum* 1975; 7:441–446.

Index